1987
YEAR BOOK OF
CARDIOLOGY®

The 1987 Year Book Series

Anesthesia: Drs. Miller, Kirby, Ostheimer, Roizen, and Stoelting

Cancer: Drs. Hickey, Saunders, Clark, and Cumley

Cardiology: Drs. Schlant, Collins, Engle, Frye, Gifford, and O'Rourke

Critical Care Medicine: Drs. Rogers, Allo, Dean, Gioia, McPherson, Michael, Miller, and Traystman

Dentistry: Drs. Cohen, Hendler, Johnson, Jordan, Moyers, Robinson, and Silverman

Dermatology: Drs. Sober and Fitzpatrick

Diagnostic Radiology: Drs. Bragg, Keats, Kieffer, Kirkpatrick, Koehler, Miller, and Sorenson

Digestive Diseases: Drs. Greenberger and Moody

Drug Therapy: Drs. Hollister and Lasagna

Emergency Medicine: Dr. Wagner

Endocrinology: Drs. Bagdade, Ryan, Molitch, Braverman, Robertson, Halter, Kornel, Horton, Korenman, Morley, Rogol, Burger, and Metz

Family Practice: Drs. Rakel, Couchman, Driscoll, Avant, and Prichard

Hand Surgery: Drs. Dobyns, Chase, and Amadio

Hematology: Drs. Spivak, Bell, Ness, Quesenberry, and Wiernik

Infectious Diseases: Drs. Wolff, Tally, Keusch, Klempner, and Snydman

Medicine: Drs. Rogers, Des Prez, Cline, Braunwald, Greenberger, Wilson, Epstein, and Malawista

Neurology and Neurosurgery: Drs. DeJong, Currier, and Crowell

Nuclear Medicine: Drs. Hoffer, Gore, Gottschalk, Sostman, and Zaret

Obstetrics and Gynecology: Drs. Mishell, Kirschbaum, and Morrow

Ophthalmology: Drs. Ernest and Deutsch

Orthopedics: Dr. Coventry

Otolaryngology—Head and Neck Surgery: Drs. Paparella and Bailey

Pathology and Clinical Pathology: Drs. Brinkhous, Dalldorf, Grisham, Langdell, and McLendon

Pediatrics: Drs. Oski and Stockman

Perinatal/Neonatal Medicine: Drs. Klaus and Fanaroff

Plastic and Reconstructive Surgery: Drs. McCoy, Brauer, Haynes, Hoehn, Miller, and Whitaker

Podiatric Medicine and Surgery: Dr. Jay

Psychiatry and Applied Mental Health: Drs. Freedman, Lourie, Meltzer, Nemiah, Talbott, and Weiner

Pulmonary Disease: Drs. Green, Ball, Menkes, Michael, Peters, Terry, Tockman, and Wise

Rehabilitation: Drs. Kaplan and Szumski

Sports Medicine: Drs. Krakauer, Shephard, and Torg, Col. Anderson, and Mr. George

Surgery: Drs. Schwartz, Jonasson, Peacock, Shires, Spencer, and Thompson

Urology: Drs. Gillenwater and Howards

Vascular Surgery: Drs. Bergan and Yao

Editor-in-Chief

Robert C. Schlant, M.D.

Professor of Medicine (Cardiology); Director, Division of Cardiology, Emory University School of Medicine, Atlanta

Editors

John J. Collins, Jr., M.D.

Chief, Division of Thoracic and Cardiac Surgery, Brigham and Women's Hospital, Boston

Mary Allen Engle, M.D.

Stavros S. Niarchos Professor of Pediatric Cardiology, Professor of Pediatrics, Director of Pediatric Cardiology, The New York Hospital–Cornell Medical Center

Robert L. Frye, M.D.

Rose Eisenberg Professor, Professor of Medicine, Mayo Clinic

Ray W. Gifford, Jr., M.D.

Senior Vice Chairman, Division of Medicine, and Senior Physician, Department of Hypertension and Nephrology, Cleveland Clinic Foundation

Robert A. O'Rourke, M.D.

Charles Conrad and Anna Sahm Brown Professor of Medicine; Director, Cardiology Division, The University of Texas Health Sciences Center, San Antonio, Texas

1987

The Year Book of
CARDIOLOGY®

Editor-in-Chief
Robert C. Schlant, M.D.

Editors
John J. Collins, Jr., M.D.
Mary Allen Engle, M.D.
Robert L. Frye, M.D.
Ray W. Gifford, Jr., M.D.
Robert A. O'Rourke, M.D.

Year Book Medical Publishers, Inc.
Chicago • London • Boca Raton

Editor-in-Chief, Year Book Publishing: Nancy Gorham
Sponsoring Editor: Cara D. Suber
Literature Surveillance Supervisor: Laura J. Shedore
Manager, Copyediting Services: Frances M. Perveiler
Assistant Manager, Copyediting Services: Elizabeth Griffith
Production Manager: H.E. Nielsen
Proofroom Supervisor: Shirley E. Taylor

Table of Contents

The material in this volume represents literature reviewed through November 1986.

Journals Represented

American Heart Journal
American Journal of Cardiology
American Journal of Emergency Medicine
American Journal of Epidemiology
American Journal of the Medical Sciences
American Journal of Medicine
American Journal of Physiology
Anesthesia and Analgesia
Annales de Radiologie
Annals of Internal Medicine
Annals of Thoracic Surgery
Archives of Internal Medicine
Archives of Surgery
British Heart Journal
British Journal of Clinical Pharmacology
British Medical Journal
Canadian Medical Association Journal
Cardiovascular Research
Circulation
Circulation Research
Clinical Pharmacology and Therapeutics
Clinical Science
European Journal of Clinical Pharmacology
Hypertension
International Journal of Cardiology
Journal of the American College of Cardiology
Journal of the American Geriatrics Society
Journal of the American Medical Association
Journal of Applied Physiology: Respiratory, Environmental, and Exercise
    Physiology
Journal of Cardiovascular Surgery
Journal of Clinical Endocrinology and Metabolism
Journal of Clinical Investigation
Journal of Consulting and Clinical Psychology
Journal of Hypertension
Journal of Surgical Research
Journal of Thoracic and Cardiovascular Surgery
Klinische Wochenschrift
Lancet
Mayo Clinic Proceedings
New England Journal of Medicine
New Zealand Medical Journal
Pediatric Cardiology
Pediatrics
Radiology
Seminars in Thrombosis and Hemostasis
Transplantation
World Journal of Surgery

Publisher's Preface

We are delighted to welcome Robert C. Schlant, M.D., and his associates, John J. Collins, Jr., M.D., Mary Allen Engle, M.D., Robert L. Frye, M.D., Ray W. Gifford, Jr., M.D., and Robert A. O'Rourke, M.D., as editors of the YEAR BOOK OF CARDIOLOGY.

This team is carrying on the tradition of distinguished editorial direction for this YEAR BOOK, commencing with the 1987 edition. We congratulate them and extend our appreciation for their superb work with the YEAR BOOK.

Introduction

This YEAR BOOK OF CARDIOLOGY, the 27th in the series, attempts to uphold and maintain the standards and traditions of previous editions. The exponentially increasing fund of basic and clinical knowledge includes all aspects of cardiovascular physiology and pathophysiology as well as clinical cardiology. This fact makes it progressively more challenging for the editors to select those articles for review and comment that they believe to be of special significance at this particular time. Although many articles are chosen to present new and exciting information potentially relative to patient management, others may be chosen to serve as a warning with regard to certain therapies or therapeutic regimens.

All of us in this challenging venture are indebted to the former editors who have participated so ably in this series: W. Proctor Harvey, John W. Kirklin, Alexander S. Nadas, Oglesby Paul, Victor E. Pollak, T. Joseph Reeves, Robert W. Wilkins, Irving S. Wright, and subsequent editors, Eugene Braunwald, Walter M. Kirkendall, Hillel Laks, Leon Resnekov, Amnon Rosenthal, and Edmund H. Sonnenblick. In the current volume, Dr. Robert A. O'Rourke has had responsibility for the section on Normal and Altered Cardiovascular Function; Dr. Mary Allen Engle has responsibility for Cardiovascular Disease in Infants and Children; I am responsible for Heart Diseases in Adults: Valvular Heart Disease, Myocardial Diseases, Pericardial Diseases, Disturbances of Cardiac Rhythm and Conduction, and Miscellaneous Topics; Dr. Robert L. Frye has responsibility for Heart Disease in Adults: Coronary Artery Disease; Dr. John J. Collins, Jr., has responsibility for Cardiac Surgery; and Dr. Ray W. Gifford, Jr., has responsibility for Hypertension. The other section editors, who have had complete freedom to select the articles for inclusion in their areas, have each done a splendid job, for which I thank them sincerely. All of the section editors would like to thank the staff at YEAR BOOK MEDICAL PUBLISHERS for their assistance, patience, and understanding. In particular, we are indebted to Ms. Nancy Gorham and Ms. Cara Suber.

It is now the joint responsibility of the current editors and the publisher to follow the outstanding course our predecessors have established, as well as to adapt, when appropriate, to new developments and techniques of communication, information storage and retrieval, and education. All of us would welcome suggestions on how we can make future volumes more useful.

Robert C. Schlant, M.D.

1 Normal and Altered Cardiovascular Function

Introduction

In this section of the YEAR BOOK OF CARDIOLOGY clinically relevant, recently published articles dealing with cardiovascular physiology, metabolism, and special cardiac techniques are reviewed. Both human and experimental animal studies are included, and a list of additional references is provided at the end of each subsection.

In the first subsection on ventricular hypertrophy, possible mechanisms for the development of impaired ventricular function subsequent to long-standing hypertrophy resulting from chronic pressure overload are reviewed. Multiple studies are currently underway to evaluate the effects of regression of ventricular hypertrophy on ventricular performance such as occurs with the successful treatment of systemic hypertension. Theoretically, the regression of hypertrophy following removal of pressure or volume overload could have either beneficial or detrimental consequences.

The exercise physiology subsection describes several studies examining the role of increments in heart rate, end-diastolic volume, and contractility in augmenting cardiac output during various types and degree of exercise. Apparent discrepancies in different exercise studies can be resolved if variations in experimental design are carefully considered. The possible role of the pericardium in limiting the left ventricular end-diastolic volume during exercise is discussed.

The subsection on ventricular diastolic function assesses the difficulty in evaluating diastolic ventricular performance in man by currently available noninvasive methods, considers the multiple hemodynamic factors influencing measurements of the isovolumic time constant for relaxation as determined invasively, and examines the effects of reduced myocardial blood flow ischemia and increased myocardial oxygen demand ischemia on diastolic properties of the left ventricle.

The measurement and usefulness of the left ventricular end-systolic pressure-volume relationship (ESPVR) are emphasized in the subsection on ventricular systolic function. Information is provided concerning the utility of this relatively load-independent measure of ventricular performance in the isolated heart and preinstrumented experimental animal, and methods for assessing end-systolic measures of segmental ventricular performance are described. Problems in acquiring noninvasive and invasive measurements of end-systolic pressure and volume in man at several levels for defining the slope of the ESPVR are detailed.

15

In the subsection on heart failure, a study assessing the effect of severe heart failure on β receptor numbers and the affinity for β receptor agonists is detailed and information pertaining to the atrial natriuretic factor is provided. The subsection on experimental myocardial ischemia/infarction includes information on the "stunned myocardium," the ability to detect subcritical coronary artery stenoses by exercise-induced abnormalities of regional wall thickening, and methods for assessing the "region at risk." Information is given concerning the use of calcium entry blockers to salvage ischemic myocardium and contradictory studies concerning the ability of enzymes that degrade free oxygen radicals to limit "infarct size."

In the subsection on myocardial metabolic studies, data are presented concerning the electrophysiologic derangements resulting from the accumulation of long-chain acyl/carnitine in hypoxic myocytes, the potentiation of thromboxane A_2 release from platelets by epinephrine, and the potential role of platelet-activating factor in coronary artery vasodilation. Also, adenosine triphosphate depletion and the accumulation of arachidonic acid in myocytes are discussed, as are the effects of alcohol on hemodynamics and membrane function.

Improved noninvasive and cineangiographic methods for determining regional ventricular function are the subject of subsection 8, and the subsequent subgroup of publications considers the multiple special cardiac techniques that have been or are being shown useful in patients with cardiac disease. Special emphasis is placed on the utility of Doppler echocardiography in determining the pressure gradient across native stenotic and prosthetic heart valves and on the great promise of fast computerized axial tomography and gated nuclear magnetic resonance as noninvasive methods for studying cardiac patients in the near future. A special article on the recommended use of the routine ECG for screening patients prior to noncardiac surgery is reviewed at some length.

The subsection of miscellaneous reports includes one manuscript review of a study demonstrating the development of systemic hypertension with aortic baroreceptor denervation in the nonhuman primate, and a second dealing with the factors influencing aortic wave propagation in man.

Robert A. O'Rourke, M.D.

Ventricular Hypertrophy

Altered Calcium Handling in Experimental Pressure-Overload Hypertrophy in the Ferret

Judith K. Gwathmey and James P. Morgan (Charles A. Dana Res. Inst. and Beth Israel Hosp. Boston)
Circ. Res. 57:836–843, December 1985   1–1

The level of contractile function in cardiac hypertrophy is dependent on many factors including the age and species of the animal studied, the duration and degree of hypertrophy, and the method by which the stimulus is applied. Because of this, contractile function in the hypertrophied heart has been reported variably to be normal, depressed, or enhanced compared with findings in controls. Many structural and functional changes occur in hypertrophy that may account for the contractile abnormalities that develop in different animal models. The calcium ion plays a major role in the contraction-relaxation cycles of cardiac muscle. Furthermore, abnormalities in calcium handling by subcellular organelles have been identified in hypertrophied cardiac muscle and correlated with changes in contractile function. The relationship between the changes in intracellular calcium handling and the functional changes that occur in cardiac hypertrophy were examined.

A model of right ventricular pressure-overload hypertrophy was developed in the ferret by critical banding of the pulmonary artery. Papillary muscles 1 mm or less in diameter were removed from ferrets with cardiac hypertrophy and from their age-matched and weight-matched controls. The muscles were loaded with the bioluminescent calcium indicator, aequorin, to record intracellular calcium transients. Compared with controls, the hypertrophied muscles demonstrated a prolonged duration of isometric contraction but a marked decrease in peak isometric tension development. The increased duration of isometric contraction in the hypertrophied muscles correlated with a similar prolongation of the calcium transient. This was interpreted to mean that the rate of sequestration and possibly release of calcium by intracellular stores was decreased in hypertrophy. Conversely, the amplitudes of the calcium transients were similar in muscles from both groups of ferrets, suggesting that the diminution in peak tension developed by the hypertrophied muscles was not because of a decreased availability of activator calcium. The prolonged time course of tension development, but not the diminished peak isometric tension response, may be related to changes in intracellular calcium handling.

▶ In experimental animals and patients with severe compensated pressure-overload left ventricular hypertrophy, the increment in wall thickness normalizes wall stress and permits the left ventricle to function normally. However, the natural history of pressure-overload hypertrophy in both animals and human beings may be described as progressive deterioration in myocardial function, resulting eventually in irreversible heart failure. There are several hypotheses concerning this sequence of events, none of which have been proven conclusively. Also, the structural and functional changes responsible for contraction abnormalities, when present, have never been fully delineated.

In the study reviewed here, the authors assessed intracellular calcium transients in papillary muscles removed from ferrets with ventricular hypertrophy. The prolonged time course of tension development in the hypertrophied papillary muscles resulting from pressure overload was probably related to a decreased rate of calcium sequestration. The changes in intracellular calcium handling may account for some, but not all, of the contraction changes seen in this model of pressure-overload hypertrophy. Additional studies using improving techniques for studying alterations in intracellular calcium, which plays a central role in the contraction-relaxation cycles of cardiac muscle, may provide additional information regarding the mechanism for the depressed ventricular performance that eventually occurs in hypertrophied cardiac muscle.—R.A. O'Rourke, M.D.

Altered Phospholipid Metabolism in Pressure-Overload Hypertrophied Hearts

Diane K. Reibel, Brian O'Rourke, Karen A. Foster, Howard Hutchinson, Cornelius E. Uboh, and Robert L. Kent (Thomas Jefferson Univ. and Temple Univ., Philadelphia)
Am. J. Physiol. 250:H1–H6, January 1986   1–2

Cardiac hypertrophy, associated with reduced myocardial contractility, develops in response to chronic pressure overloading of the heart. However, the biochemical factors and structural changes that contribute to the reduced contractility and frequent deterioration in overall function observed in pressure-overloaded hypertrophied hearts are not fully understood. Recent evidence suggests that alterations in the properties of cellular membranes occur in pressure-overloaded hearts. Although both lipid and protein components are necessary for membrane function, most studies have focused on the proteins. An attempt was made to determine the content and fatty acyl composition of phospholipids in hypertrophied hearts of animals subjected to pressure overload.

Pressure overload was induced in male Sprague-Dawley rats by abdominal aortic constriction. Twenty-one days after the constriction was created, the concentrations of myocardial phosphatidylcholine (PC), sphingomyelin, and phosphatidylinositol (Pi) were significantly elevated by 10%, 10% and 20%, respectively. However, the essential fatty acid, linoleic acid, was markedly reduced in PC, phosphatidylethanolamine (PE), Pi, and cardiolipin (CL) of hypertrophied hearts. The associated changes in fatty acyl composition were specific for the individual phospholipid class as evidenced by a significant elevation of palmitic acid in PC, docosahexaenoic acid in PE, and oleic acid in CL. Furthermore, alterations in fatty acyl composition of phospholipids were not associated with any change in the composition of cardiac triglycerides, cardiac free fatty acids, or serum lipids. The fatty acyl composition of phospholipids was also altered in pressure-overloaded hearts of cats, as shown by a reduction of linoleic acid and an increase of arachidonic acid in total phospholipids. The changes in phospholipid metabolism that occur in the pressure-overloaded mammalian heart may contribute to altered membrane function in the hypertrophied myocardium.

▶ The biochemical factors and structural changes that contribute to the impaired contractility resulting from pressure-overload hypertrophy were studied to determine the content in fatty acyl composition of phospholipids in hypertrophied hearts in animals subjected to pressure overload. Both lipid and protein components are necessary for certain membrane functions, e.g., calcium uptake by the sarcoplasmic reticulum. The fatty acyl composition of phospholipids was altered in hypertrophied ventricles because of pressure overload in both rats and cats. However, the biochemical and physiologic significance of the altered fatty acyl composition of phospholipids in pressure-overloaded myocardium requires further investigation to separate a cause and effect relationship from that of an associated finding with little hemodynamic significance.—R.A. O'Rourke, M.D.

Relationship Between Myosin Isoenzyme Composition, Hemodynamics, and Myocardial Structure in Various Forms of Human Cardiac Hypertrophy
Heinz O. Hirzel, Caspar R. Tuchschmid, Jakob Schneider, Hans P. Krayenbuehl, and Marcus C. Schaub (Univ. of Zurich)
Circ. Res. 57:729–740, November 1985   1–3

The heart adapts to altered loading conditions primarily by hypertrophy and increased muscle performance to fulfill its task of pumping blood according to the metabolic demands of the organism. The mechanism of hypertrophy in primary cardiomyopathies is not known. However, because myosin is the major contractile protein of the cardiac muscle cell producing force and shortening, it is hypothesized that changes in its isoform composition may explain the altered contractile properties in hypertrophy. Myosin has a hexameric structure consisting of two heavy chains and two pairs of light chains; various isoforms of both light and heavy chains occur. An examination was made of the changes in ventricular light chain isoform composition in relation to workload and functional states in various forms of primary and secondary hypertrophy in human beings.

Hemodynamic and angiographic parameters, muscle fiber diameter, nonmuscle tissue content, and myosin light chain isoform composition were evaluated in the left ventricle of 9 patients with primary (4 with hypertrophic, 5 with dilated cardiomyopathy) and 27 with secondary hypertrophy (11 with aortic regurgitation, 16 with aortic stenosis), 9 patients with coronary heart disease, and 7 controls. In various forms of hypertrophy, a new atrial-like light chain 1 occurred in two-dimensional electrophoresis of total tissue homogenates that amounted to 29% of total light chain 1. When related to tropomyosin, the total light chain 1 content remained constant in all groups. The mean content of this atrial light chain 1 was greatest in dilated cardiomyopathy (12.1%), less in patients with pressure (6.4%) and volume overload (2.9%), but as low in hypertrophic cardiomyopathy (0.3%) as in controls (0.4%). In patients with coronary heart disease without prior infarction, it was lower (0.6%) than with infarction (1.9%). However, its occurrence was not changed by digoxin administration. In ventricular myocardium, an atrial-like light chain 2 was not observed. The content of atrial-like light chain 1 was not related to muscle fiber diameter or nonmuscle tissue content, both of which were increased in all hypertrophy groups.

In individual cases, no firm correlation could be made between atrial-like light chain 1 content and various parameters of ventricular load and function. However, there was a significant correlation when the mean values of atrial-like light chain 1 content of each disease group were related to the respective mean values of peak circumferential wall stress. The shift of myosin light chain 1 isoforms in ventricle seems to characterize biochemically the hypertrophy process induced by mechanical stress.

▶ Multiple studies in different animal models of hypertrophy have demonstrated various alterations in myosin isoforms with differences observed even in the same animal species when hypertrophy was produced by different stimuli and at various times from the fetal stage to adulthood. In the setting described, a new atrial-like light chain 1 occurred in two-dimensional electrophoresis of total tissue homogenates. The mean content of this atrial light chain 1 was highest in hypertrophied muscle because of cardiomyopathy and lowest in patients with hypertrophic cardiomyopathy on whom its content did not differ from that in controls. Importantly, the authors found a significant correlation between the mean values of atrial-like light chain 1 content in each diseased group with the respective mean values of peak circumferential wall stress. This suggests that the shift of myosin light chain 1 isoforms in the ventricle characterizes biochemically the hypertrophy process induced by mechanical stress.—R.A. O'Rourke, M.D.

Mechanical and Inotropic Reserve in Conscious Dogs With Left Ventricular Hypertrophy

Alan M. Fujii, Stephen F. Vatner, Juan Serur, Ann Als, and Israel Mirsky (Harvard Univ., Children's Hosp., Brigham and Women's Hosp., and Beth Israel Hosp., Boston, and New England Regional Primate Res. Ctr., Southborough, Mass.)
Am. J. Physiol. 251:H815–H823, October 1986   1–4

Heart failure may develop when the hypertrophied myocardium is unable to perform additional mechanical work, or the hypertrophied heart may have reduced inotropic responsiveness to β-adrenergic receptor agonists. The extent to which left ventricular (LV) hypertrophy compensates for pressure overload from supravalvular aortic stenosis was studied at rest and with norepinephrine-induced stress in conscious instrumented dogs. Prenalterol was used to increase LV contractility with small changes in preload and afterload. Findings in animals with LV hypertrophy, produced by aortic constriction, were compared with those in sham-operated littermates within 1–2 years after the procedure.

Norepinephrine increased LV pressure from 224 mm Hg to 305 mm Hg in dogs with LV hypertrophy, compared with an increase from 121 mm Hg to 177 mm Hg in control animals. Mean systolic wall stress rose from 224 gm/sq cm to 307 gm/sq cm in the study group and from 194 gm/sq cm to 299 gm/sq cm in the control group. The responses of the differential LV pressure and velocity of circumferential fiber shortening were similar in the two groups. Animals with LV hypertrophy had normal inotropic and mechanical reserve after prenalterol administration.

Dogs with chronic, marked LV hypertrophy have normal inotropic and mechanical reserve when afterload increases and ejection-phase indices of LV function are relatively constant, or when the reverse is the case. When the LV pressure increases gradually, substantial myocardial functional reserve may be expected.

▶ In this important study, the authors studied mechanical and inotropic reserve in conscious dogs with considerable LV hypertrophy but normal resting LV performance. They tested the hypothesis that the hypertrophied myocardium may have a reduced capacity to perform additional mechanical work and may exhibit a reduced inotropic responsiveness to β-adrenergic receptor agonists. They were able to demonstrate no difference between normal animals and those with pressure-overload LV hypertrophy in the response of several measures of myocardial contractility to an infusion of norepinephrine. Also, there was no difference in the hypertrophied and nonhypertrophied LV response to infusion of the β-agonist, prenalterol. Thus, in conscious animals with severe pressure-overload hypertrophy induced by a gradual increase in LV pressure, the hypertrophied myocardium functions normally not only at rest, but also when afterload is increased while ejection phase indices remain relatively constant, or when afterload remains relatively constant while ejection phase indices are augmented.—R.A. O'Rourke, M.D.

Exercise-Induced Cardiac Hypertrophy: A Correlation of Blood Flow and Microvasculature
Eric A. Breisch, Francis C. White, Lana E. Nimmo, M. Dan McKirnan, and Colin M. Bloor (Univ. of California at San Diego)
J. Appl. Physiol. 60:1259–1267, April 1986   1–5

It is generally held that exercise training benefits the myocardium. Previous studies found that physical exercise actually reduces the incidence and severity of myocardial infarction. However, reports on the benefits of exercise in existing ischemic heart disease are limited and conflicting. An experimental study was conducted to determine how chronic exercise conditioning affects the structure and function of the myocardium. The study was done with a control group of eight normal untrained young Hampshire farm pigs and an experimental group of seven pigs that had been exercised strenuously during a 12-week period on a treadmill and subsequently experienced exercise-induced hypertrophy. All pigs were instrumented according to standard methodology.

Oxygen consumption during maximum effort on the treadmill was significantly elevated in the trained pigs. The myocyte cross-sectional area also increased significantly in the trained heart. Although severe exercise-induced cardiac hypertrophy of the left ventricle was accompanied by normal transmural coronary blood flow, coronary vascular adaptations occurred, indicating a disparity between different segments of the vascular tree. There was some evidence of limited formation of new capillaries, but the data suggest that exercise does not significantly stimulate the production of new capillaries. This lack of neovascularization is apparently offset by the capillary system's ability to increase its luminal surface area. However, formation of new arterioles was enhanced in response to exercise training. The data from this study provide anatomical verification for the blood flow changes observed in exercise-induced hypertrophy, namely, a similar increase in transmural left ventricular flow during exercise and during exercise with adenosine infusion as occurred in animals without exercise-induced ventricular hypertrophy.

▶ In this study, the authors sought to provide a morphometric explanation as to why cardiac mechanical function and myocardial blood flow at rest and during exercise are basically unaffected by chronic exercise even though exercise-induced hypertrophy results. Comparing normal and exercise-trained pigs, these investigators found an increased luminal surface area of coronary capillaries and increased number and length densities of coronary arterioles that provide a structural basis for the similar myocardial blood flow data at rest and during exercise in the normal and trained animals.—R.A. O'Rourke, M.D.

Additional recent publications that provide important information in this area include the following:

1. Anversa, P., et al.: Quantitative structured analysis of the myocardium during physiologic growth and induced cardiac hypertrophy. A review. *J. Am. Coll. Cardiol.* 7:1140–1149, 1986.
2. Cummins, P., Lambert, S.J.: Myosin transitions in the bovine and human heart. A developmental and anatomical study of heavy and light chain subunits in the atrium and ventricle. *Circ. Res.* 58:846–858, 1986.
3. Karibayashi, T., et al.: Regional differences of myocyte hypertrophy and three-dimensional deformation of the heart. *Am. J. Physiol.* 250:H378–H388, 1986.
4. Rembert, J.C., Greenfield, J.C.: Myocardial flow during tachycardia in dogs with chronic left ventricular hypertrophy. *Am. J. Physiol.* 250:H968–H973, 1986.
5. Capasso, J.M., et al.: Myocardial biochemical, contractile, and electrical performance after imposition of hypertension in young and old rats. *Circ. Res.* 58:445–460, 1986.
6. Tomanek, R.J., et al.: Morphometry of canine, coronary arteries, arterioles, and capillaries during hypertension and left ventricular hypertrophy. *Circ. Res.* 58:38–46, 1986.

Exercise Physiology

Effects of Enhanced Ventricular Filling on Cardiac Pump Performance in Exercising Dogs
Lawrence D. Horwitz and Joann Lindenfeld (Univ. of Colorado)
J. Appl. Physiol. 59:1886–1890, December 1985   1–6

Strenuous exercise with resultant improvement in cardiac output after proper training is usually linked to increased stroke volume. However, the mechanism involved in such increases is not clear. Potential factors that

Volume Loading and Severe Exercise

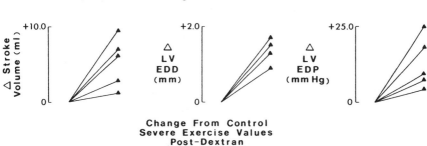

Change From Control
Severe Exercise Values
Post-Dextran

Fig 1–1.—Individual changes from control exercise results during severe exercise with dextran infusions. All dogs had increases in stroke volume, left ventricular end-diastolic left ventricular diameter, and left ventricular end-diastolic pressure in their dextran runs. (Courtesy of Horwitz, L.D., and Lindenfeld, J.: J. Appl. Physiol. 59:1886–1890, December 1985.)

could be responsible for this increase in stroke volume include an increase in myocardial contractile force, decrease in afterload, or an increase in preload. Assessment was made of the effect on stroke volume by increasing preload with dextran infusion during exercise in seven mongrel dogs weighing between 17 kg and 32 kg who were trained to run on a level treadmill.

Standard measuring devices were placed surgically around the proximal ascending aorta of each dog and baseline measurements were made of ascending aortic flow. Control exercise runs were done in a fasting state, with each dog running on a level treadmill for 3-minute periods at preselected loads of mild, moderate, or severe exertion. Each dog was given an infusion of 10% dextran in normal saline 1 hour after competion of the control run; 3 minutes later, the exercise sequences were repeated at the same loads as before.

When the data from control severe exercise runs without dextran were compared with corresponding data taken after dextran infusion, it was found that all dogs had significant increases in heart rate, stroke volume, cardiac output, and left ventricular end-diastolic pressure (Fig 1–1). The increase in stroke volume after dextran infusion was probably the result primarily of a higher preload. There is normally an increase in venous return during exercise that is partially responsible for the increase in cardiac output. In these experiments, further increments in preload during exercise could be induced by expansion of blood volume with dextran. Thus, alterations in the ability of the peripheral circulation to increase venous return to the heart is a potential means of augmenting stroke volume and cardiac output, such as with training or other interventions.

▶ There has been some controversy as to the relative importance of increases in heart rate and stroke volume and their contribution to the improvement in cardiac output that occurs during strenuous exercise. Some of this controversy is the result of differences in animal models, recording equipment, and type of exercise used in various studies. Increases in preload, decreases in afterload, or increases in contractility could each enhance stroke volume at any given exercise heart rate. In this study, the authors demonstrated that a substantial increment in stroke volume during exercise can be produced by increasing preload using dextran infusion. They were able to produce increased left ventricular filling and stroke volume during exercise with dextran as compared with control exercise results without changing isovolumic indices of myocardial contractility. Their conclusion, that an improved ability of the peripheral circulation to increase venous return to the heart during exercise could increase stroke volume and cardiac output (e.g., with dextran infusion or other interventions), is supported by the subsequent three papers (see Abstracts 1–7, 1–8, and 1–9).—R.A. O'Rourke, M.D.

Regulation of Stroke Volume During Submaximal and Maximal Upright Exercise in Normal Man

Michael B. Higginbotham, Kenneth G. Morris, R. Sanders Williams, Philip A. McHale, R. Edward Coleman, and Frederick R. Cobb (Duke Univ. and the Durham VA Med. Ctr., Durham, N.C.)
Circ. Res. 58:281–291, February 1986   1–7

   It was established in previous studies that an increase in stroke volume is an important cardiovascular adaptation to upright exercise in normal human beings. The physiologic factors that lead to this increase in stroke volume were examined by measuring pulmonary and systemic hemodynamic changes during upright bicycle exercise in 24 healthy male volunteers aged 20–50 years, who underwent simultaneous right heart catheterization, radionuclide angiography, and expired gas analysis at rest in supine and sitting positions, and while performing upright bicycle exercise to exhaustion. Although all of the participants had sedentary jobs, nine jogged regularly, but only three jogged daily.

   Oxygen consumption increased from rest to peak exercise from 0.33 L/minute to 2.55 L/minute. The arteriovenous oxygen difference increased from 5.8 vol% to 14.1 vol%. The cardiac index increased from 3.0 L/minute/sq m to 9.7 L/minute/sq m, resulting from the combination of an increase in heart rate and left ventricular (LV) stroke volume index. Whereas the linear increase in cardiac index noted during low levels of exercise was caused by both an increase in heart rate and stroke volume index, the further increases in cardiac index noted during high levels of exercise resulted entirely from an increase in heart rate alone, and the stroke volume index increased no further. The degree of increase in stroke volume index during exercise was related directly to changes in the end-diastolic and end-systolic volume indexes. The mechanism involved in the increase of LV stroke volume during upright exercise in human beings depends on the change in relationship between heart rate, LV diastolic filling, and LV contractility.

▶ This study in human volunteers during upright bicycle exercise shows that an increase in LV filling pressure and end-diastolic volume are important determinants of the stroke volume response through the Starling mechanism at low levels of exertion. At much higher levels of exertion, the increase in heart rate is accompanied by a decrease in end-diastolic volume despite a progressive increase in filling pressure, and the stroke volume must be maintained by a decrease in end-systolic volume. If one carefully considers whether upright or supine exercise is performed, as well as the relationship between heart rate, LV diastolic filling, and myocardial contractility before and at various degrees of exercise, the apparent disparities between this and other exercise studies detailed in the literature can be reconciled easily.—R.A. O'Rourke, M.D.

Effect of Isotonic Exercise Training on Left Ventricular Volume During Upright Exercise

Michael H. Crawford, Michael A. Petru, and Charles Rabinowitz, with the technical assistance of K. Wray Amon (Univ. of Texas at San Antonio, and VA Hosp., San Antonio)
Circulation 72:1237–1243, December 1985   1–8

Long-term isotonic exercise training reduces the resting heart rate and increases left ventricular (LV) end-diastolic volume, but it is not clear whether increased LV output in athletes during exercise is related merely to the larger resting end-diastolic volume or whether further increases in LV volume occur with exercise. An attempt was made to determine whether the large ventricular end-diastolic volume in a trained person can be further increased to take advantage of the less energy-consuming Frank-

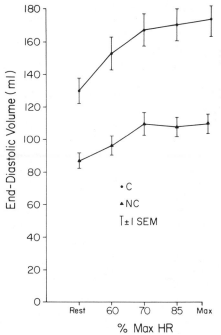

Fig 1–2.—End-diastolic volume at rest and at progressive levels of heart rate *(HR)* during exercise in competitive *(C)* and noncompetitive *(NC)* runners. (Courtesy of Crawford, M.H., et al.: Circulation 72:1237–1243, December 1985. By permission of the American Heart Association, Inc.)

Starling effect. Ten patients with angina caused by fixed coronary artery disease and 13 men with chronic stable angina served to validate the exercise two-dimensional echocardiographic technique. Thirty active normal persons, 12 of them highly trained endurance athletes, participated in bicycle exercise studies.

Isotonic exercise capacity appeared to be the chief determinant of resting LV size. Differences in LV end-diastolic volume between the competitive and noncompetitive athletes persisted during exercise (Fig 1–2) and became greater as exercise progressed. The same was true of stroke volume, but neither parameter increased significantly after 70% of maximal heart rate was achieved. The ratio of systolic blood pressure to end-systolic volume increased significantly only in the second half of maximum exercise in both groups. There were no significant group differences in ejection fraction throughout exercise. Highly trained athletes appear to make greater use of the Frank-Starling mechanism to achieve high performance levels of isotonic exercise than do less intensively trained runners.

▶ This study in competitive marathon runners and noncompetitive runners is consistent with previous observations. Left ventricular volumes were larger in the 12 competitive marathon runners. During exercise, the competitive runners exhibited larger increases in end-diastolic volume. The 18 noncompetitive athletes had a greater increase in indices of contractility. In both groups, the largest increase in end-diastolic volume occurred between the resting stage and the point during exercise when 70% of their maximum heart rate was attained. Whereas the competitive marathon runners used the Frank-Starling mechanism throughout the exercise period to a greater extent than the less conditioned athletes did, both used it to a major extent during light and moderate exercise and both tended to use an increase in contractility for any further increment in stroke volume.—R.A. O'Rourke, M.D.

The Effect of Pericardiectomy on Maximal Oxygen Consumption and Maximal Cardiac Output in Untrained Dogs

James Stray-Gunderson, Timothy I. Musch, George C. Haidet, David P. Swain, George A. Ordway, and Jere H. Mitchell (Univ. of Texas at Dallas and Southwestern Med. School, Dallas)
Circ. Res. 58:523–530, April 1986   1–9

Maximal cardiac output is a major determinant of maximal oxygen uptake, which in turn is an index of aerobic capacity. Both of these variables increase in response to a program of endurance exercise training. The training-induced increase in maximal cardiac output is totally the result of an increase in maximal stroke volume, because the maximal heart rate is unchanged or decreased by endurance training. In addition, there are data to suggest that endurance-trained athletes have larger end-diastolic volumes than do sedentary persons, which could provide for the increase in maximal stroke volume. Because the pericardium appears to exert a significant influence on the pressure-volume relationships of the left ventricle, it was hypothesized that the pericardium limits maximal oxygen consumption by limiting stroke volume and cardiac output. This hypothesis was tested in ten untrained dogs during submaximal and maximal exercise before and after pericardiectomy and in seven additional dogs before and after a sham operation. Cardiac output, heart rate, and the arteriovenous oxygen difference were measured, and oxygen consumption and stroke volume were calculated from these variables. After pericardiectomy there were significant increases in maximal oxygen consumption, maximal cardiac output, and maximal stroke volume. In addition, maximal oxygen consumption decreased markedly in the sham group. Maximal heart rate did not change after pericardiectomy, nor did maximal cardiac output, heart rate, or stroke volume change after sham operation. Both groups of dogs had similar significant decreases in hematocrit, arterial and venous oxygen contents, and the arteriovenous oxygen difference. Although neither pericardiectomy nor sham operation had any effect on oxygen consumption during submaximal exercise, the sham group had substantial increases in cardiac output and heart rate during submaximal exercise, and the pericardiectomy group tended toward increased cardiac output during submaximal exercise. These results support the hypothesis that the pericardium limits maximal oxygen consumption by limiting stroke volume and cardiac output during maximal exercise in untrained dogs. Moreover, these findings indicate that maximal oxygen consumption is limited by the oxygen transport capacity of the cardiovascular system, not by the oxidative capacity of skeletal muscle in the untrained dog.

▶ This study is of interest in relation to both the increase in left ventricular end-diastolic volume that occurs during exercise and the potential limiting effects of the pericardium on ventricular function, particularly during exercise. Interestingly, pericardiectomy produced significant increases in maximal oxygen consumption, maximal cardiac output, and maximal stroke volume with no significant change in maximal heart rate. The increments in maximal cardiac output and maximal stroke volume observed after pericardiectomy are similar to some of those observed during maximal exercise following dynamic exercise training. The results suggest that a possible adaptation to dynamic exercise training may be reflected by growth of the pericardium, and lend support to the concept that oxygen transport is the limiting component to maximal oxygen uptake.—R.A. O'Rourke, M.D.

Other important papers relevant to exercise physiology include the following:
1. Plotnick, G.D., et al.: Changes in left ventricular function during recovery from upright bicycle exercise in normal persons and patients with coronary artery disease. *Am. J. Cardiol.* 58:247–251, 1986.
2. Grover, R.F., et al.: Cardiovascular adaptation to exercise at high altitude. *Exerc. Sport Sci. Rev.* 14:269–302, 1986.
3. Kelback, H., et al.: Cardiac function and plasma catecholamines during upright exercise in healthy young subjects. *Int. J. Cardiol.* 10:223–231, 1986.
4. Hoette, C.A., et al.: Cardiac function and physical response of 146 profes-

sional football players to graded treadmill exercise tests. *J. Sports Med.* 26:34–42, 1986.

5. Vander, L.B., et al.: Acute cardiovascular responses to Nautilus exercise in cardiac patients: Implications for exercise training. *Ann. Sports Med.* 2:165–189, 1986.

Ventricular Diastolic Function

Left Ventricular Relaxation in the Filling and Nonfilling Intact Canine Heart
Edward L. Yellin, Masatsugu Hori, Chaim Yoran, Edmund H. Sonnenblick, Shlomo Gabbay, and Robert W.M. Frater (Albert Einstein College of Medicine and Bronx-Lebanon Hosp., Bronx)
Am. J. Physiol. 250:H620–H629, April 1986   1–10

There is increasing evidence that, in some heart disorders, relaxation may be impaired before contraction, thus the relaxation rate may be an early indicator of heart disease. End-systolic volume clamping was used to determine whether isovolumic relaxation is monoexponential, and to demonstrate that the left ventricle may relax to a negative pressure asymptote. Left ventricular relaxation was studied in the filling and transiently nonfilling working hearts of open-chest dogs by totally occluding the mitral anulus during one systole.

In the completely isovolumic nonfilling cycle, the ventricle relaxed to a lower pressure minimum than normal, usually to a negative level. When the ventricle was clamped at end systole, late relaxation was more rapid than predicted by a monoexponential relationship. The monoexponential time constant (T) nevertheless is a useful index of relaxation, correlating well with other temporal indices. When it is calculated from a filling cycle by assuming a zero pressure asymptote, there is no significant difference from the true value based on the nonfilling cycle.

▶ It is well established that abnormalities of left ventricular (LV) diastolic function frequently preceded impaired LV systolic function in patients with cardiac disease. This is particularly relevant to those with systemic hypertension and/or ischemic heart disease who frequently have signs and symptoms caused by pulmonary venous hypertension at rest or during exercise when measurements of LV systolic function are normal.

Current methods used to measure LV diastolic performance are less than satisfactory. In the experimental animal and in patients undergoing cardiac catheterization, the time constant of isovolumic relaxation, T, has been used to assess diastolic performance. Also, the LV end-diastolic pressure-volume relationship has been used to assess LV diastolic performance, and the peak rate of diastolic LV filling has been measured by noninvasive techniques as an indicator of diastolic performance in patients with various kinds of cardiac disease.

This study by Yellin and associates is important. The conventional monoexponential time constant, T, is not significantly different either physiologically or statistically from a more accurately derived time constant. Also, because the deviation of the exponential curve of pressure decline is not drastically different from the isovolumic pressure curve, it remains a good first approximation to the relaxation process and is useful in analysis of LV filling and diastolic properties.—R.A. O'Rourke, M.D.

Left Ventricular Filling Dynamics: Influence of Left Ventricular Relaxation and Left Atrial Pressure

Yoshio Ishida, Jay S. Meisner, Katsuhiko Tsujioka, Jose I. Gallo, Chaim Yoran, Robert W.M. Frater, and Edward L. Yellin (Albert Einstein College of Medicine, Bronx)
Circulation 74:187–196, July 1986   1–11

In many diseases, relaxation abnormalities are among the earliest manifestations of cardiac dysfunction. In fact, the time constant *(T)* of an assumed exponential isovolumetric pressure decline has been accepted as a good indicator of early cardiac function and is frequently measured during cardiac catheterization to evaluate left ventricular (LV) relaxation. Because this direct index of isovolumetric relaxation requires invasive measurement of LV pressure, it is assumed that LV relaxation can be measured indirectly by estimation of early diastolic filling. It was hypothesized that an early filling rate is a function of the atrioventricular pressure difference and, hence, is influenced by the left atrial pressure as well as by the rate of LV relaxation.

Research was carried out using eight large mongrel dogs. As indices the authors chose the left atrial pressure at the atrioventricular pressure crossover (PCO) and the *T* of an assumed exponential decline in left ventricular pressure. The magnitude and timing of filling parameters in conscious dogs was determined accurately by direct measurement of phasic mitral flow and high-fidelity chamber pressures. Loading conditions were altered by infusions of volume and angiotensin II to obtain a diverse hemodynamic data base. Angiotensin II was administered to cause a change in LV pressure of less than 35% (A-1) or a change in peak LV pressure of more than 35% (A-2). The peak rapid filling rate (PRFR) increased with volume loading, was unchanged with A-1, and was decreased with A-2, whereas *T* and PCO increased in all three groups. The PRFR correlated weakly with both *T* and PCO, and strongly with the diastolic atrioventricular pressure difference at the time of PRFR. The correlation improved significantly when *T* and PCO were both included in the multivariate regression. The PRFR is determined by both the left atrial pressure and the LV relaxation rate and should be used with caution as an index of LV diastolic function.

▶ The PRFR during diastole is frequently used clinically as an index for LV relaxation because it can be determined by noninvasive techniques, including echocardiography and radionuclide ventriculography. Many studies have used this measurement by noninvasive techniques to assess alterations in diastolic function produced by cardiac disease and by medical or surgical interventions.

This important study shows that the peak rapid ventricular filling rate is determined not only by the LV relaxation rate, but also by the left atrial pressure. The PRFR is determined by the driving atrioventricular (AV) pressure differences, and alterations in left atrial pressure can minimize or overcome the effects on early diastolic filling of changes in LV relaxation. The PRFR correlated strongly with the diastolic AV pressure difference at the time of PRFR and weakly with both T and the AV pressure crossover. Thus, PRFR should be used with caution as an index of LV diastolic function.—R.A. O'Rourke, M.D.

Myocardial Relaxation: Effects of Preload on the Time Course of Isovolumetric Relaxation
William H. Gaasch, John D. Carroll, Alvin S. Blaustein, and Oscar H.L. Bing (Tufts Univ. and VA Med. Ctr., Boston)
Circulation 73:1037–1041, May 1986   1–12

The time course of left ventricular (LV) isovolumetric pressure decline is set by a series of interacting factors including loading conditions, the inactivation rate of individual fibers, and the degree of fiber inhomogeneity within the wall of the ventricle. Because these factors are continuously modulated by autonomic tone and metabolic events, it is difficult to interpret some of the reported changes in the LV isovolumetric relaxation rate. At present there are no published studies defining the effects of an isolated increase in LV preload on isovolumetric relaxation. The effect of a pure increase in preload on isovolumetric relaxation was assessed in the intact dog heart and isometric relaxation in isolated cardiac muscle preparations.

The study used eight anesthetized dogs and rats. In the dogs 8–12 ml of blood was infused into the left ventricle during a single diastole, and the exponential time constant (T) of isovolumetric relaxation was determined in 62 single-beat experiments in which the LV systolic pressure increased (mean, 112 mm Hg to 128 mm Hg). In a second set of 23 experiments, the LV systolic pressure was held constant (mean, 109 mm Hg to 107 mm Hg) by simultaneous ventricular infusion and aortic unloading. During the first protocol, T increased from 28.0 msec to 30.7 msec, whereas in the second protocol (constant systolic pressure) there was no change in T. In addition, the time course of isometric relaxation was evaluated in the LV papillary muscles of six rats and in the right ventricular trabecular muscles of four dogs. Preload varied from 30% to 100% of the peak of the isometric length-tension curve in each muscle. In this range of preload, the isometric force decline recordings were superimposable as long as the comparisons were made at equal levels of total load. An isolated increase in preload apparently does not influence the time course of isovolumetric relaxation.

► For several years there have been multiple studies designed to define which hemodynamic alterations cause changes in the time constant (T) of LV isovolumetric pressure decline. In this study the authors demonstrate conclusively that isolated changes in preload do not affect a change in T, nor influence the time course of isometric relaxation in isolated heart muscles.—R.A. O'Rourke, M.D.

The Relationship of High Energy Phosphates, Tissue pH, and Regional Blood Flow to Diastolic Distensibility in the Ischemic Dog Myocardium
Shin-ichi Momomura, Joanne S. Ingwall, J. Anthony Parker, Peter Sahagian, James J. Ferguson, and William Grossman (Beth Israel Hosp., Brigham and Women's Hosp., and Harvard Univ., Boston)
Circ. Res. 57:822–835, December 1985   1–13

A reversible increase in left ventricular (LV) diastolic pressure relative to chamber volume is a frequent observation in patients with angina pectoris. Moreover, recently a similar upward shift in LV diastolic pressure-segment length relationships was observed in dogs with critical coronary stenoses during ischemia induced by pacing tachycardia. Conversely, primary myocardial ischemia caused by brief occlusion of a coronary artery or global reduction in coronary blood flow failed to produce an upward shift in LV diastolic pressure-volume or pressure-segment length relationships. At present, there is no clear explanation for the differences in diastolic distensibility in these two different types of ischemia. Assessment was made of the relationship between myocardial diastolic function and metabolism by measuring the myocardial high-energy phosphate content, tissue pH, and regional blood flow during ischemia caused by increased oxygen demand compared with primary ischemia of comparable duration caused by coronary occlusion.

Studies were performed using open-chest dogs. After 3 minutes of pacing tachycardia in dogs with critical coronary stenoses (demand-type ischemia in 14), regional systolic function was mildly depressed, whereas LV diastolic pressure-segment length relationships shifted upward, demonstrating decreased distensibility of the ischemic myocardial segment. In association with these changes in function, the subendocardial adenosine triphosphate (ATP) content dropped significantly, as did the creatine phosphate level, and myocardial pH declined only slightly. Conversely, at 3 minutes of coronary artery occlusion (primary ischemia in 14 dogs), regional segment shortening was replaced by systolic bulging, and neither LV pressure-segment length relationships nor diastolic distensibility of the ischemic segment were changed. During coronary artery occlusion, the subendocardial ATP content declined slightly, whereas the creatine phosphate level decreased markedly and the myocardial pH fell substantially. The decline in pH was 236% of that seen with demand-type ischemia. The regional myocardial blood flow revealed a decreased endocardial epicardial ratio and a decreased absolute subendocardial flow with demand-type ischemia. Subendocardial blood flow in demand-type ischemia was still much greater than flow during coronary artery occlusion.

Diastolic dysfunction could not be explained simply by ATP depletion, which was modest and similar with both types of ischemia. It is likely that protection against diastolic dysfunction in primary ischemia may be the result of the combined effects of hydrogen ion accumulation, loss of coronary vascular turgor, and repeated systolic stretch of the ischemic segment.

▶ Several recent studies support a causative role for demand ischemia in producing impaired ventricular diastolic relaxation and decreased regional myocardial distensibility. In this animal study, myocardial ischemia caused by 3 minutes of complete coronary occlusion produced dominant systolic dysfunction of the ventricle with mild diastolic impairment. There was a fall in myocardial pH with preservation of a nearly normal ATP concentration. However, with myocardial ischemia caused by coronary stenosis plus tachycardia for 3 minutes, impaired diastolic function was predominant. In this situation, the ATP content was mildly depleted, but the decline in pH was much smaller. These differences in ATP depletion and acidosis may explain why diastolic abnormalities predominate in the model of ischemia produced by increasing myocardial oxygen demand.—R.A. O'Rourke, M.D.

Effects of Verapamil on Regional Myocardial Diastolic Function in Pacing-Induced Ischemia in Dogs

Patrick D. Bourdillon, Walter J. Paulus, Takashi Serizawa, and William Grossman (Harvard Univ., Brigham and Women's Hosp., and Beth Israel Hosp., Boston)
Am. J. Physiol. 251:H834–H840, October 1986   1–14

An upward shift in the left ventricular (LV) diastolic pressure-volume relationship is noted during pacing-induced angina and after pacing tachycardia in dogs with fixed coronary stenoses. Caffeine, which potentiates this shift, prolongs intracellular calcium availability, suggesting that calcium channel blockade might counter its effect on the diastolic pressure-volume relationship. The effects of verapamil were studied in dogs with fixed coronary stenoses subjected to pacing tachycardia. A dose of 0.08 mg/kg, equivalent to that used clinically, was administered; also the effect of verapamil pretreatment was studied in dogs given caffeine intravenously to lower the systolic blood pressure by 20%.

Verapamil treatment led to a fall in arterial pressure and had some negative inotropic effect at rest. An upward shift of the LV diastolic pressure-segment length relationship was observed during pacing tachycardia, with or without verapamil pretreatment. Caffeine injection led to marked exacerbation of the upward shift of the LV diastolic pressure-segment length relationship on pacing, and pretreatment with verapamil did not significantly diminish this effect.

Verapamil does not prevent the upward shift of the LV diastolic pressure segment-length relationship accompanying pacing-induced ischemia in dogs with coronary stenoses, nor did it prevent exacerbation of the upward shift caused by caffeine. Intracellular calcium homeostasis presumably is impaired in this setting. It is possible that increased calcium influx via separate channels could operate with decreased calcium sequestration by the sarcoplasmic reticulum to produce increased cytosolic calcium and result in incomplete diastolic relaxation or partial inactivation. The result might be superimposition of an "active" stiffness on the passive elasticity of the ventricular myocardium.

▶ The direct effect of calcium entry blockade on the diastolic properties of the ventricle is controversial. Previous studies found that calcium entry blockade, using doses of calcium blockers that do not alter importantly systolic function, results in prolongation of the time constant of isovolumic relaxation. This was true both in normal animals and in animals in which myocardial ischemia resulted in prolongation of isovolumic relaxation before administration of calcium entry blockers.

Several clinical studies from Boston have suggested that calcium entry blockade actually improves diastolic properties in patients with ischemic heart disease and in those with hypertrophic cardiomyopathy.

In the present study in dogs with 90% stenoses of the left anterior descending and circumflex coronary arteries, the abnormal rise in LV end-diastolic pressure for any LV wall segment length was not altered by pretreatment with verapamil. Because the upward shift in the diastolic pressure-segment length relationship with pacing-induced ischemnia was not prevented by calcium entry blockade with verapamil, it is unlikely that this upward shift during myocardial ischemia is mediated by increased transmembrane calcium flux.—R.A. O'Rourke, M.D.

Noninvasive Assessment of Left Ventricular Diastolic Function: Comparative Analysis of Doppler Echocardiographic and Radionuclide Angiographic Techniques

Paolo Spirito, Barry J. Maron, and Robert O. Bonow (Natl. Insts. of Health, Bethesda, Md.)
J. Am. Coll. Cardiol. 7:518–526, March 1986   1–15

Doppler echocardiography provides important clinical information about valvular stenosis and regurgitation, intracardiac shunts, and cardiac output. Recently, the left ventricular (LV) diastolic flow velocity waveform obtained with Doppler recording, in combination with a two-dimensional echocardiographic assessment of mitral valve area and LV volume, was used to estimate instantaneous diastolic flow. Thus, the Doppler diastolic flow velocity waveform may provide measurements of LV diastolic function. However, the complexity of the measurements is increased by the need for quantitative echocardiographic determination of mitral valve area and LV volume. Preliminary studies have indicated that variables obtained solely from the Doppler LV diastolic flow velocity waveform could be used to obtain an indirect assessment of diastolic function. An attempt was made to verify whether this method allows a valid assessment of diastolic function.

Measurements of diastolic flow velocity obtained by Doppler echocardiography were compared with volumetric determinations of LV diastolic filling obtained by radionuclide angiography in 12 patients without cardiac disease and in 25 patients with a variety of cardiac diseases. The two methods were in agreement in distinguishing normal from abnormal diastolic function in 21 (84%) of the 25 patients with cardiac disease, identifying diastolic function as normal in 8 and abnormal in 13 of these patients. Furthermore, good correlations were observed between certain Doppler variables of LV diastolic flow velocity and radionuclide angiographic variables of LV filling. The time interval from the aortic closing component of the second heart sound to the end of the early diastolic flow velocity peak, measured by Doppler echocardiography, was in close agreement with the time interval from end systole to the end of rapid filling determined by radionuclide angiography. In addition, descent of the Doppler early diastolic flow velocity peak correlated with the radionuclide angiographic peak filling rate. The ratio between the heights of the early and late peaks of diastolic flow velocity exhibited good correlation with the ratio between percent of LV filling during rapid filling and during atrial systole.

The LV diastolic flow velocity profile obtained with Doppler echocardiography compares closely with radionuclide angiographic variables in evaluation of LV diastolic function. Because of this, indexes derived directly from the Doppler diastolic flow velocity waveform may be useful in providing a noninvasive, reliable, and easily obtained estimate of diastolic performance in patients with cardiac disease.

▶ There has been great interest in developing noninvasive methods for the initial and serial evaluation of diastolic performance in patients with cardiac disease. Both radionuclide ventriculography and two-dimensional echocardiography have been used for this purpose. It was proposed more recently that Doppler mitral valve velocity recordings might be useful for this purpose.

In the study reviewed here, Doppler echocardiographic and radionuclide ventriculographic measurements of diastolic flow velocity were compared in a laboratory where the radionuclide ventriculography technique is performed well. Good correlations were observed between certain Doppler measures of LV diastolic flow velocity and radionuclide measurements. However, despite good corelation coefficients for LV diastolic flow velocity by the two techniques, the standard error of the estimate is relatively large. Thus, in any individual case, one technique is likely to over- or underestimate severely the actual measurement of LV diastolic filling as compared with the alternate technique. The authors appropriately indicate that LV diastolic filling is a complex phenomenon determined by multiple factors, including LV relaxation, intrinsic myocardial muscle properties, and loading conditions of the left ventricle.—R.A. O'Rourke, M.D.

Additional interesting publications concerning LV diastolic function include the following:
1. Nakamura, Y., et al.: Measurement of relaxation in isolated rat ventricular myocardium during hypoxia and reoxygenation. *Cardiovasc. Res.* 20:690–697, 1986.

2. Chemla, D., et al.: Relationship between inotropy and relaxation in rat myocardium. *Am. J. Physiol.* 250:H1008–H1016, 1986.
3. Miller, T.R., et al.: Left ventricular diastolic filling and its association with age. *Am. J. Cardiol.* 58:531–535, 1986.
4. Kettunen, R., et al.: Time constant of isovolumic pressure fall in the intact canine left ventricle. *Cardiovasc. Res.* 20:698–704, 1986.
5. Lawson, W.E., et al.: A new use for M-mode echocardiography in detecting left ventricular dysfunction in coronary artery disease. *Am. J. Cardiol.* 58:210–213, 1986.
6. Lorell, B.H., et al.: The influence of pressure overload left ventricular hypertrophy on diastolic properties during hypoxia in isovolumically contracting rat hearts. *Circ. Res.* 58:653–663, 1986.

Ventricular Systolic Function

Effect of Alteration of Left Ventricular Activation Sequence on the Left Ventricular End-Systolic Pressure-Volume Relation in Closed-Chest Dogs

R. Conrad Park, William C. Little, and Robert A. O'Rourke (Univ. of Texas at San Antonio)

Circ. Res. 57:706–717, November 1985   1–16

The left ventricular (LV) end-systolic pressure-volume relationship is a sensitive index of LV systolic function that is relatively independent of loading conditions. The slope of this relationship is sensitive to changes in ventricular performance, but it has not yet been determined whether dyssynchronous activation of the left ventricle affects LV systolic performance independent of changes in loading conditions. The effect of alterations of the LV activation sequence produced by ventricular pacing on the LV end-systolic pressure-volume relationship were examined in chronically instrumented dogs.

Ten healthy adult mongrel dogs underwent pacing of the heart, initially from the atrium, followed by pacing from each of the ventricular epicardial and/or endocardial sites in random order. The animals were sacrificed at the completion of the study to verify proper positioning of the instruments.

Hemodynamic data from the steady-state periods during pacing from the atria and various ventricular epicardial sites indicated that alterations of the normal LV activation sequence depress LV systolic pumping function, resulting in a rightward shift of the LV end-systolic pressure-volume relationship. The data further indicate that the extent of the rightward shift of the pressure-volume relationship seems to be in proportion to the degree of dyssynchronous activation of the LV. The decreased stroke volume during ventricular pacing is caused by both a decrease in LV end-diastolic volume and a rightward shift of the LV end-systolic pressure-volume relationship.

▶ The LV end-systolic pressure-volume relationship is linear in normal contracting isolated canine hearts, chronically instrumented dogs, and man. The slope of the relationship is sensitive to changes in ventricular performance resulting from global interventions; it increases in response to positive inotropic manipulations and decreases with negative inotropic interventions.

Several clinical implications result from the foregoing study. First, any disturbance of ventricular activation caused by ventricular pacing or conduction system abnormalities must be considered when interpreting the LV end-systolic pressure-volume relationship. Also, ventricular pacing appears to depress LV pumping performance in addition to the impairment of ventricular diastolic filling that usually results from loss of a properly timed atrial systole.—R.A. O'Rourke, M.D.

Influence of Pacing Site on Canine Left Ventricular Contraction
Daniel Burkhoff, Robert Y. Oikawa, and Kiichi Sagawa, with the technical assistance of Kenneth Rent (Johns Hopkins Univ.)
Am. J. Physiol. 251:H428–H435, August 1986   1–17

The influence of pacing site on various aspects of left ventricular (LV) performance was examined to investigate the hypothesis that the effective ventricular muscle mass that participates in generation of active contractile strength is reduced when the pacing site is moved from the atrium to the ventricle. Studies were performed on isolated canine hearts constrained to contract isovolumically to allow for study of LV properties. The LV pressure waves were recorded in eight isolated hearts paced at 130 beats per minute. Pacing was done epicardially from the atrium, LV apex, LV free wall (LVFW), and right ventricular (RV) free wall, and endocardially from the RV endocardium.

Peak isovolumic pressures were smaller with ventricular pacing than with atrial pacing. Moreover, pacing from different myocardial sites produced different levels of contractile strength, with beats from the atrium the strongest and beats from the LVFW the weakest. There was little influence on contraction duration or on the time-course of chamber stiffening and relaxation, as judged from the similarity of the shapes of the isovolumic pressure waves. A highly significant, linear, negative correlation was noted between peak isovolumic pressure and duration of the QRS complex of an epicardial surface electrogram. In comparison with atrial pacing, the slope of the end-systolic pressure-volume relationship was decreased with ventricular pacing, but the volume axis intercept was relatively constant. Reduced ventricular oxygen consumption was noted in association with reduced ventricular strength resulting from ventricular pacing so that metabolic efficiency was preserved. These data support the above-stated hypothesis.

▶ These studies in isolated supported canine hearts that contracted isovolumically suggest that the effective mass of muscle that participates in chamber contraction is reduced with ventricular pacing. The data from this group differ somewhat from findings reported previously by Park et al. (Abstract 1–16). In the current study the slope of the end-systolic pressure-volume relationship was decreased with ventricular pacing, but the volume intercept was relatively constant. These differing findings may result from some altered properties of the electrical activation system created when the heart is studied in isolation.— R.A. O'Rourke, M.D.

End-Systolic Measures of Regional Ventricular Performance

Thomas Aversano, W. Lowell Maughan, William C. Hunter, David Kass, and Lewis C. Becker (Johns Hopkins Univ.)
Circulation 73:938–950, May 1986   1–18

It is often of interest to know the regional myocardial contractile state. Current methods available to determine this parameter include measurement of dimension changes, either absolute or percent wall thickening (ΔT or $\%\Delta T$) or segment length shortening (ΔL or $\%\Delta L$). When these values change, it is assumed that this indicates a change in regional contractile state or performance. However, dimension change measures of regional myocardial performance are highly load dependent, and it is likely that simple dimension change measures can be unreliable estimates of the regional myocardial contractile state. It was hypothesized that end-systolic pressure-thickness and end-systolic pressure-length relationships (ESPTR, ESPLR) are more load-independent measures of regional function.

In 16 anesthetized mongrel dogs, ESPTR and ESPLR could be measured without detectable baroreceptor-mediated reflex changes in the cardiac contractile state. However, systemic administration of dobutamine shifted the ESPTR to the right and the ESPLR to the left of control, largely because of a change in the slope (Ees) of the relationships. It was observed that both ΔT, $\%\Delta T$ and ΔL, $\%\Delta L$ failed to detect the positive inotropic effect of dobutamine because of an associated reduction in preload. Nevertheless, with systemic administration of propranolol, ESPTR, ESPLR, ΔT, $\%\Delta T$, and ΔL, $\%\Delta L$ all detected the negative inotropic effect. Propranolol given systemically shifted the ESPTR to the left and the ESPLR to the right of control, primarily the result of a change in Ees. The regional administration of dobutamine shifted the ESPTR and the ESPLR in the direction of positive contractility in the region the received the drug; however, simple dimension change measures of regional function did not detect the inotropic effect because preload fell and the timing of regional end-systole was changed. With regional propranolol, both the ESPTR, ESPLR, and simple dimension change measures were able to detect the negative inotropic effect. Determination of the ESPTR and ESPLR is a reliable measure of regional ventricular function that may be better than simple dimension change measures of regional function, especially when the loading conditions or timing of regional systole are changed by an intervention.

▶ These studies of 16 anesthetized mongrel dogs suggests that the ESPTR and ESPLR are reliable measures of regional ventricular performance and may be better than simple dimension change measures of regional function during interventions than are change loading conditions or synchrony of regional contraction. These indices appear to be less load-dependent measures of regional function than are percent changes in wall thickening or segmental shortening. Although the ESPTR and ESPLR are useful in detecting and defining changes in contractile performance, they have not been normalized, making comparison of absolute values between animals difficult to interpret.—R.A. O'Rourke, M.D.

Assessment of Slope of End-Systolic Pressure-Volume Line of In Situ Dog Heart
Yuichiro Igarashi and Hiroyuki Suga (Natl. Cardiovascular Ctr. Res. Inst., Osaka, Japan)
Am. J. Physiol. 250:H685–H692, 1986   1–19

The end-systolic pressure-volume relationship line that passes through the left upper corners of the pressure-volume loops of steady-state contractions during variable loading is reported to be nearly independent of preload, afterload, and heart rate in a given constant contractile state in the excised cross-circulated canine left ventricle. However, it is difficult to maintain a constant contractile state in an in situ heart while variable loading conditions are produced. A method of determining in situ slope was developed by producing an isovolumic contraction through abrupt occlusion of the ascending aorta after steady-state ejecting contractions in anesthetized open-chest dogs.

Left ventricular pressure was measured with a catheter tip micromanometer and plotted against the time integral of aortic flow, which was measured with an electromagnetic flowmeter at the last ejecting and the first isovolumic contraction. The same end-diastolic volume was assumed. Both pacing and infusion of isoproterenol were used. The end-systolic pressure-volume curve was drawn from the peak isovolumic pressure-volume point tangential to the left upper corner of the pressure-volume loop of the ejecting contraction. The control slope of 16.4 mm Hg/ml was increased 59% by isoproterenol administration and reduced 47% by propranolol. Atrial pacing led to little change in the slope. This method of aortic occlusion is useful in assessing left ventricular contractility in the in situ canine heart.

▶ In this study, the authors examine a new method of evaluating E_{max} to the in situ heart. Using abrupt aortic occlusion, they measure left ventricular pressure and aortic flow and assume the same left ventricular end-diastolic volume. Ventricular pressure and aortic flow trajectories of these contractions are superimposed in the same pressure-volume diagram to determine the end-systolic pressure-volume line. The slope of this line sensitively reflected acute changes in contractile state and was constant despite heart rate changes induced by atrial pacing. This approach has promise as a simple new method for assessment of ventricular contractile state in the in situ heart.—R.A. O'Rourke, M.D.

Assessment of the End-Systolic Pressure-Volume Relationship in Human Beings With the Use of a Time-Varying Elastance Model

Raymond G. McKay, Julian M. Aroesty, Gary V. Heller, Henry D. Royal, Sanford E. Warren, and William Grossman (Beth Israel Hosp. and Harvard Univ.)
Circulation 74:97–104, July 1986   1–20

Considerable evidence has indicated that the end-systolic pressure-volume relationship is linear over a physiologic range of loading conditions and is a sensitive indicator of left ventricular (LV) contractile function. However, analysis of these relationships in human beings has been hindered by the lack of a practical method of serial volume assessment and by an imprecise definition of end-systole. Modifications of the end-systolic relationship to circumvent these difficulties have included the use of single-point end-systolic pressure-volume ratios, the use of peak systolic pressure/minimum ventricular volume points for end-systolic points, and the use of end-ejection as a marker for end-systole. The correlation was assessed between the parameters generated by these modifications with the slope (E_{max}) and intercept (V_o) of the end-systolic line as defined by Sagawa's model of time-varying elastance.

The study group consisted of 26 patients (17 men) whose mean age was 60 years; all were undergoing cardiac catheterization. Left ventricular pressure and gated radionuclide volume were measured simultaneously under various loading conditions, and pressure-volume diagrams were constructed for each loading condition from 32 simultaneous pressure-volume coordinates. There were two pressure-volume diagrams recorded from 14 patients and three pressure-volume diagrams from 12. The E_{max} and V_o were evaluated in all patients from the elastance as described by Sagawa's model; these were designated true E_{max} computed from a single-point end-systolic ratio, from peak systolic pressure/minimum systolic volume points, and from end-ejection pressure-volume points marked by peak negative differential LV pressure.

The parameters E_{max} and V_o of a time-varying elastance model of the end-systolic pressure-volume relationship can be constructed for human beings using simultaneous LV pressure measurements and gated radionuclide ventriculography. Moreover, true E_{max}, when calculated by this method, is reasonably approximated by single-point pressure-volume ratios and peak systolic end-ejection measurements.

▶ This patient study used measurements of the end-systolic pressure-volume relationship (ESPVR) obtained using simultaneous LV pressure measurements and gated radionuclide ventriculography. The true E_{max} calculated by this method appears reasonably approximated by single point pressure-volume ratios and peak systolic and end-ejection measurements.

Use of LV ESPVRs in man to assess LV performance has been desirable, but the need to alter the end-systolic pressure using drugs that either increase systemic vascular resistance or cause arterial vasodilatation while obtaining only two or three points over a limited range of pressure has been a problem. Also important has been the need to assess LV volume at end systole using a reliable method that has minimal error. Current techniques are suboptimal. The use of vasodilators or vasopressors may change the slope of the ESPVR without altering contractility, and it is desirable to obtain multiple points to construct the most appropriate line indicating the slope of this relationship. In the present study, as in most clinical studies, the linearity of the end-systolic relationship was approximated using pressure-volume relationships over a limited range of pressures. A second assumption is that there is a constant inotropic state at baseline and after pharmacologic manipulation. The possibility of a centrally mediated reflex change in contractility cannot be ruled out.

A recent study by Freeman and associates (*Circulation* 74:1107–1113, 1986) in preinstrumented conscious dogs indicates that the ESPVR obtained by pharmacologic alteration of load is different from that obtained using rapid inferior vena cava occlusion and is dependent on the vasoactivation used. Methoxamine shifted the relationship to the left and nitroprusside shifted it to the right. The composite ESPVRs in animals given angiotensin II had a steeper slope and were shifted to the right compared with those generated by control caval occlusion. The composite relationships in animals given methoxamine had a flatter slope with no significant differences in V_o compared with control caval occlusion. These factors must be considered when interpreting the findings of studies using ESPVR, particularly in patients to whom one drug is given to obtain a point at a higher end-systolic pressure and another drug is given to obtain a end-systolic volume point at a lower systolic pressure.—R.A. O'Rourke, M.D.

Other publications concerning LV systolic performance include the following:
1. Suga, H., et al.: Peak isovolumic pressure-volume relation of puppy left ventricle. *Am. J. Physiol.* 250:H167–H172, 1986.
2. Kil, P.J.M., Schiereck, P.: End-systolic pressure-volume relations of isolated ejecting rabbit left ventricles after quick diastolic volume changes. *Cardiovasc. Res.* 19:782–792, 1986.
3. Iskandrian, A.S., Heo, J.: Left ventricular pressure/volume relationship in coronary artery disease. *Am. Heart J.* 112:375–381, 1986.
4. Way, B., et al.: Hysteresis of left ventricular end ejection pressure dimension relations after acute pressure loading in the intact canine heart. *Cardiovasc. Res.* 20:440–447, 1986.
5. Schorten, V.J.A., Terkeurs, H.E.D.J.: The force-frequency relationship in rat myocardium. *Pflugers Arch.* 407:14–17, 1986.
6. Teplick, R., et al.: Time dependence of the oxygen cost of force development during systole in the canine left ventricle. *Circ. Res.* 59:27–38, 1986.

Heart Failure

Loss of High Affinity Cardiac Beta Adrenergic Receptors in Dogs With Heart Failure
Dorothy E. Vatner, Stephen F. Vatner, Alan M. Fujii, and Charles J. Homcy (Harvard Univ., Massachusetts Gen. Hosp., and Brigham and Women's Hosp., Boston, and New England Primate Res. Ctr., Southborough, Mass.)
J. Clin. Invest. 76:2259–2264, December 1985   1–21

There have been several disorders of autonomic cardiovascular control described in experimental animals and in patients with heart failure. It is possible that the mechanism of altered autonomic control of the heart involves changes in receptor regulation. Several studies have examined β-adrenergic receptor regulation in heart failure with conflicting results reported. However, no previous study has systematically evaluated the changes in β-adrenergic receptor density and affinity, using agonist and antagonist ligand binding studies in combination with measurement of adenylate cyclase activity in an experimental large mammalian model of left ventricular (LV) failure. β-Adrenergic and muscarinic receptor regulation was examined in dogs with pressure overload-induced LV failure.

Left ventricular failure was characterized by a doubling of LV weight-body weight ratio and elevation of LV end-diastolic pressure. Despite a 44% increase in receptor density as measured by antagonist binding studies with [^{3}H]dihydroalprenolol, there was a twofold decrease in receptor affinity, e.g., an increased dissociation constant (K_d) in heart failure. Agonist displacement of [^{3}H]dihydroalprenolol binding with isoproterenol in the presence and absence of 5'-guanylylimidodiphosphate [Gpp(NH)p] showed a marked decrease of high affinity binding sites in heart failure. Similarly, β-adrenergic receptor-mediated stimulation of adenylate cyclase and maximal stimulation with Gpp(NH)p or sodium fluoride was also depressed in heart failure. In addition, there was a concomitant drop in muscarinic receptor density (242 fmole/mg vs. 111 fmole/mg).

Whereas muscarinic receptor density dropped, β-adrenergic receptor density actually increased during LV failure. However, a larger portion of the β-adrenergic receptors are not functionally coupled to the GTP-stimulating protein, as shown by the decrease in the fraction of receptors that bind agonist with high affinity.

▶ There has been considerable interest in the status of β-adrenergic receptor density and affinity in patients with congestive heart failure. In fact, a decrease in β-receptor number in patients with heart failure has been attributed to long-standing catecholamine stimulation, resulting in "down-regulation." This is proposed as the reason why there is no improvement in long-term survival in patients treated with chronic β-agonists in attempts to improve myocardial contractility long term. Also, some have suggested using β-adrenergic blocking agents to treat patients with severe dilated cardiomyopathy in an effort to improve long-term survival either by causing "up-regulation" of β receptors, thus improving the response to catecholamines and/or by preventing potentially fatal arrhythmias.

In this important study in dogs with LV failure produced by chronic pressure load, there was actually an increased β-adrenergic receptor number. However, a larger proportion of the β-adrenergic receptors were not functionally coupled to the GTP-stimulatory protein, as indicated by a decreased percentage of the receptors that bound agonists with high affinity. In contrast, the muscarinic receptor number was reduced by 50% in the left ventricles with heart failure. This may result from loss of sympathetic prejunctional neurons in heart failure, as occurs with cardiac denervation. The results of this study are consistent with clinical observations in man regarding the use of β receptor agonists and antagonists, and clarify the previous controversy concerning the effect of chronic heart failure on β receptor numbers and affinity.—R.A. O'Rourke, M.D.

The Relationship Between Plasma Levels of Immunoreactive Atrial Natriuretic Hormone and Hemodynamic Function in Man

Eric R. Bates, Yoram Shenker, and Roger J. Grekin (VA Med. Ctr., Ann Arbor)
Circulation 73:1155–1161, June 1986   1–22

Atrial peptides, termed atrial natriuretic hormone (ANH), are released from atrial myocytes and induce diuresis, natriuresis, and vasorelaxation in man. A radioimmunoassay for human plasma immunoreactive ANH was used to examine relationships between plasma levels and various hemodynamic parameters in 34 patients having right heart catheterization, 21 of whom also had left heart catheterization. Blood was sampled for ANH determination before contrast injection.

Right atrial and pulmonary wedge pressures, mean arterial pressure, and heart rate were independent and significant predictors of central plasma immunoreactive ANH levels. Correlation with right atrial pressure was closest, and this parameter also correlated significantly with peripheral ANH levels. In patients with left ventricular failure, the plasma ANH level was elevated out of proportion to the right atrial pressure. Pulmonary wedge pressure also correlated significantly with peripheral ANH levels. Mean central ANH levels were twice the peripheral levels.

It would appear that distention of either the left or right atrium may be a potent stimulus to immunoreactive ANH release in man. However, circulating levels may be ineffective in producing diuresis and natriuresis. It is possible that inactive forms of ANH are secreted, or that the sympathetic vasoconstrictor tone or the renin-aldosterone system overrides the natriuretic-diuretic effects of physiologic levels of ANH in states of volume overload. Further studies of the mechanisms regulating ANH secretion in man should include atrial pressure estimates.

▶ There has been many recent basic and clinical studies concerning the atrial natriuretic factor. Atrial peptides released from secretory granules located in atrial myocytes induce diuresis, natriuresis, and vasorelaxation in animals and man. Atrial distention appears to be the predominant stimulus that triggers release of ANH in rats.

In the present study, the relationship between plasma levels of immunoreactive ANH and different hemodynamic parameters were assessed in 34 patients undergoing right heart catheterization. Patients with volume overload states had elevated levels of ANH with distention of either atrium acting as the potent stimulus for release of this hormone. However, the presence of prominent edema despite high ANH levels suggests that circulating ANH is ineffective in producing diuresis and natriuresis in patients with chronic congestive heart failure.

This is just one of many studies of ANH performed in patients with heart failure. Considerable new information concerning regulation of ANH secretion and its effect on hemodynamics, including myocardial contractility, should be forthcoming in the near future.—R.A. O'Rourke, M.D.

Other relevant recent publications include the following:

1. Ballerman, B. J., Brenner, B. J.: Role of atrial peptides in body fluid homostasis. *Circ. Res.* 58:619–630, 1986.
2. Rodeheffer, R. J., et al.: Atrial pressure and secretion of atrial natriuretic factor into the human central circulation. *J. Am. Coll. Cardiol.* 8:18–26, 1986.

Experimental Myocardial Ischemia/Infarction

Reversal of Dysfunction in Postischemic Stunned Myocardium by Epinephrine and Postextrasystolic Potentiation
Lewis C. Becker, Joseph H. Levine, Anthony F. DiPaula, Thomas Guarnieri, and Thomas Aversano (Johns Hopkins Univ.)
J. Am. Coll. Cardiol. 7:580–589, March 1986   1–23

Although coronary reperfusion is able to salvage ischemic myocardium anatomically, function may remain depressed even in the absence of infarction after normal flow is restored. Salvaged myocardium that exhibits prolonged impairment of function after ischemia is referred to as "stunned." In animal studies it has been demonstrated that administration of catecholamines can produce at least a short-term functional improvement in stunned myocardium. Dysfunction in stunned myocardium may result from a deficiency of adenosine triphosphate and high energy phosphate precursors. An attempt was made to learn whether sufficient functional and metabolic reserve exists in stunned myocardium to sustain a prolonged, maximal inotropic response to epinephrine and postextrasystolic potentiation.

The study was performed using 11 open-chest dogs in which the left anterior descending coronary artery was occluded for 5 minutes, followed by 10 minutes of reflow; this was repeated 12 times with a final 1-hour recovery period. Regional myocardial function was assessed using pairs of ultrasonic dimension crystals implanted in ischemic and nonischemic zones. During repetitive reflows, a progressive decrease in mean systolic segment shortening occurred: baseline, 21.8%; first reflow, 15.2%; twelfth reflow, 4.3%; and 1-hour recovery, 7.9%. When intravenously administered epinephrine was titrated to produce a maximal inotropic response, it caused segment shortening to increase to 21.6% after 10 minutes and to 24.8% after 1 hour of infusion despite a 20-mm Hg increase in systolic pressure. The same dose of epinephrine given prior to ischemia increased segment shortening to 30.5%. In six dogs, postextrasystolic potentiation before ischemia increased segment shortening from 21.8% to 31.1%, and after 1 hour of recovery from ischemia, from 7.9% to 24.8%. In nonischemic segments there were lesser increases in segment shortening.

The present data demonstrate that the stunned myocardium possesses considerable functional reserve. Deficient energy stores are not likely to be the basis for the depressed function seen at rest in stunned myocardium.

▶ Myocardium salvaged after normal myocardial blood flow is restored, but demonstrating prolonged impairment of function after ischemia, is often called "stunned" myocardium. In the current study, the finding that both postextrasystolic potentiation and systemic epinephrine both caused a marked and quantitatively similar improvement in postischemic function suggests that β-adrenergic stimulation is not a necessary condition for this improvement.

The studies also indicate that repetitive brief periods of ischemia can lead to cumulative impairment in myocardial function. Recovery of function in salvaged myocardium after reperfusing in the setting of acute myocardial infarction may be delayed by hours or days. An earlier assessment of the amount of salvage achieved may be possible by measuring regional inotropic reserve with catecholamine infusion or postextrasystolic potentiation; such information could be important in deciding whether to perform coronary angioplasty on the infarct-related vessel.—R.A. O'Rourke, M.D.

Exercise-Induced Regional Dysfunction With Subcritical Coronary Stenosis
Jong-Dae Lee, Tsukasa Tajimi, Brian Guth, Rainald Seitelberger, Mark Miller, and John Ross, Jr. (Univ. of California at San Diego, LaJolla)
Circulation 73:596–605, March 1986   1–24

Exercise-induced ischemia has been studied extensively using analyses of regional myocardial blood flow (MBF), regional contraction, and overall left ventricular (LV) function. Regional contractile function is responsive to reductions in MBF, particularly to the subendocardium. In human beings, global or regional LV function, as determined by radionuclide imaging or two-dimensional echocardiography during exercise testing, is abnormal in some patients with coronary heart disease. However, little is known about the sensitivity of abnormal regional wall motion for identifying mild abnormalities of subendocardial blood flow induced by exercise stress. The hypothesis that regional myocardial contractile dysfunction can detect subtle regional coronary blood flow maldistribution induced by exercise was examined in seven dogs in which LV pressure, regional systolic wall thickening (WTh), and MBF were measured when mild degrees of coronary artery stenosis were produced during treadmill exercise.

During exercise without coronary stenosis, WTh increased by a mean of 21% and transmural MBF increased uniformly. Subsequently, in each dog two levels of coronary stenosis were produced during exercise: (1) St-Ex 1, where WTh during exercise failed to increase significantly and (2) St-Ex II, where WTh during exercise decreased moderately from the resting control value. In the potentially ischemic zone, coronary hyperemia occurred with each run: The mean resting subendocardial MBF was 1.09 ml/gm/minute, and it was 3.04 ml/gm/minute during control exercise; it was 2.48 ml/gm/minute during St-Ex 1, and 1.55 ml/gm/minute during St-Ex II. Furthermore, the subendocardial-subepicardial blood flow ratio fell from a mean of 1.32 during control exercise to 1.07 during St-Ex 1, and 0.64 with St-Ex II. Changes in the subendocardial electrogram and reactive hyperemia were found more consistently during St-Ex II than during St-Ex I.

Thus, failure of regional function to increase during exercise detected a slight maldistribution of regional MBF, whereas reduction of regional function during exercise of 10% or more below the resting value was a reliable marker of a regional flow defect and was consistently associated with other evidence of ischemia. Regional dysfunction during exercise can detect subcritical but functionally significant coronary stenosis, which may permit regional wall motion to be used to detect coronary artery disease at an early stage.

▶ In this important exercise study in dogs, regional myocardial dysfunction could be demonstrated during subtle regional myocardial blood flow maldistribution induced by exercise. At the mildest level of coronary artery stenosis, regional systolic wall thickening during exercise failed to increase significantly and with more severe coronary stenosis, wall thickening during exercise decreased moderately from the resting value. The findings indicate that regional wall motion is reliable for detecting subcritical coronary stenosis during exercise, with coronary flow maldistribution and other evidence of ischemia developing when a definite decrease in wall motion below the resting level occurs. Thus, a decrease in regional wall motion of 10% or more during exercise indicates inadequate subendocardial perfusion. However, the modest abnormalities in regional contraction function observed in this study during exercise in animals with ultrasound crystals used to detect changes in wall thickness would be difficult to detect by the conventional noninvasive techniques that are used in man. Nevertheless, newer techniques (e.g., tomographic gated blood pool radionuclide ventriculography, or nuclear magnetic resonance imaging) applied during exercise or hyperemia eventually may permit reliable detection of such minor contraction abnormalities in patients with subcritical coronary artery stenosis.—R.A. O'Rourke, M.D.

Premortem Assessment of Myocardial Area at Risk With the Use of Intracoronary Technetium Macroaggregated Albumin and Gated Nuclear Imaging
Andrew J. Feiring, Philip Bruch, Tarek S. Husayni, Peter T. Kirchner, and Melvin L. Marcus (Univ. of Iowa)
Circulation 73:551–561, March 1986   1–25

It has been generally believed that the extent of myocardial necrosis after acute coronary artery occlusion could be predicted accurately simply by angiographic identification of the site of obstruction. However, there is evidence that the size of the vascular bed at risk is the primary determinant of infarct size. The importance of defining the area at risk before evaluating infarct-limiting agents has been well documented in animal studies. A method was developed for assessing the area at risk in 18 closed-chest dogs undergoing acute coronary artery occlusion. Subsequently,

^{99m}Tc (15 mCi)-labeled macroaggregated albumin was injected through an angiographic catheter into the left main coronary artery. Gated nuclear images were obtained in left anterior oblique views in 11 dogs with left anterior descending occlusions and in right anterior oblique views in 7 dogs with circumflex artery occlusions; the corresponding end-diastolic images were examined. The heart was then excised and the autoradiographic area at risk in the left ventricle was assessed.

The theoretical advantage of the use of gated acquisition for determination of the area at risk over the use of nongated acquisition was evaluated. Studies in five control dogs in which concomitant left atrial and intracoronary injection of different radioactive-labeled macroaggregates had been used showed no false positive defects and similar, relatively homogeneous radionuclide distribution. The postmortem autoradiographic area at risk ranged from 3.8% to 36.3% of the left ventricular mass, whereas end-diastolic areas at risk in vivo correlated well with those determined by the postmortem autoradiographic method. In addition the area at risk in vivo with the nongated image correlated well with the postmortem area at risk. Nongated imaging was less sensitive and accurate than gated imaging and resulted in three false negative studies, as well as poorer correlation with results of postmortem autoradiography.

The premortem canine area at risk can be accurately and reproducibly assessed using this nuclear imaging technique. Gated nuclear imaging substantially enhances the sensitivity of determination of area at risk as compared with static image acquisition. Because intracoronary ^{99m}Tc-labeled albumin macroaggregates are well tolerated in man, this technique may be useful in assessing the area at risk in clinical studies of invasive coronary artery reperfusion.

▶ The amount of left ventricular dysfunction resulting from acute myocardial infarction (AMI) is dependent on the extent of "infarct size." The goal of early aggressive therapy in patients with AMI is to reduce the extent of myocardial necrosis by either improving coronary blood flow to areas of still viable myocardium or decreasing the oxygen demands, or both. To assess the salutory effect of any potentially useful therapeutic agent in patients with myocardial infarction it is necessary to compare the area of risk with the actual size of a completed myocardial infarction in the patient being treated with intervention, or to assess "infarct size" and mortality in large numbers of patients receiving a therapeutic intervention as compared with a control group receiving a placebo in a blinded, randomized fashion.

The importance of defining the area at risk before evaluating infarct-limiting agents has been well documented in animal studies. However, despite many investigative studies, no intervention has been demonstrated conclusively to limit infarct size in patients. In this animal study, the premortem determination of the area at risk after acute coronary artery occlusion could be accurately and reproducibly quantified in dogs with the use of intracoronary technetium-99m-labeled macroaggregates of albumin (MAA). Gated imaging with isolation and analysis of the end-diastolic frame permitted clear delineation of the area at risk without motion artifact, and intracoronary ^{99m}Tc-MAA is well tolerated in human beings. This technique may prove useful in evaluating the outcome of invasive attempts at coronary artery reperfusion (e.g., coronary angioplasty) in patients with AMI. However, this method requires the use of intracoronary isotope injection, and the search for noninvasive methods for determining the area at risk and the actual "infarct size" continue.—R.A. O'Rourke, M.D.

Enhancement of Salvage of Reperfused Ischemic Myocardium by Diltiazem

Robert M. Knabb, Thomas L. Rosamond, Keith A.A. Fox, Burton E. Sobel, and Steven R. Bergmann (Washington Univ.)
J. Am. Coll. Cardiol. 8:861–871, October 1986   1–26

Calcium channel blockade offers promise in helping salvage ischemic myocardium in patients having coronary thrombolysis because of the adverse effects of calcium influx accompanying reperfusion. The value of diltiazem was examined in dogs with thrombotic coronary occlusion in which thrombolysis was induced by streptokinase infusion. Intracoronary thrombolysis was begun 2 hours after occlusion of the left anterior descending coronary artery. Study animals received diltiazem, 15 μg/kg, intravenously, starting 90 minutes after coronary occlusion. Myocardial blood flow was studied by the microsphere method, and metabolism was assessed by positron emission tomography (PET).

Intracoronary infusion of streptokinase consistently restored coronary patency. Administration of diltiazem did not alter the heart rate or blood pressure before reperfusion, or the extent of ischemia. Infarct size was decreased the most in diltiazem-treated animals. When PET was used to determine infarct size, in terms of the extent of myocardium with less than 50% of peak ^{11}C-palmitate uptake 24 hours after occlusion, the percent of region at risk was significantly reduced by reperfusion alone and was further reduced in dilitazem-treated dogs.

Diltiazem, given before coronary thrombolysis, promotes myocardial salvage in dogs. Calcium channel blockers hold promise for enhancing myocardial salvage and warrant a trial in patients having coronary thrombolysis. Also, PET is a useful means of evaluating adjunctive pharmacologic therapy in the setting of coronary thrombolysis.

▶ Experimental animal studies have documented myocardial salvage after coronary thrombolysis and suggest that it may be facilitated by concomitant administration of pharmacologic agents. Early coronary thrombolytic therapy is being initiated in an increasing number of patients with acute myocardial infarction. The coincident use of calcium entry blockers might offset the potentially deleterious effects of the intracellular influx of calcium that accompanies reperfusion.

Using PET for the noninvasive assessment of myocardial perfusion and extent of infarction and measurement of creatine kinase activity in myocardial homogenates, the authors demonstrated that the concomitant administration of the calcium blocker, diltiazem, markedly enhances salvage of reperfused myocardial after coronary thrombolysis in dogs with induced thrombotic coronary occlusion. These results merit further studies on the usefulness of calcium entry blockers with coronary thrombolysis in patients who present within the first few hours after acute myocardial infarction.—R.A. O'Rourke, M.D.

Protective Effects of N-2-Mercaptopropionyl Glycine Against Myocardial Reperfusion Injury After Neutrophil Depletion In the Dog: Evidence for the Role of Intracellular-Derived Free Radicals

Stephanie E. Mitsos, Timothy E. Askew, Joseph C. Fantone, Steven L. Kunkel, Gerald D. Abrams, Anthony Schork, and Benedict R. Lucchesi (Univ. of Michigan)
Circulation 73:1077–1086, May 1986   1–27

Reperfusion of the ischemic myocardium can salvage tissue, but oxygen-derived free radicals may contribute to cell injury after reperfusion. The roles of intracellular-derived and neutrophil-derived oxygen metabolites in reperfusion injury were studied by administering the free-radical scavenger N-2-mercaptopropionyl glycine (MPG) to dogs that were depleted of circulating neutrophils with specific antisera. Ischemia was produced for 90 minutes by occluding the left circumflex coronary artery, and 6 hours of reperfusion followed. The MPG was given intra-arterially in a dose of 20 mg/kg for 1 hour, starting 15 minutes before the start of reperfusion.

Infarction size was reduced by one third in animals given neutrophil antiserum, compared with those given nonimmune serum. The combined use of neutrophil antiserum and MPG reduced infarction size by nearly two thirds of the area at risk, a significantly greater effect than occurred with antiserum alone. The area at risk was similar in all groups of animals. Hemodynamic differences did not account for the myocardial protection observed.

Oxygen free radicals derived from both extracellular and intracellular sources appear to contribute to reperfusion injury of the myocardium. Salvage may be enhanced by using free-radical scavengers and by altering leukocyte function. This approach may be useful in patients undergoing coronary bypass surgery and in patients with acute myocardial infarction with early reperfusion.

▶ Reperfusion of ischemic myocardium is associated with a number of potentially deleterious effects and oxygen-derived free radicals may be important mediators of the myocardial injury associated with reperfusion. This currently is an area of extensive investigation and the importance of these substances is unproven. A potential source of these reactive oxygen species is the activated neutrophil that mediates tissue injury through release of oxygen radicals. Moreover, neutrophil depletion appears to be associated with a significant reduction in the extent of irreversible myocardial injury.

In this dog study, the combination of MPG and neutrophil antiserum reduced "infarct size" more than neutrophil antiserum alone did, suggesting that both extramyocardial- and intramyocardial-derived oxygen free radicals contribute significantly to reperfusion-induced myocardial injury in this experimental model of acute ischemia followed by 6 hours of reperfusion. Longer follow-up studies, and the importance of these observations to patients undergoing treatment for acute myocardial infarction with or without aggressive interventional therapy, are important considerations.—R.A. O'Rourke, M.D.

Failure of Superoxide Dismutase and Catalase To Alter Size or Infarction in Conscious Dogs After 3 Hours of Occlusion Followed by Reperfusion
Kim P. Gallagher, Andrew J. Buda, Diane Pace, Richard A. Gerren, and Marshal Shlafer (Univ. of Michigan)
Circulation 73:1065–1076, 1986   1–28

Enzymes that degrade free oxygen radicals are under study for reducing myocardial reperfusion injury. The effects of superoxide dismutase and catalase, which degrade superoxide anion and hydrogen peroxide, respectively, were examined in anesthetized open-chest dogs subjected to occlusion of the left circumflex artery for 3 hours, followed by 24 hours of reperfusion. Regional wall thickness was estimated by sonomicrometry. Infusions were begun 15 minutes before reperfusion and continued for 45 minutes of reperfusion. Both enzymes were given in doses of 5 mg/kg. Myocardial blood flow was measured by the labeled microsphere technique, and infarct size was determined by Evans blue and triphenyl tetrazolium staining.

Similar patterns of systolic wall thinning were seen in the treated and control animals. Myocardial blood flow also was similar in all groups. No myocardial protection was evident in terms of infarct size. There was no relationship between the size of the area at risk and infarct size. The pressure-rate product also failed to correlate closely with infarct size, but collateral blood flow correlated reasonably well.

Myocardial protection by superoxide dismutase and catalase appears to be model dependent. No significant change in infarct size was observed in conscious dogs subjected to coronary occlusion for 3 hours and reperfusion for 24 hours. The clinical circumstances under which these enzymes might prove useful remain to be defined.

▶ In contrast to prior studies in different animal models, this investigation in conscious dogs subjected to 3 hours of coronary occlusion followed by reperfusion failed to demonstrate any alteration in "infarct size" with either superoxide dismutase or catalase, enzymes that degrade the oxygen radicals superoxide anion and hydrogen peroxide.

This study indicates that additional investigations are necessary to define conclusively which patients, it any, are likely to benefit from the use of agents that reduce oxygen free radicals, in the setting of acute myocardial infarction.—R.A. O'Rourke, M.D.

Additional recent relevant publications include the following:
1. Zalewski, A., et al.: Relation of myocardial salvage to size of myocardium at risk in dogs. *Am. J. Cardiol.* 56:974–977, 1985.
2. Anversa, P., et al.: Myocardial infarction in rats. Infarct size, myocyte hypertrophy and capillary growth. *Circ. Res.* 58:26–37, 1986.
3. Vik-Mo, H., et al: Limitation of myocardial infarct size by metabolic interventions that reduce accumulation of fatty acid metabolites in ischemic myocardium. *Am. Heart J.* 111:1048–1054, 1986.
4. Todd, G. L., et al.: Protective effects of slow channel calcium antagonists on noradrenaline induced myocardial necrosis. *Cardiovasc. Res.* 20:645–651, 1986.
5. Przyklenk, K., Kloner, R. A.: Superoxide dismutase plus catalase improve contractile function in the canine model of the "stunned myocardium." *Circ. Res.* 58:148–156, 1986.
6. Prigent, F., et al.: Noninvasive quantitation of the extent of jeopardized myocardium in patients with single-vessel coronary disease by thallium-201 SPECT. *Am. Heart J.* 111:578–586, 1986.
7. Jugdutt, B. I., Amy, R. W.: Healing after myocardial infarction in the dog: Changes in infarct hydroxyproline and tomography. *J. Am. Coll. Cardiol.* 7:91–102, 1986.

Myocardial Metabolic Studies

The Dependence of Electrophysiological Derangements on Accumulation of Endogenous Long-Chain Acyl Carnitine in Hypoxic Neonatal Rat Myocytes

Maureen T. Knabb, Jeffrey E. Saffitz, Peter B. Corr, and Burton E. Sobel (Washington Univ.)

Circ. Res. 58:230–240, February 1986   1–29

Endogenous cardiac amphiphiles [e.g., lysophosphoglycerides and long-chain acyl carnitines (LCA)] accumulate in the ischemic myocardium and induce electrophysiologic alterations in vitro that resemble those seen in ischemic myocardium in vivo. Although it is thought that their amphiphilic properties may facilitate their incorporation into sarcolemma with consequent perturbation of ion transport, little direct information is available regarding the potential redistribution and accumulation of endogenous LCA in sarcolemma of hypoxic cells. The extent that electrophysiologic derangements induced by hypoxia depend on accumulation of endogenous amphiphiles in sarcolemma has not been elucidated. An attempt was made to characterize the subcellular distribution and concentration of endogenous LCA in rat neonatal myocytes superfused with normoxic or hypoxic solutions.

Hypoxia increased LCA more than fivefold, and a carnitine acyltransferase inhibitor precluded this accumulation. Tissue was prepared for electron microscopy using a procedure specifically developed for selective extraction of endogenous short-chain and free carnitine but retention of endogenous LCA. In normoxic-perfused cells, LCA was concentrated in mitochondria and cytoplasmic membranous components, with only small amounts present in the sarcolemma. However, hypoxia increased mitochondrial LCA by tenfold and sarcolemmal LCA by 70-fold. After 60 minutes of hypoxia, sarcolemma contained 1.4×10^7 LCA molecules per cu μm of membrane volume, a value corresponding to approximately 3.5% of total sarcolemmal phospholipid. Also, hypoxia substantially decreased the maximum diastolic potential, action potential amplitude, and maximum upstroke velocity of phase 0. The carnitine acyltransferase inhibitor strongly blocked accumulation of LCA in each subcellular compartment and prevented the decrease of electrophysiologic function induced by hypoxia. Endogenous LCA is likely to be a mediator of the electrophysiologic alterations induced by hypoxia.

▶ This study demonstrates a 70-fold increase of endogenous LCA in sarcolemma of hypoxic myocytes and provides direct evidence that the accumulation of endogenous LCA contributes to electrophysiologic derangements induced by hypoxia. The electrophysiologic depression observed in this study was proportional to the magnitude of the increase of LCA, and phenylalkyloxirane carboxylic acid, an inhibitor of carnitine acyltransferase, attenuated the electrophysiologic depression induced by hypoxia.—R.A. O'Rourke, M.D.

Physiological Concentrations of Epinephrine Potentiate Thromboxane A$_2$ Release From Platelets in the Isolated Rat Heart

Maryann Purchase, Gregory J. Dusting, Dennis M.F. Li, and Mark A. Read (Austin Hosp., Heidelberg, Victoria, Australia)
Circ. Res. 58:172–176, January 1986   1–30

It is well established that epinephrine induces direct aggregation of human blood platelets at concentrations in the micromolar range and potentiates platelet aggregation to other agonists at somewhat lower concentrations. Nevertheless, the lowest concentrations at which epinephrine interacts with other agonists are still two orders of magnitude higher than the normal blood concentrations achieved during pathologic stress. The effect of very low concentrations of epinephrine on thromboxane $A_2 (TxA_2)$ release from platelets was examined in the isolated rat heart perfused with washed platelets.

In hearts perfused with rabbit or human platelets, injection of sodium arachidonate caused release of both prostacyclin and TxA_2. However, when hearts were perfused with aspirin-treated platelets, arachidonate caused the release of only prostacyclin, indicating that TxA_2 originates largely in the platelets. When epinephrine (0.6–6 nmole/L) was infused through the heart, the arachidonate-induced release of TxA_2 was potentiated. Similar potentiation of TxA_2 release was demonstrated in rat hearts perfused with either rabbit or human platelets and in rabbit hearts perfused with rabbit platelets. Conversely, when rabbit platelets were infused through an incubation coil of tubing rather than the heart, epinephrine did not change TxA_2 release. There was no substantial loss of rabbit platelets on perfusion through rat hearts, nor were aggregates observed in the effluent either before or immediately after arachidonate injections, even in the presence of epinephrine. Thus, the epinephrine-induced potentiation of TxA$_2$ release could not be explained by aggregation.

Physiologic concentrations of epinephrine can potentiate TxA$_2$ release from platelets when they are stimulated by arachidonic acid within the heart. This could result from redirection of arachidonate metabolism to a local potentiating factor within the vessel wall. It is possible that potentiation of TxA$_2$ release might contribute to myocardial ischemia associated with platelet activation.

▶ The important finding in this study is that low concentrations of epinephrine, in the physiologic range of circulating blood levels, can potentiate the release of TxA$_2$ from platelets. This finding of thromboxane potentiation provides a new explanation for the deleterious effects of circulating epinephrine released following myocardial ischemia, smoking, and physiological stress, and the platelet hyperactivity observed after myocardial infarction. These findings also explain elevation of the coronary sinus thromboxane B$_2$ level measured during and after episodes of myocardial ischemia in experimental animals and in man.—R.A. O'Rourke, M.D.

Platelet-Activating Factor and the Release of a Platelet-Derived Coronary Artery Vasodilator Substance in the Canine
Charles V. Jackson, William A. Schumacher, Steven L. Kunkel, Edward M. Driscoll, and Benedict R. Lucchesi (Univ. of Michigan)
Circ. Res. 58:218–229, February 1986   1–31

Platelets and leukocytes produce a unique phospholipid, acetyl-glyceryl-ether-phosphorylcholine (AGEPC), also referred to as platelet-activating-factor (PAF). Acetyl-glyceryl-ether-phosphorylcholine causes platelet and leukocyte aggregation, as well as thromboxane and leukotriene synthesis. It also has diverse hemodynamic effects, including constriction of the pulmonary and coronary vasculature in porcine, guinea pig, and canine hearts, and enhancement of vascular permeability in rabbits and guinea pigs. Acetyl-glyceryl-ether-phosphorylcholine can produce hypotension in spontaneously hypertensive and normotensive rats. Because of these findings, it was hypothesized that AGEPC is an important modulator of vasomotor and inflammatory reactions in the cardiovascular system. An effort was made to characterize the hemodynamic effects of intracoronary injection of AGEPC and the influences of pharmacologic blockade and platelet depletion on its activity in male mongrel dogs.

Intracoronary injections of AGEPC produced maximum increases in the left circumflex coronary artery blood flow of 55 ml/minute, 52 ml/minute/ and 52 ml/minute at 0.5 nM, 1.0 nM, and 2.0 nM, respectively. In contrast, there were only modest changes in systemic arterial blood pressure and regional developed isometric contractile force under the same experimental conditions. The increase in left circumflex coronary artery blood flow in response to AGEPC was attenuated (44%), but not prevented, by pretreatment with diphenhydramine (4 mg/kg intravenously), and was not affected by pretreatment with aspirin (20 mg/kg intrvenously) or the systemic administration of the serotonin receptor antagonist, methysergide. However, the coronary vasodilator response to AGEPC was markedly decreased by the induction of thrombocytopenia (95% platelet depletion) through the administration of sheep-derived canine platelet antiserum. Intracoronary artery injection of platelet-rich plasma activated with AGEPC into thrombocytopenic dogs caused a substantially greater increase in coronary artery blood flow than injection of either nonactivated platelet-rich plasma or platelet-depleted plasma supplemented with AGEPC. However, similar changes in coronary artery blood flow could be obtained after the intracoronary artery injection of cell-free supernates from washed platelets activated with AGEPC.

When exposed to AGEPC, circulating platelets can release a coronary dilator substance. Coronary artery dilation is not prevented by pharmacologic receptor antagonists for histamine, serotonin, or inhibitors of cyclooxygenase.

▶ This study indicates that platelet-activating factor (AGEPC) is capable of eliciting a coronary artery vasodilator response to the release of a platelet-derived factor that has yet to be identified. The observation that platelets can participate in producing coronary artery relaxation in the presence of a normal endothelium may have significance with respect to the pathophysiologic mechanism(s) by which coronary vasospasm might be facilitated when endothelial damage has occurred. Platelet aggregation at a site devoid of endothelium might favor local vasoconstriction caused by the release of thromboxane A_2. The role of platelet-derived factors and endothelial factors in producing coronary vasoconstriction or coronary artery dilatation in normal coronary artery endothelial tissue and in the presence of coronary atherosclerosis needs further investigation. The clinical relevance of many of these observed changes remains to be demonstrated.—R.A. O'Rourke, M.D.

Mechanisms of Accumulation of Arachidonic Acid in Cultured Myocardial Cells During ATP Depletion
Michael D. Gunn, Anjan Sen, Anthony Chang, James T. Willerson, L. Maximillian Buja, and Kenneth R. Chien (University of Texas at Dallas and Southwestern Med. School, Dallas)
Am. J. Physiol. 249:H1188–H1194, 1985   1–32

The metabolism of arachidonic acid and its conversion to prostaglandins and other oxygenated metabolites may be of major importance in the pathophysiology of myocardial ischemia. Both prostaglandins and leukotrienes have substantial effects on platelet aggregation and coronary blood flow during normoxia and ischemia. In perfused heart and in vivo myocardial models there is an increase in the release of unesterified arachidonic acid during myocardial ischemia. Also, the degradation of membrane phospholipids and accumulation of arachidonic acid are associated with the loss of cell viability. There is also increased release of prostaglandins into the coronary venous effluent after myocardial ischemia. Although the importance of arachidonic acid in the pathogenesis of myocardial ischemia has been suggested, the biochemical mechanisms regulating the release of arachidonic acid are not known. An attempt was made to determine whether release of arachidonic acid from myocardial cells was more dependent on the extent of adenosine triphosphate (ATP) depletion than on the inhibition of fatty acid oxidation. These studies were also designed to assess whether arachidonic acid release only occurred when ATP was depleted beyond a critical threshold level.

To evaluate the relationship between arachidonic acid release and ATP depletion, cultured myocardial cells from neonatal rat hearts were labeled with [^{3}H]arachidonate and [^{14}C]palmitate. Both [^{3}H]arachidonic acid and [^{14}C]palmitic acid were released from membrane phospholipids in response to ATP depletion with various metabolic inhibitors. The major esterified sources of the arachidonate were phosphatidylcholine, phosphatidylethanolamine, and phosphatidic acid. The release of both fatty acids was related to the extent of ATP depletion and not to whether a glycolytic or respiratory inhibitor was used. When various combinations and doses of metabolic inhibitors were used, experimental conditions that produced a decrease of more than 75% in ATP content were associated with accumulation of arachidonic acid.

An ATP-dependent step may be linked to the accumulation of arachidonic acid during myocardial ATP depletion. It is hypothesized that myocardial cells may release arachidonic acid directly in response to ATP depletion.

▶ The metabolism of arachidonic acid and its conversion to prostaglandins and other oxygenated metabolites may be of major importance in the pathophysiology of myocardial ischemia. Prostaglandins and leukotrienes have marked effects on platelet aggregation and coronary blood flow. There appears to be an increase in the release of unesterifed arachidonic acid during myocardial ischemia. If the response of cultured myocardial cells is similar to intact myocardium, the results suggest the myocardial cells are a major source of arachidonic acid release during ischemia and that a potential stimulus may be ATP depletion.

Recently, Revtyak and associates found that ATP-depleted cultured myocardial cells release arachidonic acid that is not converted to cyclooxygenase or lipoxygenase products, and that arachidonic acid released during ATP depletion may be metabolized by circulating platelets or adjacent and adherent cells (Revtyak, G.E., et al.: *J. Am. Coll. Cardiol.* 9(suppl. A):186A, 1987).—R.A. O'Rourke, M.D.

Excitation-Contraction Coupling in Rat Myocardium: Alterations With Long Term Ethanol Consumption

David Tepper, Joseph M. Capasso, and Edmund H. Sonnenblick (Albert Einstein College of Medicine, New York)
Cardiovasc. Res. 20:369–374, May 1986   1–33

It has long been thought that alcohol may adversely affect the heart, and a syndrome called alcoholic heart disease has been described that is associated with depressed myocardial function and arrhythmias. If alcohol consumption continues, these symptoms may progress to severe myocardial failure. The mechanisms underlying these alterations have not been defined, but ethanol appears to induce a wide range of alterations in cardiac function and structure in various animal models. However, the functional abnormalities are variable and difficult to relate to the pathogenesis of the overall cardiac depression seen in patients with cardiac heart disease. The effects of chronic alcohol consumption on the contractile and electrical characteristics of left ventricular papillary muscles in male Wistar rats were investigated.

The mechanical and electrical effects of chronic ethanol consumption were studied in rats maintained with 40% ethanol and water solution for a 30-week study period and in controls. The left ventricular papillary muscles were studied by myography at 30 C, 0.1-Hz stimulation, and external calcium concentration of 2.4 mmole/L. There were no significant differences between alcoholic and control rats with regard to resting tension. Nevertheless, developed tension, time to peak tension, time to one half relaxation, and time to peak shortening were markedly depressed in preparations from the study animals. In addition, the velocity of shortening and relengthening at all relative loads were depressed in alcoholic preparations. There was no significant difference in action potential between the two groups with regard to resting membrane potential, action potential amplitude, overshoot, or maximum rate of rise of the upstroke. Conversely, the duration at 50% and 75% of total repolarization was markedly shorter for action potential in the alcoholic group than in controls. Chronic ethanol ingestion leads to an inability to develop normal levels of force, a depressed force-velocity relationship, and shortening of action potential duration.

▶ There has been a long-term interest in the effects of chronic alcohol use on cardiac function and structure, and this has been studied in various animal models. The present study showed a consistent decrease in developed tension by isolated papillary muscles with chronic alcoholism as well as shorter membrane action potential in alcoholic rats. The electrophysiologic changes produced by chronic alcoholism may help to explain the contractile modifications during chronic alcohol ingestion. However, further studies are indicated to delineate more clearly the role played by the membrane as indicated by alterations in the transmembrane action potential.—R.A. O'Rourke, M.D.

Sodium Nuclear Magnetic Resonance Imaging of Myocardial Tissue of Dogs After Coronary Artery Occlusion and Reperfusion
Paul J. Cannon, Andrew A. Maudsley, Sadek K. Hilal, Howard E. Simon, and Frederick Cassidy (Columbia Univ.)
J. Am. Coll. Cardiol. 7:573–579, March 1986   1–34

The development of thrombolytic therapy has stimulated efforts to find a noninvasive method to detect, localize, and measure areas of myocardial ischemic injury distal to coronary artery obstruction. Several different studies have suggested that sequential measurements of the intracellular sodium content might be useful as a guide to the extent and reversibility of ischemic damage. Although it provides only a weak signal, tissue sodium in the brains of animals and man can be imaged in vivo using high magnetic field nuclear magnetic resonance (NMR) imaging systems. The feasibility of visualizing sodium-23 in normal and ischemic tissue of the excised canine heart was examined.

To produce a region of ischemia and infarction in the myocardium, a coronary artery was subjected to 1 hour of surgical occlusion followed by 1 hour of reperfusion in six dogs. The dogs were killed and sodium-23 NMR images of the excised hearts were obtained using a high field NMR imaging system. These images were compared with tissue sodium contents measured by flame photometry. The regions of ischemic damage were clearly visible as areas of an increased sodium NMR signal on the three-dimensional images. Furthermore, there was good agreement between the relative intensity of the sodium signals and the sodium contents of normal myocardium and myocardium subjected to coronary artery occlusion and reperfusion. Imaging with NMR sodium may be a useful means of detecting the location and extent of myocardial damage in patients with coronary artery disease.

▶ Some alterations of the present sodium NMR imaging approach used above may be needed to obtain useful measurements of ischemic damage in patients with heart disease. However, if NMR shift reagents can be developed that are safe for patients, it is possible that NMR imaging and intracellular sodium can be used to monitor regional alterations of myocardial tissue in response to ischemia and reperfusion.—R.A. O'Rourke, M.D.

Other recent publications of interest include the following:

1. Vermylen, J., et al.: Role of platelet activation and fibrin formation in thrombogenesis. *J. Am. Coll. Cardiol.* 8:2B–9B, 1986.
2. Sparks, H. V., Bardenheyer, H.: Regulation of adenosine by the heart. *Circ. Res.* 58:193–201, 1986.
3. Shephard, J. T., Vanhoutt, D. M.: Mechanisms responsible for coronary vasospasm. *J. Am. Coll. Cardiol.* 8:50A–54A, 1986.
4. Adkonizio, V. P., et al.: Effects of verapamil and diltiazem on platelet function. *Am. J. Physiol.* 250:H366–H371, 1986.
5. Jaschonek, K., et al.: Platelet prostacyclin binding in coronary artery disease. *J. Am. Coll. Cardiol.* 8:259–266, 1986.

Regional Ventricular Function

Regional Myocardial Dysfunction: Evaluation of Patients With Prior Myocardial Infarction With Fast CT

Martin J. Lipton, Donald W. Farmer, Ellen J. Killebrew, Alain Bouchard, Peter

B. Dean, Hans G. Ringertz, and Charles B. Higgins (Univ. of California at San Francisco)
Radiology 157:735–740, December 1985   1–35

Computed tomography (CT) is capable of defining regional myocardial dysfunction when ischemia is present and also of demonstrating regional myocardial abnormalities in human beings who have had prior infarctions. However, because prolonged breath holding is required during ECG-gated CT, this method has not been widely used for assessing heart disease. An ultrafast CT scanner designed specifically for cardiac imaging was used to avoid problems of prolonged breath holding associated with standard CT scanning techniques.

The study comprised 18 male and 3 female patients aged 42–73 years who had a history of prior myocardial infarction. A control group of five patients did not have a history of coronary artery disease but had left ventricular hypertrophic disease. None of the patients was taking a medication that could depress the myocardium. A prototype CT scanner with a 50-msec exposure time (cine-CT) was used to examine all participants, and cine-CT scans were compared with standard left ventriculographic images obtained from conventional angiocardiography. The anterior, apical, septal, and lateral wall regions showed the best results in the cross-sectional CT scans (Fig 1–3), but the posterior and inferior walls could not be evaluated consistently.

The cine-CT scans were adequate in 23 of 26 patients (88%). Computed tomographic image quality was good in 18 patients and acceptable in 5. Findings in the other three patients were excluded from the results for technical reasons. At rapid speed (20 scans per second) cine-CT provides useful data concerning regional ventricular wall motion. A good correlation exists between this technique and conventional angiocardiography.

▶ Accurate and reliable techniques for assessing regional left ventricular per-

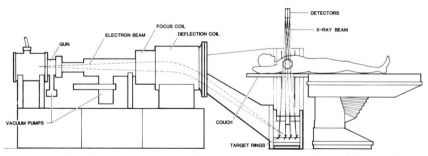

Fig 1–3.—Cine-CT images obtained with 50-msec exposures in a control group patient with good left ventricular function but left ventricular hypertrophic disease. Changes in the left ventricular cavity and wall dimensions during the cardiac cycle are apparent. (Courtesy of Lipton, M.J., et al.: Radiology 157:735–740, December 1985. Reproduced with permission of the Radiological Society of North America.)

formance in patients with coronary artery disease are still being sought. Current techniques, including left ventricular cineangiography, provide less than optimal information and are primarily qualitative rather than quantitative. The study reviewed above used rapid cine-CT to assess wall motion in a group of patients with prior myocardial infarction. In this preliminary study, the qualitative analysis revealed a good correlation between fast cine-CT and left ventriculography in assessing segmental left ventricular wall motion. The spatial resolution of CT is considerably greater than that of radionuclide ventriculography or two-dimensional echocardiography. The development of this and other better imaging techniques should allow more reliable assessment of segmental wall motion caused by ischemic heart disease and be helpful in making decisions, e.g., in which areas of myocardium is improvement in contractility likely with coronary artery reperfusion.—R.A. O'Rourke, M.D.

Reversibility of Cardiac Wall-Motion Abnormalities Predicted by Positron Tomography

Jan Tillisch, Richard Brunken, Robert Marshall, Markus Schwaiger, Mark Mandelkern, Michael Phelps, and Heinrich Schelbert (Univ. of California at Los Angeles)
N. Engl. J. Med. 314:884–888, Apr. 3, 1986   1–36

After restoration of adequate blood flow, regional myocardial contractile dysfunction at rest improves. In the clinical setting, abnormalities in regional resting cardiac wall motion are thought to result from persistently depressed blood flow, prolonged myocardial cellular dysfunction after transient ischemia, or myocardial infarction. To determine whether revascularization improves abnormal resting wall motion, it was necessary previously to demonstrate reversible flow abnormalities on exercise thallium-201 scans or to provide evidence of improved wall motion after nitroglycerin administration. However, these techniques present potential problems with regard to sensitivity and specificity. Preserved myocardial uptake of fluorine-18-deoxyglucose (^{18}FDG), associated with decreased uptake of the blood-flow indicator nitrogen-13-ammonia (^{13}NH$_3$) as determined by positron emission tomography (PET), correlates with angiographic evidence of severe multivessel coronary disease. Whether preserved myocardial uptake of ^{18}FDG in a region with abnormal wall motion at rest is an indication of myocardial metabolic viability was investigated, and whether reversibility of the wall- motion disturbance by adequate surgical revascularization could be predicted with these criteria was examined. The series included 17 patients who underwent coronary artery bypass surgery and PET studies. Abnormalities were quantified using radionuclide or contrast angiography, or both, before and after grafting; the PET images were obtained preoperatively.

Abnormal wall motion in regions in which PET images showed preserved glucose uptake was predicted to be reversible; however, abnormal motion in regions with depressed glucose uptake was predicted to be irreversible.

According to these criteria, abnormal contraction in 35 of 41 segments was accurately predicted to be reversible (85%), and abnormal contraction in 24 of 26 regions was accurately predicted to be irreversible (92%). Conversely, ECGs demonstrating pathologic Q waves in the region of asynergy predicted irreversibility in only 43% of regions. Imaging with PET and $^{13}NH_3$ to measure blood flow and ^{18}FDG to measure metabolic viability of the myocardium is an accurate method of predicting the potential reversibility of wall motion abnormalities after surgical revascularization.

▶ During low-flow ischemia, glucose metabolism is increased relative to fatty acid oxidation until the flow is too low to permit washout of inhibitory endproducts of glucose metabolism. At this point, glycolysis ceases and cellular entry begins. Thus, continuation of glucose metabolism with critical reduction of blood flow may support cellular viability despite decreased regional myocardial contractility. Based on this concept, the authors undertook PET studies using ^{18}FDG uptake to indicate preserved glucose metabolism in areas of the ventricles supplied by stenotic coronary arteries associated with wall motion abnormalities. The results of the studies detailed above indicate a great potential for the use of PET and metabolic imaging in patients with coronary artery disease before and after reperfusion therapy.—R.A. O'Rourke, M.D.

Advantages and Applications of the Centerline Method for Characterizing Regional Ventricular Function
Florence H. Sheehan, Edward L. Bolson, Harold T. Dodge, Detlef G. Mathey, Joachim Schofer, and Hok-Wai Woo (Univ. of Washington, and Univ. Hosp. Eppendorf, Hamburg, FRG)
Circulation 74:293–305, August 1986   1–37

Currently, in clinical practice, wall motion is assessed subjectively from contrast ventriculograms. However, these qualitative evaluations are unreliable. This has led to the development of quantitative methods that measure the extent of wall motion at 4–100 points around the endocardial contour. Because recent studies have questioned the assumptions on which many of these methods are based, the centerline method of measuring regional wall motion was developed. Its sensitivity and specificity in detecting abnormal regional function compare favorably with those of other methods, and its reliability has been demonstrated. The theoretical advantages and applications of the centerline method for quantitative assessment of regional myocardial function were evaluated.

Motion was assessed along 100 chords constructed perpendicular to a centerline drawn midway between the end-diastolic and end-systolic contours and normalized for heart size. Abnormality was expressed in units of SDs from the mean motion in a normal reference population to provide an index of both the severity and the significance of the wall motion abnormality. The mean abnormality averaged more than 100 chords and correlated highly with the area ejection fraction. The centerline method uses a "sliding window" to assess motion where it is abnormal because assessment of wall motion in predefined regions of the ventricular contour underestimates abnormality. In addition, the extent (percent of contour) of regional abnormalities can be determined from the 100 data points. The severity of hypokinesis at the site of acute myocardial infarction correlated better with infarct size estimated from creatine kinase release than did the ejection fraction or the circumferential extent of hypokinesis. Because the centerline method measures motion along locally determined vectors and requires no apex, origin, coordinate system, or geometric reference figure, it can be applied to contours as dissimilar as the 60-degree left anterior oblique projection of the left ventricle and the 75-degree left anterior oblique projection of the right ventricle.

▶ The authors have studied a method for quantitating regional wall motion from left ventricular cineangiograms that is designed to measure not only the severity of any abnormality but also its significance in quantitative terms. Unfortunately, a standard for assessing methods of wall motion measurement is lacking. At the same time, measuring regional ventricular function is important for determining the effects of therapeutic interventions designed to salvage ventricular function in patients with acute ischemic syndromes. The "centerline method" is an excellent approach to the problem of measuring regional wall motion and is being used in the current National Heart, Lung, and Blood Institute study of coronary thrombolysis in patients treated early after an acute myocardial infarction.—R.A. O'Rourke, M.D.

Quantitative Assessment of Regional Left Ventricular Motion Using Endocardial Landmarks

Cornelis J. Slager, Ton E.H. Hooghoudt, Patrick W. Serruys, Johan C.H. Schuurbiers, Johan H.C. Reiber, Geert T. Meester, Pieter D. Verdouw, and Paul G. Hugenholtz (Erasmus Univ., Rotterdam)
J. Am. Coll. Cardiol. 7:317–326, February 1986   1–38

Although there are several methods available for analyzing left ventricular (LV) wall motion from contrast angiograms, there is no exact generally accepted procedure for tracking fixed points along the endocardial wall. In animals, specific sites of the endocardium can be followed with endocardially implanted metal clips and roentgen cinematography; however, endocardial markers have not been inserted in human beings. Because major differences exist in extent and direction among the movements of neighboring endocardial, midwall, and epicardial sites as the wall thickens, none of these methods can provide an accurate description of endocardial wall motion. A method was developed to assess LV endocardial wall motion in human beings from the pathways of anatomical landmarks recognizable on the endocardial border.

To test the theory that the motion pattern of small anatomical landmarks, recognizable at the LV endocardial border in the contrast angiocardiogram, reflects wall motion, minute metal markers were inserted in the endocardium of eight pigs using a novel retrograde transvascular approach. Subsequently, marker motion was recorded with roentgen cinematography and compared with the motion of landmarks on the endocardial contours detected from the contrast ventriculogram with an automated contour detection system. Linear regression analysis of the directions of the systolic metal marker and endocardial landmark pathways revealed a high level of correlation. In addition, landmark pathways were also assessed in 23 normal human left ventriculograms. Normal LV endocardial wall motion during systole, as observed in the 30-degree right anterior oblique view, is characterized by a dominant inward transverse motion of the opposite anterior and inferoposterior walls and a descent of the base toward the apex, with the apex itself being almost stationary.

The motion pattern of landmarks appearing at the endocardial border, as detected with an automated technique for analysis of cineangiograms, appears to reflect the motion pattern of actual anatomical structures. From the analysis of results of normal landmark motion, it is possible to derive a generalized model for endocardial wall motion that aids the further development of methods to quantify regional LV function in clinical practice.

▶ From the analysis of cineangiographic results assessing landmark motion in pigs after metal marker insertion, a generalized model for endocardial wall motion was derived to be used for further development of this approach to the quantitative assessment of regional LV function designed to obviate the multiple problems involved. This study uses a method of regional wall motion analysis that more closely approximates the visual subjective assessment obtained by viewing an LV cineangiogram. It uses the detectable endocardial features on the angiographic silhouette to "track" identified ranges of the myocardium through the cardiac cycle. Sophisticated computer-assisted analysis is used to "track" these endocardial landmarks, and the method has been carefully validated by comparing derived data with the fixed endocardial marker data in the animal experiments.—R.A. O'Rourke, M.D.

In addition, the following recent publications on regional wall motion are of interest:

1. Grossman, W.: Editorial comment. Assessment of regional myocardial function. *J. Am. Coll. Cardiol.* 8:327–328, 1986.
2. Geffin, G. A., et al.: Effect of preload on ischemic and nonischemic left ventricular regional function. *Cardiovasc. Res.* 20:415–427, 1986.
3. Lanzer, P., et al.: Quantitation of regional myocardial function by cine computed tomography. Pharmacologic changes in wall thickness. *J. Am. Coll. Cardiol.* 8:682–692, 1986.
4. Buda, A. J., Zota, R. J.: Serial assessment of circumferential regional left ventricular function following complete coronary occlusion. *Am. Heart J.* 112:447–452, 1986.
5. Guyer, D. E., et al.: An echocardiographic technique for quantifying and displaying the extent of regional left ventricular dyssynergy. *J. Am. Coll. Cardiol.* 8:830–835, 1986.

Myocardial Perfusion Imaging

Reverse Redistribution of Thallium-201: A Sign of Nontransmural Myocardial Infarction With Patency of the Infarct-Related Coronary Artery

A. Teddy Weiss, Jamshid Maddahi, Allan S. Lew, P.K. Shah, William Ganz, H.J.C. Swan, and Daniel S. Berman (Cedars-Sinai Med. Ctr. and Univ. of California, Los Angeles)

J. Am. Coll. Cardiol. 7:61–67, January 1986   1–39

The characteristic pattern of thallium-201 scintigrams in myocardial ischemia is a perfusion defect noted on early postinjection images. The defect is seen either at rest or during stress, and it is usually normalized after a time delay of several hours ("reversible defect"). Conversely, a region with myocardial infarction typically exhibits a perfusion defect that remains unchanged ("persistent defect"). However, occasionally a perfusion defect may appear or become more obvious on the delayed rather than on the early image. This is the pattern of "reverse redistribution" on stress redistribution thallium-201 images; although it has been reported previously, its etiology, significance, and clinical implications are not known. The frequency of this thallium-201 reverse redistribution pattern was assessed in patients with an acute myocardial infarction who received streptokinase therapy; clinical significance was evaluated with respect in patency of the infarct-related coronary artery and the presence of viable myocardium in the reperfused region as indicated by regional wall motion and poststreptokinase therapy decrease in thallium-201 defect size.

The study population consisted of 67 consecutive patients who underwent streptokinase therapy, had resting thallium-201 studies before intervention, and underwent resting thallium-201 and radionuclide ventriculographic studies 7–10 days after the intervention. In 50 patients (75%) the reverse redistribution pattern was seen in the day-10 thallium-201 study (group 1); 9 (13%) had a nonreversible defect (group II), and the remaining 8 (12%) had normal findings or a reversible defect (group III). The reverse redistribution pattern was associated with patency of the infarct-related artery (100%), quantitative improvement in resting thallium-201 defect size from day-1 to day-10 study (94%), and normal or near-normal wall motion on day-10 radionuclide ventriculography (80% of segments with substantial and 54% of those with mild reverse redistribution). Conversely, nonreversible defects were associated with markedly less frequent patency of the infarct-related artery (67%), improvement in defect size (11%), and normal or near-normal wall motion (21%). With respect to these variables, findings in group I patients were similar to those in group III patients. The quantitated thallium-201 percent washout was higher in regions with the reverse redistribution pattern (49%) relative to the contralateral normal zone (24%). The reverse redistribution pattern results from a higher than normal washout rate of thallium-201. This pattern may be a sign of nontransmural myocardial infarction with a patent infarct-related coronary artery.

▶ During thallium-201 scintigraphy a perfusion defect sometimes appears or becomes more obvious on the delayed images. This study indicates that one of the causes of a reversed distribution pattern is a higher-than-normal washout rate of thallium in patients undergoing successful thrombolysis with a patent infarct-related coronary artery and a non-Q wave myocardial infarction as a result. However, it must be emphasized that this finding may also occur because of inhomogeneous washout of thallium as a normal variant, and that its incidence in patients with acute myocardial infarction not receiving thrombolytic therapy and in patients with unstable angina, many of whom also have coronary artery thrombosis producing myocardial ischemia, is unknown at the present time.—R.A. O'Rourke, M.D.

Thallium-201 Myocardial Imaging During Pharmacologic Coronary Vasodilation: Comparison of Oral and Intravenous Administration of Dipyridamole
Raymond Taillefer, Jean Lette, Denis-Carl Phaneuf, Jean Léveillé, François Lemire, and Richard Essiambre (Hôpital Hôtel-Dieu de Montréal)
J. Am. Coll. Cardiol. 8:76–83, July 1986   1–40

A comparison was made of the diagnostic accuracy of thallium-201 myocardial imaging after the intravenous and oral administration of dipyridamole. Two different oral regimens were used to find the optimal dipyridamole dose. Oral and intravenous studies were performed at 1-week intervals and within 3 weeks of coronary angiography and left ventriculography.

Studies were done in 35 men and 15 women aged 34–70 years who complained of chest pain. They were divided randomly into two groups of 25 each. Group I was given 200 mg of dipyridamole orally, and group II received 400 mg of dipyridamole orally, prior to thallium-201 stress testing. In each group, heart rate and systolic and diastolic blood pressure were recorded after oral and intravenous administration of dipyridamole.

In group I, thallium-201 imaging detected one or more perfusion defects in the initial images in 13 of the 20 patients with coronary artery disease, for a sensitivity of 65% in the 200-mg oral study, and in 17 of the 20 patients for a sensitivity of 85% after intravenous administration. In group II, coronary artery disease was diagnosed in 16 of 19 patients, for a sensitivity of 84% in the 400-mg oral study, and in 15 of 19 patients for a sensitivity of 79% in the intravenous study. Thus, the results with the 400-mg oral dose were significantly better than those with the 200-mg oral dose, and sensitivity was equal to that after intravenous administration. There were no serious complications, e.g., arrhythmia, myocardial infarction, or death. Minor complications included headache and nausea, but side effects were less severe and less frequent with the oral doses than with the intravenous dose. Thallium-201 myocardial imaging during coronary vasodilation induced with 400 mg of dipyridamole orally is safe and reliable.

▶ Methods for using thallium-201 myocardial imaging to detect ischemia in patients unable to exercise are definitely needed. Several studies have demonstrated the usefulness of thallium-201 myocardial imaging after the intravenous administration of dipyridamole, an agent that causes arteriole dilatation and redistribution of flow to normal areas, away from areas with severe coronary artery stenosis.

The current study suggests that thallium-201 myocardial imaging during pharmacologically induced coronary dilation using an oral dose of dipyridamole is a safe and reliable alternative for evaluation of coronary artery disease in patients unable to achieve adequate exercise levels. However, the number of patients with no coronary artery disease in this study was too small to draw conclusions on the true specificity of the test, and further studies comparing the usefulness of oral dipyridamole during thallium-201 myocardial imaging are needed with comparisons to thallium imaging during treadmill exercise testing or arm crank exercise as well as versus the intravenous form.—R.A. O'Rourke, M.D.

Additional publications of interest in this area include the following:

1. Kirkecide, R. L., et al.: Assessment of coronary stenoses by myocardial perfusion imaging during pharmacologic vasodilation. VII. Validation of coronary flow reserve as a single integrated functional measure of stenosis severity reflecting all its geometric dimensions. *J. Am. Coll. Cardiol.* 7:103–115, 1986.

2. Picano, E., et al.: Role of dipyridamole-echocardiography test in electrocardiophically silent effort ischemia. *Am. J. Cardiol.* 58:235–238, 1986.

3. Gould, K. L., et al.: Noninvasive assessment of coronary stenosis by myocardial perfusion imaging during pharmacologic coronary vasodilation. VIII. Clinical feasibility of positron cardiac imaging without a cyclotron using generator-produced rubidium-82. *J. Am. Coll. Cardiol.* 7:775–789, 1986.

Special Cardiac Techniques

Instantaneous Pressure Gradient: A Simultaneous Doppler and Dual Catheter Correlative Study

Philip J. Currie, Donald J. Hagler, James B. Seward, Guy S. Reeder, Derek A. Fyfe, Alfred A. Bove, and A. Jamil Tajik (Mayo Clinic and Found.)
J. Am. Coll. Cardiol. 7:800–806, April 1986   1–41

Pressure gradients can be estimated noninvasively using continuous-wave Doppler echocardiography. The accuracy and validity of continuous-wave Doppler estimation of pressure gradients was assessed in a wide variety of right ventricular (RV) and left ventricular (LV) outflow stenotic lesions, with simultaneous Doppler and dual catheter pressure measurements. The dual catheter technique was used to determine more precisely peak-to-peak and instantaneous pressure gradients.

The study population consisted of 95 consecutive patients with RV or LV outflow obstructive lesions in whom simultaneous Doppler and dual catheter pressure measurements were made during clinically indicated cardiac catheterization. There were 38 RV and 62 LV outflow obstructive lesions. In addition, 49 patients had a nonsimultaneous Doppler study performed within 7 days prior to catheterization. The simultaneous pressure waveforms and Doppler spectral velocity profiles were digitized at 10-msec intervals to derive maximal, mean, and instantaneous gradients (mm Hg). The correlation coefficient for simultaneous maximal Doppler and catheter gradient measurements was 0.95; for Doppler and catheter mean gradients, it was 0.94; and for maximal Doppler and peak-to-peak catheter gradients, it was 0.92. The correlation of maximal and mean Doppler gradients with the respective catheter gradients was similarly high when the RV and LV outflow lesions were analyzed separately; however, the maximal Doppler gradient was markedly higher than the peak-to-peak catheter gradient. The latter finding was more noticeable with LV outflow stenotic lesions. The correlation of the outpatient maximal Doppler and catheter gradients was significantly lower than the simultaneous correlation in the 49 patients with the two Doppler studies.

Continuous-wave Doppler echocardiography accurately measures the instantaneous pressure gradient across both LV and RV outflow obstructive lesions. However, the maximal Doppler gradient should not be equated with the peak-to-peak catheter gradient. Further, because Doppler echocardiography measures instantaneous pressure gradients, it should not be compared directly with nonsimultaneous events.

▶ Continuous-wave Doppler echocardiography is now commonly used to make noninvasive estimates of pressure gradients across semilunar and atrioventricular valves. In adults, it is commonly used to estimate the severity of the LV outflow gradient in patients with aortic stenosis, other techniques being less applicable and often inaccurate, particularly in patients who are elderly with a systolic murmur suggesting aortic stenosis. The Doppler gradient across a stenosis is usually calculated using a modified Bernoulli equation in which the gradient in mm Hg is related to four times the square of the instantaneous velocity in meters/second.

In a relatively large number of patients with LV or RV outflow tract obstruction, the authors demonstrated an excellent correlation between the simultaneously recorded transvalvular gradient determined by cardiac catheterization and that predicted by Doppler echocardiography. However, it should be emphasized that the standard error of the estimate is relatively large, and this may represent an important problem in decision making in the patient in whom noninvasive measurement of the pressure gradient is borderline with regard to a recommendation for surgery (e.g., a Doppler estimated aortic valve gradient of 45 mm Hg). Doppler echocardiography is the most reliable noninvasive technique for estimating the degree of aortic or pulmonic valve stenosis, but it should be emphasized that the simultaneous determination of cardiac output, heart rate, and ventricular ejection time with measurement of the mean pressure gradient is necessary to determine the semilunar valve area, which may or may not be reflected by a large or small pressure gradient, depending on the values for stroke volume and ejection time.—R.A. O'Rourke, M.D.

Correlation of Continuous Wave Doppler Velocities With Cardiac Catheterization Gradients: An Experimental Model of Aortic Stenosis

Mikel D. Smith, Philip L. Dawson, Jonathan L. Elion, David C. Booth, Rodney Handshoe, Oi Ling Kwan, Gary F. Earle, and Anthony N. DeMaria (Univ. of Kentucky and VA Med. Ctr., Lexington)

J. Am. Coll. Cardiol. 6:1306–1314, December 1985   1–42

It is difficult to assess the severity of aortic stenosis accurately by clinical examination alone. Although various noninvasive techniques (e.g., two-dimensional and M-mode echocardiography) are available potentially to measure aortic obstruction, none is satisfactory. An experimental study was performed in dogs to compare simultaneously recorded Doppler spectral signals with high-fidelity catheter pressures in a model of aortic stenosis.

A rubber band that could be progressively tightened circumferentially was placed around the aorta to invoke aortic stenosis in six anesthetized dogs weighing 21–26 kg. In all, 88 different pressure gradients, ranging from 5 mm Hg to 160 mm Hg, were thus produced. Continuous-wave Doppler recordings were obtained at baseline and simultaneously with catheterization gradients at each level of induced stenosis.

There was excellent linear correlation between the maximal instantaneous Doppler gradient and the maximal instantaneous catheterization gradient. However, measurement of the Doppler gradient at midsystole resulted in a more accurate correlation with the peak-to-peak catheterization gradient. Although an excellent correlation was observed between the Doppler gradient and the mean catheterization-derived gradient, correlations between Doppler and catheterization ejection and acceleration times were only fair. A useful estimate of peak-to-peak catheterization gradient can best be derived by measuring the Doppler velocity at midsystole.

▶ In this animal study, 88 different pressure gradients over a wide range were assessed by Doppler echocardiography across the aortic valves of six dogs. The correlations between the maximal instantaneous Doppler gradient and the maximal catheterization gradient, and between the mean Doppler gradient and mean catheterization gradient, were better in this animal study than in the previous study in patients with naturally occurring disease. The standard of the error of the estimate was much smaller than in human studies. However, it must be emphasized that the experimental preparation used most closely resembled supravalvular aortic stenosis rather than valvular aortic stenosis, and that these measurements were obtained under nearly ideal conditions.—R.A. O'Rourke, M.D.

Doppler Echocardiographic Evaluation of Hancock and Björk-Shiley Prosthetic Valves

Kiran B. Sagar, L. Samuel Wann, Walter H.J. Paulsen, and Donald W. Rom-

hilt (Med. College of Virginia, Richmond, and Med. College of Wisconsin, Milwaukee)
J. Am. Coll. Cardiol. 7:681–687, March 1986 1–43

Although the design and durability of prosthetic valves has improved markedly malfunction still occurs. The most useful means of documenting prosthetic valve dysfunction is cardiac catheterization; however, reliable hemodynamic data may be difficult to obtain in some patients when it is undesirable to place a catheter through the prosthetic valve, or when both mitral and aortic prostheses are present. Although currently available noninvasive methods (e.g., phonocardiography, echocardiography, and cinefluoroscopy) are helpful, they are not reliable. Several studies suggested that Doppler echocardiography may be useful to detect and quantitate native valve dysfunction. Because of this, it was hypothesized that Doppler echocardiography may be useful to detect and quantitate prosthetic valve dysfunction. The characteristics of the normally functioning Hancock (porcine) and Björk-Shiley (tilting disk) prostheses were examined and the accuracy of Doppler echocardiography defined in detection or malfunction of these prostheses in the mitral and aortic positions.

The study group consisted of 50 patients with normally functioning Hancock and Björk-Shiley mitral and aortic valves and 46 with suspected malfunction of such valves who subsequently underwent cardiac catheterization. The Doppler echocardiographic characteristics were studied in all 96 patients; the mean gradients were estimated for both mitral and aortic valve prostheses, and the valve area was calculated for the mitral prostheses. The Doppler prosthetic mitral valve gradient and valve area showed good correlation with values obtained with cardiac catheterization for both types of prosthetic valves. Furthermore, the correlation coefficient for the mean prosthetic aortic valve gradient was also good ($r = 0.93$), although Doppler echocardiography tended to overestimate the mean gradient at lower degrees of obstruction. Regurgitation of Hancock and Björk-Shiley prostheses in the mitral and aortic positions was accurately diagnosed. Doppler echocardiography appears to be a reliable method for the characterization of normal and abnormal prosthetic valve function.

▶ Doppler echocardiography appears to be the best noninvasive technique currently available for detecting prosthetic valve dysfunction. Doppler echocardiography provided an accurate estimation of the transprosthetic valve gradient in both patients with aortic and mitral valve prostheses. The pressure half-time method was used to calculate the prosthetic mitral valve gradient. Mild to severe prosthetic valve regurgitation was also detected in some of the patients with prosthetic valves. However, no correlations are given for the semiquantitative measurement of valvular regurgitant by Doppler echocardiography and a quantitative angiographic measurement of prosthetic valve regurgitation, e.g., the calculated regurgitant fraction. Whether or not Doppler echcoardiography is as good for quantitating regurgitation as for stenosis across prosthetic valves remains to be determined.—R.A. O'Rourke, M.D.

The Influence of Preload and Heart Rate on Doppler Echocardiographic Indexes of Left Ventricular Performance: Comparison With Invasive Indexes in an Experimental Preparation

Kenneth Wallmeyer, L. Samuel Wann, Kiran B. Sagar, John Kalbfleisch, and H. Sidney Klopfenstein (Med. College of Wisconsin, Milwaukee)

Circulation 74:181–186, July 1986

1–44

It is important to assess left ventricular (LV) performance to determine the presence and prognosis of many forms of heart disease as well as to monitor the effectiveness of therapeutic interventions. However, conventional invasive techniques are limited by high cost, the risk of possible complications, and technical difficulties in assessing performance during dynamic states, e.g., exercise. Doppler echocardiography offers a reliable method with which to measure aortic blood flow velocity and acceleration noninvasively. The ability of Doppler echocardiography to assess LV performance in six open-chest dogs was evaluated.

Preload was varied by intravenous infusions of nitroglycerin, heart rate was controlled by atrial pacing, and changes in inotropic state were induced by two different doses of dobutamine and administration of propranolol. The length of the LV anterior wall myocardial segment was used as an index of preload. The maximum aortic blood flow, the peak acceleration of aortic blood flow, and differential LV pressure (dP/dt) were assessed with an electromagnetic flow probe around the ascending aorta and a high-fidelity pressure transducer in the left ventricle. A continuous-wave Doppler transducer applied to the aortic arch was used to determine peak aortic blood velocity, mean acceleration, time to peak velocity, and the systolic velocity integral.

The differences between mean values obtained under different inotropic conditions were significant for peak velocity and for mean acceleration. Furthermore, within a given animal, Doppler measurements of peak velocity correlated closely with maximum aortic flow, maximum acceleration of aortic flow, and maximum dP/dt. In addition, mean acceleration measured by Doppler echocardiography was also in close agreement with conventional indexes but was subject to greater interobserver variability. Conversely, Doppler measurements of time to peak and the systolic velocity integral correlated less well with conventional hemodynamic indexes. Doppler measurements of peak aortic blood velocity and mean acceleration offer an effective means to assess noninvasively short-term changes in LV performance under conditions of varying preload, heart rate, and inotropic state.

▶ Most prior studies using Doppler echocardiography to assess LV performance have focused on the noninvasive measurement of cardiac output by this technique at rest or with exercise. This study in dogs shows the potential of using Doppler measurements of peak aortic flow velocity and mean acceleration in the same individual to show changes occurring in ventricular performance during short-term interventions. However, these measurements are likely to be no better (and probably not as good) than other noninvasive measurements of ventricular performance (e.g., ejection fraction by radionuclide techniques or echocardiography) for distinguishing normal persons from patients with impaired LV performance. Also, because the measurements obtained depend on the rate of ejection of blood from the ventricle, they are likely to be influenced by afterload (not measured in this study) as well as being an index of the inotropic state.—R.A. O'Rourke, M.D.

Comparison of Bipolar and Unipolar Programmed Electrical Stimulation for the Initiation of Ventricular Arrhythmias: Significance of Anodal Excitation During Bipolar Stimulation
William G. Stevenson, Isaac Wiener, and James N. Weiss (Univ. of California at Los Angeles)
Circulation 73:693–700, April 1986   1–45

A comparison was made of the initiation of either clinically important sustained monomorphic ventricular tachycardia (VT) or less specific arrhythmias by using both bipolar and cathodal unipolar programmed ventricular stimulation to ascertain whether anodal excitation during bipolar stimulation facilitates initiation of such arrhythmias. The series included 28 patients seen for evaluation of spontaneous sustained ventricular fibrillation (VF) (11 patients), nonsustained tachycardia (8), or syncope (9). All patients underwent both bipolar and cathodal unipolar programmed ventricular stimulation with one to three extrastimuli delivered during ventricular pacing at two rates from the right ventricular apex.

There were no differences between unipolar and bipolar stimulation with regard to the late diastolic threshold or refractory periods of the basic drive, first, or second extrastimuli. Six patients experienced sustained monomorphic VF. Four patients experienced tachycardia, initiated by both bipolar and unipolar stimulation with the same number of extrastimuli, whereas in only two patients was tachycardia initiated by unipolar stimulation and in one by bipolar stimulation. No difference in the incidence of initiation of sustained monomorphic VT, polymorphic VT, or repetitive ventricular responses was noted in the groups with and without evidence of anodal excitation during bipolar pacing. The risk of initiation of either nonsustained polymorphic VT or repetitive ventricular responses in patients with anodal excitation during bipolar stimulation was not higher than the risk during unipolar stimulation despite the fact that anodal excitation was associated with a shorter ventricular refractory period.

▶ Programmed ventricular stimulation continues to be an important technique for inducing monomorphic sustained VT in patients with spontaneous VT in the electrophysiology laboratory. Despite theoretical considerations to the contrary, the risk of initiation of either nonsustained polymorphic VT or repetitive ventricular responses in patients with anodal excitation during bipolar stimulation was no greater than that during unipolar stimulation in this study.—R.A. O'Rourke, M.D.

In Vivo Measurement of Myocardial Mass Using Nuclear Magnetic Resonance Imaging

Andrew M. Keller, Ronald M. Peshock, Craig R. Malloy, L. Maximilian Buja, Ray Nunnally, Robert W. Parkey, and James T. Willerson (Univ. of Texas at Dallas and Southwestern Med. School, Dallas)
J. Am. Coll. Cardiol. 8:113–117, July 1986   1–46

Nuclear magnetic resonance (NMR) imaging has been used successfully to calculate left ventricular (LV) mass in vitro. An experimental study was undertaken to determine whether NMR can be used to calculate accurately the LV mass in vivo using ten mongrel dogs weighing between 5 kg and 30 kg. Imaging was done with NMR techniques. The LV mass was measured by computing the volume of myocardium in each slice from the known volume element (voxel) dimension, using the average voxel count for each slice. Left ventricular myocardial volume was measured in five short-axis end-diastolic images that spanned the left ventricle. The LV mass was then calculated from the LV myocardial volume and compared with the weight of the left ventricle after formalin immersion-fixation.

Linear regression analysis showed that LV mass as determined with NMR imaging was only slightly higher than that obtained from LV weight estimation. Thus, NMR imaging overestimated the myocardial mass, probably because of partial volume effects and difficulty with border definition. Thus, NMR imaging can accurately assess the myocardial mass in vivo in a canine model.

▶ Current noninvasive and invasive methods for measuring LV mass are suboptimal. Particularly, they are of limited value in patients with ischemic heart disease and asymmetric cardiomyopathy. Both contrast ventriculography and echocardiography use assumptions regarding LV geometry, and thallium-201 single-photon emission CT requires normal myocardial perfusion for thallium-201 distribution to assess LV mass. Measurements of LV mass by CT or dynamic spatial reconstruction require the use of significant doses of ionizing radiation and the intravenous administration of contrast agents. Nuclear magnetic resonance (NMR) imaging is becoming available at many medical centers. In this study in ten dogs without LV hypertrophy, there was excellent correlation between the NMR-determined mass and LV weight at post mortem examination. Also, interobserver variation was low and reproducibility was good. Preliminary results suggest that, in the near future, NMR may become an important tool in assessment of myocardial mass in patients with cardiac disease.—R.A. O'Rourke, M.D.

Utility of the Routine Electrocardiogram Before Surgery and on General Hospital Admission: Critical Review and New Guidelines

Ary L. Goldberger and Mark O'Konski (Harvard Univ. and Univ. of California at San Diego)
Ann. Intern. Med. 105:552–557, October 1986   1–47

Although a 12-lead ECG is recommended for adults on general hospital admission and before various operations involving the use of general or regional anesthesia, the benefits of this test are controversial. Furthermore, this problem may have important implications for the cost and quality of health care. The indications for the routine use of the ECG preoperatively and on general hospital admission were reassessed.

Several studies on the yield of routine preoperative ECGs found that abnormalities are relatively common and that a major determinant of their prevalence is patient age (Fig 1–4). The major positive effect of a preoperative ECG is related to the detection of previously unrecognized myocardial infarction. This is important, because careful intraoperative and postoperative management may reduce the complication rate in high-risk patients. In addition, certain patients may attain long-term benefits from treatment with β-blocking drugs, and postponement of elective surgery in patients with recent infarction may decrease the operative risk. However, whereas the ECG may provide major information relative to the diagnosis of a recent myocardial infarction, it does not indicate the timing of the event.

Aside from the diagnosis of unrecognized myocardial infarction, the ECG has been of small benefit in detecting certain arrhythmias associated with increased perioperative risk. However, the yield is greatest in patients with the highest risk of arrhythmias, including asymptomatic older patients and those with a positive cardiovascular history or physical findings. The major negative effect of a preoperative ECG stems from the fact that routine application of a test with limited specificity for a disease leads to the generation of abnormal results in patients who do not have the disease. There is no evidence to support obtaining an ECG in all patients on a

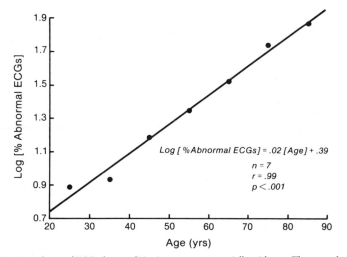

Fig 1–4.—Prevalence of ECG abnormalities increases exponentially with age. The mean frequency of abnormal ECG findings in seven age groups, weighted by the total number of patients in each population in four studies is plotted. (Courtesy of Goldberger, A.L., et al.: Ann Intern. Med. 105:552–557, October 1986.)

routine basis preoperatively as a baseline for comparison, and little evidence exists to support the practice of performing an ECG in patients without apparent heart disease when they are admitted to the hospital.

► The ECG continues to be an extremely useful technique in the diagnosis of cardiac disease (often silent) and in determining the effects of various types of cardiac disease on chamber size and wall thickness, cardiac rhythm, and the conduction system. It is by far the least expensive of currently available non-invasive and invasive cardiac tests. However, the routine use of any medical test, particularly in low-risk patients, must be considered in relation to the cost-effective practice of medicine. The preceding paper was commissioned by the Blue Cross and Blue Shield Medical Necessity Project under the auspices of the Socity for Research and Education in Primary Care Internal Medicine.—R.A. O'Rourke, M.D.

Risks for Renal Dysfunction With Cardiac Angiography
Charles P. Taliercio, Ronald E. Vlietstra, Lloyd D. Fisher, and John C. Burnett (Mayo Clinic and Found.)
Ann. Intern. Med. 104:501–504, April 1986   1–48

It is generally accepted that preexisting renal insufficiency is a source of increased risk for acute renal dysfunction after the use of contrast media and these agents accounts for approximately 10% of all patients with hospital-acquired acute renal failure. The incidence of contrast medium-associated nephropathy was studied retrospectively in a group of high-risk patients who underwent cardiac angiography using patient records spanning a 10-year period. All patients with baseline serum creatinine levels of at least 2.0 mg/dl prior to undergoing cardiac angiography were identified. The criterion for a diagnosis of contrast medium-associated nephropathy was a rise in the serum creatinine level of more than 1 mg/dl within 1–5 days after cardiac angiography when compared with baseline levels. Of 17,000 cardiac angiographic studies done during the study period, 104 male and 35 female patients who underwent a total of 141 cardiac angiographic examinations were found to have preexisting abnormal renal function and serum creatinine levels of at least 2.0 mg/dl. An additional 43 patients met the study criteria, but they were excluded from analysis because of inadequate follow-up of renal status. Patients with functional class IV heart failure were divided into subgroups with and without low cardiac output.

Of 139 patients, 32 (23%) had contrast medium nephropathy. Anuria or oliguria developed in 13 of the 32 patients, and 2 required dialysis. Renal function returned to baseline levels in 25 patients. Contrast medium nephropathy was associated independently with class IV heart failure in patients with low cardiac output (71%), more than one radiocontrast study in a given patient within a 72-hour period (50%), and insulin-dependent diabetes mellitus (44%), but not with age, hypertension, or hyperuricemia. Also, the dosage of radiocontrast material used was significantly associated with the subsequent development of nephropathy, with a 2% incidence in patients who received less than 125 ml of contrast material and a 19% incidence in those given at least 125 ml. Familiarity with the risk factors associated with preexisting renal dysfunction may minimize the occurrence of acute renal dysfunction after cardiac angiography.

▶ Contrast ventriculography and selective coronary arteriography are performed in a large number of patients with definite or suspected cardiac disease, many of whom have underlying renal disease. This retrospective analysis during a 10-year period shows the importance of various risk factors in the development of contrast nephropathy after cardiac angiography. In patients who are at an increased risk of sustaining greater impairment of renal function, several alternative noninvasive techniques are available for assessing left ventricular performance without the need for injecting contrast material. Determination of the left ventricular ejection fraction by radionuclide ventriculography or two-dimensional echocardiography is recommended for patients at high risk, many of whom may need only hemodynamic measurements and selective coronary arteriography at the time of cardiac catheterization.—R.A. O'Rourke, M.D.

Some of the many recent publications concerning special cardiac techniques are as follows:

1. Johnston, D.L., et al.: Magnetic resonance imaging during acute myocardial infarction. *Am. J. Cardiol.* 57:1059–1065, 1986.
2. Florentine, M.S., et al.: Measurement of left ventricular mass using gated nuclear magnetic resonance. *J. Am. Coll. Cardiol.* 8:107–112, 1986.
3. Rich, S., et al.: Determination of left ventricular ejection fraction using ultrafast computed tomography. *Am. Heart J.* 112:392–396, 1986.
4. Raichler, J.S., et al.: Dynamic three-dimensional reconstruction of the left ventricle from two-dimensional echocardiograms. *J. Am. Coll. Cardiol.* 8:364–370, 1986.
5. Valdex-Cruz, L.M., et al.: Studies in vitro of the relationship between ultrasound and laser Doppler velocimetry and applicability of the simplified Bernoulli relationship. *Circulation* 73:300–308, 1986.
6. Levy, R.D., et al.: Continuous ambulatory pulmonary artery pressure monitoring. A new method using a transducer tipped catheter and a simple recording system. *Br. Heart J.* 55:336–343, 1986.
7. Lambert, C.R., et al.: Low-frequency requirements for recording ischemic ST-segment abnormalities in coronary artery disease. *Am. J. Cardiol.* 58:225–226, 1986.
8. Bryg, R.J., et al.: Effect of coronary artery disease on Doppler-derived parameters of aortic flow during upright exercise. *Am. J. Cardiol.* 58:H-19, 1986.
9. Myers, J.H., et al.: Direct measurement of inner and outer wall thickening dynamics with epicardial echocardiography. *Circulation* 74:164–172, 1986.
10. Kemper, A.J., et al.: In vivo prediction of the transmural extent of experimental acute myocardial infarction using contrast echocardiography. *J. Am. Coll. Cardiol.* 8:143–149, 1986.

Miscellaneous Topics

Aortic Baroreceptor Deafferentation in the Baboon

Vernon S. Bishop, Joseph R. Haywood, Robert E. Shade, Michael Siegel, and Carolyn Hamm (Univ. of Texas at San Antonio and Southwest Found. for Biomedical Res., San Antonio)

J. Appl. Physiol. 60:798–801, March 1986   1–49

Results of animal studies suggest that there is a quantitative difference in the response of arterial pressure and baroreflex function to denervation of the aortic and carotid baroreceptors. Aortic baroreceptor denervation causes mild hypertension and a reduced ability to buffer hypotensive stimuli, whereas carotid sinus denervation does not cause a chronic increase in arterial pressure in the dog. These findings indicate that, in the absence of functional carotid sinus reflexes, the aortic baroreceptors may effectively buffer decreases in arterial pressure. There is little information available about the separate role of the aortic and carotid sinus baroreceptors in the regulation of arterial pressure. An examination was made of the hypothesis that, in the nonhuman primate, the carotid sinus baroreceptors can effectively regulate arterial pressure in the absence of aortic baroreceptors.

Adult male baboons (18–22 kg) were chronically maintained on a tether system that permitted them to move freely about their cage. This allowed continuous monitoring of arterial pressure and heart rate over 24-hour periods with periodic drug administration to test cardiovascular function. Mean control values of arterial pressure and heart rate were 86 mm Hg and 77.5 beats per minute, respectively. After the aortic baroreceptors were removed, the mean arterial pressure rose to 105 mm Hg and the heart rate increased to 118 beats per minute. The variability of these parameters did not change after denervation. However, there was suppression of the arterial pressure-heart period relationship and augmentation of the depressor response to ganglionic blockade with hexamethonium. Removal of the aortic baroreceptors causes a reduction in the sensitivity of the heart rate baroreflex and a subsequent increase in arterial pressure that is a result of an increased sympathetic nervous system function.

▶ Previous studies in dogs and rats have shown that selective denervation of aortic baroreceptors leads to mild hypertension. This implies that reflexes from the aortic baroreceptors participate in the regulation of arterial pressure under normal basal conditions. In this study, denervation of aortic baroreceptors produced substantial increases in the mean arterial pressure in the awake baboon. The resulting hypertension was characterized by the absence of lability and a significant reduction in baroreflex function, resulting in elevations of sympathetic activity. The implications from this study relative to baroreceptor responsiveness in patients with essential hypertension remain to be determined.— R.A. O'Rourke, M.D.

Regional Wave Travel and Reflections Along the Human Aorta: A Study With Six Simultaneous Micromanometric Pressures
Ricky D. Latham, Nico Westerhof, Pieter Sipkema, Bernard J. Rubal, Peter Reuderink, and Joseph P. Murgo (Brooke Army Med. Ctr., Fort Sam Houston, Tex., and Free Univ., Amsterdam)
Circulation 72:1257–1269, December 1985   1–50

Although alterations in the contour of the pressure wave along the aorta have been observed for many years, the mechanisms responsible for these changes have not been identified. Most of the previous laboratory investigations have been in animal preparations, in which the proximal aortic pulse contour differs from that in man in most cases. The entire human aorta and its terminal branches were investigated with simultaneous equidistant (10 cm) micromanometric pressure measurements to determine regional pulse wave velocities, identify the major arterial reflection site(s), and assess the influence of clinical maneuvers on reflected waves.

The study was carried out using normal individuals who were undergoing elective cardiac catheterization. A specially designed catheter with six micromanometers equally spaced at 10-cm intervals was positioned with the tip sensor in the distal external iliac artery and the proximal sensor in the aortic arch; simultaneous pressures were obtained and analyzed for foot-to-foot wave velocity, and apparent phase velocity was derived by Fourier analysis. These quantities were determined during nine control, eight Valsalva, and four Muller maneuvers, and in eight instances during femoral artery occlusion by bilateral manual compression. The local reflection coefficient in the proximal descending aorta, at the junction of the renal arteries, and at the terminal aortic bifurcation was calculated from regional cross-sectional areas, determined from aortography, and regional foot-to-foot pulse wave velocities during control. To determine whether significant reflections originate in the aorta at the level of the renal arteries, aortograms were used to design a latex tube model with geometric properties similar to the descending aorta, and the velocities and reflection characteristics in the model and in vivo were compared.

Thoracic aortic pressures under control conditions revealed a reflected wave originating from the region of the aorta at the level of the renal arterial branches, whereas abdominal pressures exhibited reflection from a site peripheral to the terminal aortic bifurcation. However, in the low-frequency range, apparent phase velocity was higher proximal to the renal arteries when compared with distal sites. The minimum value occurred at a higher frequency in the lower thoracic aorta than at more distal sites. The effects of reflection on apparent wave velocity in the tube model were consistent with data obtained in vivo. The Valsalva maneuver decreased the reflection from the aortic region of the renal arteries, thereby allowing the distal reflected wave to become more evident on the thoracic pressure waveforms. The bilateral femoral artery occlusion usually enhanced the distal reflection and the Müller maneuver usually led to a small increase in reflection.

The geometric and elastic nonuniformity of the aorta often results in two major sites of arterial wave reflection that influence aortic pressure waveforms in man. The first major reflection site is located at the aortic level of the renal arterial branch, and the second is found distal to the terminal aortic bifurcation.

▶ The mechanisms responsible for the changes in the contour of the pressure wave along the aorta have not been fully delineated. Previous investigations have shown that clinical interventions in man influence wave reflections. The authors have shown that the Valsalva maneuver diminishes reflection from the proximal reflection site, which appears to be at the aortic level of the renal artery branches; that the Müller maneuver effects reflection to a limited extent; and that femoral artery occlusion increases aortic reflection from the distal site that is beyond the terminal aortic bifurcation. These studies provide a basis for additional investigation of wave propagation characteristics and vasculature architecture that should provide the physician with greater insight into the physiologic interpretation of pressure wave shapes routinely measured in the proximal aorta.—R.A. O'Rourke, M.D.

2 Cardiovascular Disease in Infants and Children

Development of the Heart

Quantitative Morphology of the Aortic Arch in Neonatal Coarctation
W. Robert Morrow, James C. Huhta, Daniel J. Murphy, Jr., and Dan G. McNamara (Baylor Univ. and Texas Children's Hosp., Houston)
J. Am. Coll. Cardiol. 8:616–620, September 1986   2–1

Neonates with coarctation of the aorta are frequently seen with severe congestive failure. Postnatal constriction of the aortic isthmus and ductus arteriosus has been implicated, but aortic arch hypoplasia is present in some affected neonates and is presumed to be caused by decreased arch blood flow in utero. Morphometric analysis of the great vessels was carried out with two-dimensional echocardiography in 14 neonates with isolated coarctation and 14 normal neonates younger than age 1 month to estimate the degree of aortic arch hypoplasia and analyze the distribution of blood flow. All infants were of term gestation.

Measurements to within 0.5 mm showed that the transverse aortic arch and isthmus in infants with coarctation were significantly smaller than in control neonates. The pulmonary valve and main pulmonary artery diameters were significantly greater in neonates with coarctation than in the normal infants. The left carotid artery was also significantly enlarged in neonates with coarctaton. No differences were observed in descending aortic or left subclavian artery diameters.

Segmental hypoplasia of the aortic arch is useful in the echocardiographic diagnosis of coarctation in neonates. Pulmonary valve and pulmonary artery enlargement in the absence of an intracardiac shunt should suggest coarctation. Duct flow is increased, and blood flow in the ascending aorta and aortic arch is reduced in coarctation. Nevertheless, the carotid and innominate arteries are enlarged. Increased carotid flow may result from coarctation in utero, possibly contributing to cerebral circulatory abnormalities and to cerebral complications in adulthood.

▶ Discussion about the causes of coarctation of the aorta have long caused debate between those favoring the hypothesis that coarctation occurs because of migration of ductal tissue into the juxtaductal aorta and those who think that this cannot explain all of the features known about coarctation. The ductus-migration theory proposes that when the ductus undergoes normal postnatal constriction and obliteration, it pulls in the aorta, creating a shelf and the constriction in the aorta that we call coarctation. That theory does not explain coarctation at sites other than juxtaductal, however, nor is it consistent with the observations made by these authors implying prenatal redistribution of blood flow that favors right heart output through the open ductus to the descending aorta. Hypoplasia of the ascending and transverse aortic arch are present very early in life, as this study documents. Therefore, coarctation of the aorta is not simply a postnatal event resulting from constriction of migrated ductal tissue.—M.A. Engle. M.D.

Developmental Considerations of Mitral Valve Anomalies

A.C.G. Wenink, A.C. Gittenberger-de Groot, and A.G. Brom (Univ. of Leiden, The Netherlands)
Int. J. Cardiol. 11:85–98, April 1986   2–2

Previously conducted embryologic studies enabled identification of a spectrum of congenital valve anomalies reflecting valvular development and maldevelopment. In particular, detailed study of mitral valve embryology allowed recognition of various forms of mitral valve pathology, each of which has its own specific developmental history.

Two aspects are fundamental to atrioventricular valve development: one, the principle of junctional invagination and myocardial undermining, and, two, the principle of topographically related morphogenesis. Two groups of malformations can be distinguished. Disturbances of the general principle include the parachute valve in which myocardial undermining may proceed to fusion of the papillary muscles, or the hammock valve in which the already small orifice is further compromised by an unduly large mass of papillary muscles, leaving extremely small openings between leaflet and muscle tissue. The second type of topographic malformations involves abnormalities of septation and valve formation. A prime example is the atrioventricular septal defect in which there is a clear relationship between valve pathology and abnormal septation. In atrioventricular septal defect, a principal characteristic is deficiency of the inlet septum, which at its fusion site does not reach the aortic root; because of this the undermining process of the primary fold may not easily continue onto the inlet component of the septum. Rather, the process occurs independently at antero-superior and posteroinferior sites, producing the well-recognized superior and inferior bridging leaflets. Another example is the straddling mitral valve, which often accompanies an outlet malalignment defect of the Taussig Bing type. Interestingly, the development of the mitral valve itself provides no clues as to the understanding of mitral atresia. Further research is needed to clarify details of its morphogenesis.

▶ Wenink, Gittenberger-de Groot, and Brom focus on the basis for anomalies of the mitral valve and they illustrate their points beautifully in diagrams and photographs. In so doing they not only clarify the two major processes involved, but they also correct certain errors in terminology that have crept into usage.

One of these is the term "endocardial cushion defect." They point out how-little the endocardial cushions contribute to atrioventricular (AV) valve development. The mitral and tricuspid valves and their tension apparatus are formed from the inner layer of the walls of the inlet portions of the left and right ventricles. The undermining process is supported by invagination of the AV sulcus, which provides the necessary fibrous tissue. The role of the endocardial tissue is inconspicuous. The ventricular myocardium is of prime importance.

A second misnomer is the so-called cleft of the aortic leaflet of the mitral valve in AV septal defect. They call this opening between the superior and inferior bridging leaflets a "gap," related to improper fusion of inlet and primary septal components. They distinguish the gap of the mitral valve in AV septal defect from the much less common isolated cleft of the left AV valve.

Furthermore, they point to the frequent association of mitral valve anomalies and septational disorders, making the point that one should be alert to that possibility when evaluating a patient with a seemingly straightforward diagnosis, e.g., central muscular ventricular septal defect.—M.A. Engle, M.D.

Abnormalities of the Mitral Valve in Congenitally Corrected Transposition (Discordant Atrioventricular and Ventriculoarterial Connections)

Leon M. Gerlis, Neil Wilson, and David F. Dickinson (Killingbeck Hosp., Leeds, England)
Br. Heart J. 55:475–479, May 1986   2–3

Hearts with congenitally corrected transposition often have abnormalities of the tricuspid valve, the pulmonary valve, and the subpulmonary area. The aortic valve may also be abnormal, but there has been no systematic study of or reference to abnormalities of the mitral valve in this condition. The prevalence and nature of these abnormalities was documented in 29 hearts with congenitally corrected transposition. All were examined for evidence of abnormality of the mitral valve.

Mitral valve defects were found in 16 (55%) of the 29 specimens. These abnormalities were most commonly of cusp number (21%) and tension apparatus (21%). A less common finding was valve dysplasia (10%). Other abnormalities identified included common valve, stenosis, and cleft valve. Several specimens had more than one morphological abnormality. The median age at death of patients with mitral valve abnormalities (mean, 6.5 years; range, 1 day to 24 years) was markedly higher than that of patients without these abnormalities (mean, 1.9 years; range, 1 day to 11 years). There were more females than males with affected valves (ratio, 2:1). Certain malformations (e.g., ventricular septal defect and tricuspid or pulmonary valve anomalies) were represented in similar proportions in hearts with and without mitral anomalies. Ventricular septal defects were present in 23 patients (79%). Pulmonary stenosis was present in 10 and pulmonary atresia in 9 of the 23 specimens. In congenitally corrected transposition of the great arteries, whereas abnormalities of the mitral valve are common, the described anomalies minor.

▶ Gerlis and associates looked for and found abnormalities of the mitral valve (the right-sided, bicuspid valve) in more than half of the specimens of ventricular inversion that they examined. Unlike the common and well-known associated anomalies of pulmonic stenosis or atresia, and of downward displacement of the left-sided atrioventricular valve (left-sided Ebstein's anomaly of the tricuspid valve), the developmental abnormalities of the mitral valve were of minor physiologic importance. It is unlikely that they contributed much to the life or death of these patients.—M.A. Engle, M.D.

Congenital Heart Disease

Natural History

Importance of (Perimembranous) Ventricular Septal Aneurysm in the Natural History of Isolated Perimembranous Ventricular Septal Defect

Claudio Ramaciotti, Andre Keren, and Norman H. Silverman (Univ. of California at San Francisco)

Am. J. Cardiol. 57:268–272, Feb. 1, 1986   2–4

Many isolated ventricular septal defects (VSDs) either close or diminish in size spontaneously. Perimembranous ventricular septal aneurysm (VSA) tissue is thought to be responsible for this spontaneous process, but the actual incidence of VSA involvement is unknown. A review was made of the records of 247 patients with isolated VSDs to assess the frequency of VSA in this patient group by means of cross-sectional echocardiography.

On the basis of echocardiographic findings, the patients were divided into two groups: group A consisted of 190 patients with an associated VSA (Fig 2–1), and group B, 57 patients without an associated VSA. The VSD was further assessed on the basis of clinical and hemodynamic criteria. Follow-up ranged from 3 months to 25 years.

In group A, the VSD closed spontaneously in 11% of the patients, improved clinically without surgery in 33%, and necessitated surgery in 11%. In contrast, 47% of group B patients required surgery, whereas the VSD closed spontaneously in only 2% and improved clinically without surgery in 16%. The VSA was found on the first echocardiographic examination in 94% of the patients. Analysis of data just on the larger VSDs showed that 28% of the patients in group A had surgery, as did 84% of those in group B.

Ventricular septal aneurysms constitute an important mechanism of closure in patients with VSD. They occur early and they impart a more favorable prognosis than in patients without an aneurysm.

▶ Cardiologists have known for the past 30 years that some VSDs decrease in size spontaneously and may even close, any time from early infancy well into adult life. Aneurysm-like formation that involves the septal leaflet of the tricuspid valve adjacent to the defect brings about the improvement, even in large defects that cause cardiac failure in the first few months of life. What initiates the process and carries it along until the defect is partially or completely closed is unknown. This echocardiographic study, corroborated by findings at cardiac

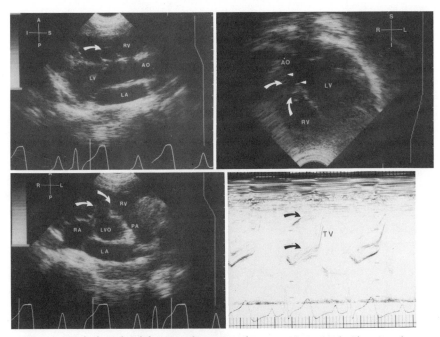

Fig 2–1.—Methods used to define a pseudoaneurysm *(large arrows)* associated with perimembranous ventricular septal defect (VSD) from a patient with an associated ventricular septal aneurysm, a moderate-sized shunt, and relatively normal pulmonary arterial pressure. **Top left,** parasternal long-axis view; **bottom left,** parasternal short-axis view; **top right,** apical four-chamber view in anatomical orientation, with *small arrowheads* indicating the base of the VSD and adherence of the base of the pseudoaneurysm to it; **bottom right,** M-mode recording generated from the parasternal short-axis plane with the beam passing through the right ventricle *(RV)*, pseudoaneurysm, tricuspid valve leaflet *(TV)*, and right atrium *(RA)*. A indicates anterior; *AO,* aorta; I, inferior, *L,* left, *LA,* left atrium; *LV;* left ventricle; *LVO,* left ventricular outflow; *P,* posterior; *R,* right; *S,* superior.

(Courtesy of Ramaciotti, C., et al.: Am. J. Cardiol. 57:268–272, Feb. 1, 1986.)

catheterization in 69 of the 247 patients, provides new information on the subject by demonstrating that VSAs occur early. The study confirms the beneficial effect of the aneurysm in decreasing the effective size of the defect, and it implies that one might defer surgery on the child with aneurysm formation and, instead, follow the patient closely and with echocardiography, hoping for and expecting spontaneous improvement that might eliminate the need for an operation.—M.A. Engle, M.D.

Incidence & Prenatal Screening

Prenatal Screening for Congenital Heart Disease
Lindsay D. Allan, Diane C. Crawford, Sunder K. Chita, and Michael J. Tynan (Guy's Hosp., London)
Br. Med. J. 292:1717–1719, June 28, 1986   2–5

Congenital heart disease, the most common severe congenital abnormality, causes more than half of the deaths from congenital anomalies. To

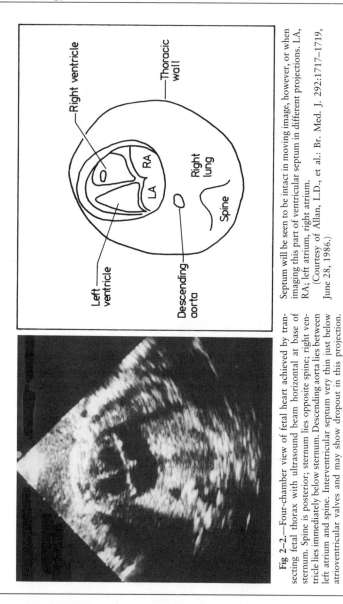

Fig 2–2.—Four-chamber view of fetal heart achieved by transecting fetal thorax with ultrasound beam horizontal at base of sternum. Spine is posterior; sternum lies opposite spine; right ventricle lies immediately below sternum. Descending aorta lies between left atrium and spine. Interventricular septum very thin just below atrioventricular valves and may show dropout in this projection. Septum will be seen to be intact in moving image, however, or when imaging this part of ventricular septum in different projections. LA, RA; left atrium, right atrium.

(Courtesy of Allan, L.D., et al.: Br. Med. J. 292:1717–1719, June 28, 1986.)

aid in routine ultrasound screening procedures, a simplified approach to fetal cardiac screening was developed that can be used in gestations of 16 weeks or more. Use of the four-chamber view of the heart is readily and quickly achieved, and a normal appearance excludes most severe congenital anomalies. The four-chamber view is shown in Figure 2–2. Referral center data for cardiac abnormalities seen in a 5-year period are summarized in the table. The increase in absolute numbers reflects increased referrals of high-risk pregnancies to the center; however, the proportion of affected

CASES OF CONGENITAL HEART DISEASE DETECTED PRENATALLY IN
REFERRAL CENTER AND PROPORTIONS SUSPECTED BY REFERRING
ULTRASONOGRAPHERS (JANUARY 1980 TO OCTOBER 1985)

	1980	81	82	83	84	85	Total
No detected in referral centre	3	10	7	13	24	32	89
No suspected before referral			3	4	11	22	40

(Courtesy Allan, L.D., et al.: Br. Med. J. 292:1717–1719, June 28, 1986.)

pregnancies rose from 1 in 50 in 1980 to 1 in 12 currently. Suspected cardiac abnormalities were confirmed in more than 80% of the patients.

These data show that such routine examination is feasible and can readily distinguish most severe abnormalities in the fetal heart. The technique is already in use on a limited basis; more than 80% of the pregnant women in England receive at least one obstetric screening, and this could include a four-chamber view of the heart. Scanning between 16 and 20 weeks of gestation is ideal for determination of cardiac abnormalities. Early detection allows referral for echocardiography at a time when various options are still open. The parent can be counseled on the prospects of long-term survival or advised as to termination of the pregnancy. For the types of gross abnormality seen on these scans, the prognosis is usually poor. If the pregnancy is continued, optimum antenatal care can be planned in advance.

Abnormalities detectable by the four-chamber view alone include hypoplastic left heart syndrome; mitral, pulmonary, or tricuspid atresia; and double inlet ventricle. Roughly three cardiac abnormalities per 1,000 live births present in infancy. Of these, it is predicted that 2/1,000 live births could be detected by the four-chamber view. This screening program should detect more than 60% of severe structural defects of the heart that are seen in the first year of life; moreover, use of this procedure would not require a change in resources or personnel. Experience suggests that screening also would not result in large numbers of anxious patients being referred needlessly for a second opinion, because most suspected congenital heart defects were confirmed, and false positive results were uncommon. Such prenatal screening could have profound implications for the practice and organization of pediatric cardiology.

▶ One of the early applications for echocardiography was in the detection of congenital heart disease in the fetus. Fetal echocardiography is now a combined obstetric-pediatric cardiologic service in many cardiac centers. The authors have become expert in the diagnosis of fetal cardiac abnormalities. In this article they propose the addition of cardiac screening by the four-chamber view to the obstetric ultrasound screening that is so prevalent in pregnant women. Those women suspected to be carrying a fetus with a cardiac abnormality could then be referred to a pediatric cardiac diagnostic center for confirmation and for options in a plan of management. Recommendations could be made based on the specific anomaly and results of medical and/or surgical therapy.

Humanitarian and ethical concerns are raised by this new diagnostic capability, and these require the same kind of thoughtful deliberation and analysis as were given to development of the technique itself.—M.A. Engle, M.D.

Spectrum of Congenital Heart Disease Detected Echocardiographically in Prenatal Life
Lindsey D. Allan, Diane C. Crawford, Robert H. Anderson, and Michael Tynan (Guy's Hosp. and Brompton Hosp., London)
Br. Heart J. 54:523–526, November 1985   2–6

Based on 5 years' experience with fetal echocardiography in the prenatal detection of congenital heart disease (CHD); the authors hypothesized that a higher proportion of affected infants with the diagnosis made in utero have had severe malformations than is the case in children presenting in infancy. Furthermore, cardiac abnormalities found in aborted fetuses and stillborn infants were more severe than those abnormalities diagnosed after birth. This hypothesis was tested by review of cardiac anomalies encountered in 72 fetuses with malformed hearts identified by echoardiography.

Patients were referred for fetal echocardiography for a variety of reasons, among them a family history of congenital heart disease, exposure to a teratogen in early pregnancy, the detection of nonimmune hydrops fetalis, fetal arrhythmia, or an extracardiac anomaly, e.g., exomphalos, neural tube defects, or renal abnormalities. Patients were also referred because a possible cardiac anomaly was reported after obstetric ultrasonography. A cardiac malformation was noted by fetal echocardiography in 72 fetuses, 67 of which died. There were 34 terminations of pregnancy, 13 intrauterine deaths, and 20 neonatal deaths. There were five survivors, including three not yet delivered and two who underwent surgery. Of the two infants operated on, one had complete transposition and the other had aortic coarctation. When the diagnoses in the entire group were compared with the diagnoses in infants with CHD seen during the first year of life, certain differences became obvious. In the 72 fetuses in the present series there was a relative paucity of ventricular septal defects, pulmonary stenosis, atrial septal defects, and total anomalous pulmonary venous connection, but there was an excess of absent left atrioventricular connection, interrupted aortic arch, pulmonary atresia with intact septum, atrioventricular septal defect, myocardial disease, Ebstein's anomaly, and cardiac tumor.

Many of the differences between the series can probably be accounted for by the selection of patients for referral for fetal echocardiography. Thus, few mothers who have had children with mild heart disease (e.g., septal defects or pulmonary stenosis) are referred for examination. It is the mothers who have already had a child die of a major congenital heart disease who are far more likely to be referred. There are major differences in the spectrum of congenital heart disease seen prenatally and postnatally, complex defects being more common prenatally. An accurate picture of the true prevalence of congenital heart disease requires a large prospective study of an unselected series of pregnancies.

▶ Traditionally, the term congenital heart disease implies a cardiovascular anomaly present *at* birth. Development of fetal echocardiography permits discussion of anomalies present *before* birth. This paper teaches us that the latter tend to be more severe and to result in fetal loss. The authors reviewed reports of spontaneous abortions, which also included a larger number of severe anomalies. Thus, the incidence of cardiac defects in the first trimester of pregnancy must be higher than the commonly quoted figure of 6 to 8 per 1,000 live births. The frequency of malformations preterm is higher than at birth.

A feature to be highly commended in this paper is the authors' great diagnostic accuracy in using the echocardiogram to study the fetal heart. Remarkably, they reported that in the 67 fetuses that died, "in all the malformation was confirmed at necropsy."—M.A. Engle, M.D.

Congenital Heart Malformations in the First Year of Life: A Necropsy Study
Anita S. Hegerty, Robert H. Anderson, and Siew Yen Ho (Cardiothoracic Inst., London, England)
Br. Heart J. 54:583–592, December 1985   2–7

The most common cardiac condition of childhood is congenital heart disease. It may affect as many as 2% of live births, and many of these infants die within the first few weeks of life. More die, with or without surgical intervention, before the end of their first year. A systematic sequential segmented approach was used to analyze findings in a large series of necropsy patients aged 1 year or younger collected during a 10-year period.

The hearts from 291 infants with congenital heart disease were examined systematically to assess which lesions were present and which of several was the primary defect. There was an abnormal connection between cardiac segments in one third of the infants. However, patent ductus arteriosus, usually a common defect, was not a prominent finding at necropsy, whereas the common arterial trunk, usually a rare defect was found in 10% of the hearts. The clinical and necropsy incidence of complete transposition (7.3% in the first month, 10% in the group aged 1–12 months) was in agreement with findings from other studies. Notably, the incidence of certain lesions present at necropsy (e.g., Fallot's tetralogy) has changed in the past 10 years, perhaps because of advances in treatment. A decline in the frequency with which a lesion is detected at necropsy may also relate to differences in classification. The presence of additional lesions influences the prognosis and subcategorization within the major defect grouping and gives some insight into the cause of death in many instances.

▶ It has long been recognized that the greatest risk of dying for one born with a congenital malformation is before the first birthday. This present series, based on necropsies performed at one cardiac center between 1974 and 1984, affirms that this continues to be true, despite the emphasis since 1970 on early diagnosis and treatment of the newborn with congenital heart disease.

Of the 291 specimens in this study, death occurred in the first month in approximately one third, between the first month and first birthday in one third, and in the remaining years of childhood in one third.

This study identified 13 primary lesions, and though that anomaly might not have been the principal cause of death, in each instance it contributed to the premature death. In the first month of life, the most common anomalies in this necropsy series were common arterial trunk and mitral and/or aortic atresia (9.9% for both) and univentricular atrioventricular connection and arch hypoplasia, including coarctation (9.3% for both). Tetralogy of Fallot accounted for no cases in the first month but 4.3% after 1 month. After the first month the most common anomaly was atrioventricular septal defect (15%) and complete transposition (10%). The most commonly diagnosed anomaly clinically, namely, ventricular septal defect (VSD), was not common in either age group at necropsy (4.6% and 5%).

The authors compare their findings with those of the New England Regional Infant Cardiac Program of 1969–1974 with 2,381 infants studied (Fyler, D.C., et al.: *Pediatrics* 65:376–461, 1980) and the Bohemian study by Samanek and coworkers in Prague of 2,257 autopsies in 1952–1979 (Samanek, M., et al.: *Int. J. Cardiol.* 8:235–248, 1985). The incidence of the clinical diagnosis of VSD was 15.7% in the former study and 22.6% by autopsy diagnosis in the latter.

The authors commented that two other anomalies common in clinical practice were not found at necropsy: pulmonic stenosis and aortic stenosis. They considered it disturbing that three malformations with a low natural incidence (complete transposition, intraventricular antrioventricular connection, and arch malformations) are the most frequently referred complex malformations and are dominant in the necropsy material, despite surgical intervention.—M.A. Engle, M.D.

▶ ↓ We know so woefully little about the causes of congenital heart disease that we need all the clues we can get to propose some reasonable hypotheses to account for the approximately 95% of instances of congenital heart disease that are still unexplained as to causation.

The two following papers offer two postulates: one, genetic, affecting a large racial group, the Chinese, and the other, a common pathogenetic pathway for the simultaneous occurrence of two conditions in the rare DiGeorge syndrome.—M.A. Engle, M.D.

Frequency of Various Congenital Heart Diseases in Chinese Adults: Analysis of 926 Consecutive Patients Over 13 Years of Age
Wen-Pin Lien, Jin-Jer Chen, Jyh-Hong Chen, Jiunn-Lee Lin, Yen-Yaw Hsieh, Teh-Lu Wu, Shu-Hsun Chu, and Chi-Ren Hung (Natl. Taiwan Univ. Hosp., Taipei City)
Am. J. Cardiol. 57:840–844, April 1986   2–8

The incidence rates of congenital heart disease in various parts of the world are not consistent. In some areas, including various Asian countries, low incidence rates have been reported. These low figures could be the result of either incomplete data or ethnic differences, but the latter variable may be overestimated. A retrospective analysis was made of records from a Chinese population in Taiwan with diagnosed congenital heart disease.

The study group comprised 926 consecutive patients aged 14–68 years who, in a 24-year period, had been given a diagnosis of congenital heart disease and had undergone cardiac catheterization. Approximately 60% of the patients had undergone surgery after diagnosis. Children under the age of 14 years were excluded.

Ventricular septal defect (VSD) was seen in 24.4% of the patients, atrial septal defect in 21.6%, tetralogy of Fallot truncus arteriosus in 0.3%. Furthermore, the type of VSD was different in the Chinese when compared with series of Caucasians. A muscular outlet type of VSD was far more common in the Chinese (38%) than in the others (4% to 8%). Membranous VSD occurred in 70% to 83% of patients reported in the United States, but in 62% of the Chinese series.

Congenital aortic valvular stenosis and coarctation of the aorta are uncommon in Chinese adults in comparison with the incidence rates in Western countries, whereas aneurysm of the sinus of Valsalva was more commonly seen in the Chinese study population. Genetic factors, rather than environmental differences or dietary habits, may explain these differences.

▶ It is remarkable that common kinds of congenital heart disease are common the world over, in human beings and even in some studies in animals (Taussig, H.B.: *Am. J. Cardiol.* 50:544–549, 1982). This analysis of Chinese adults confirms that the five most frequent anomalies were the same as in most large series from Western countries. Notable exceptions, however, were two lesions that obstruct left ventricular outflow (coarctation of the aorta and aortic stenosis) that are common in the Western world but rare in Chinese. Another interesting difference is the much greater frequency of subpulmonic ventricular septal defect in the Chinese, an uncommon condition in Caucasians. Environmental factors are unlikely to have any influence on these three unusual circumstances, because the incidence of the other conditions was about the same in this Taiwanese study as in other reports from other countries. It is surely tempting to ascribe a genetic cause. It will be interesting to see Chinese studies on the offspring of these adults with congenital heart disease and to note the incidence and varieties of cardiac anomalies in the children.—M.A. Engle, M.D.

Cardiovascular Anomalies in DiGeorge Syndrome and Importance of Neural Crest as a Possible Pathogenetic Factor
Lodewyk H.S. Van Mierop and Lynn M. Kutsche (Univ. of Florida)
Am. J. Cardiol. 58:133–137, July 1, 1986   2–9

The DiGeorge syndrome is a rare immunodeficiency disorder with a distinct pattern of inheritance that is often associated with cardiovascular malformations. A review was made of the data concerning 161 patients with DiGeorge syndrome, 111 of whom were reported previously and 50 with newly diagnosed disease. Cardiac catheterization and angiocardiography were used to determine the occurrence and type of cardiovascular anomalies.

The major cardiovascular anomaly in 32 of the 50 new patients was interrupted aortic arch (IAA) type B or persistent truncus arteriosus (TA). Tetralogy of Fallot was seen in another ten patients, whereas four had a ventricular septal defect and three had transposition of the great arteries. The remaining patient in this group had a normal heart. In 28 patients associated anomalies were present, mainly of the head and face, but also involving major organ systems.

These data confirm previous reported findings of the strong predominance of IAA type B and TA as the major cardiovascular anomalies in patients with DiGeorge syndrome. These anomalies involved the aortic arch system and the arterial pole of the heart. Neural crest cells play a crucial role in the development of these structures as well as the thymus, a pharyngeal pouch derivative. An abnormality in the neural crest is postulated to account for these cardiac anomalies and thymic-dependent cellular immunodeficiency.

▶ In this rare syndrome, characterized by immunodeficiency and congenital heart disease affecting the aortic arch and arterial pole of the heart, the authors point out that an event that interfered with the neural crest could result in both of these features. They noted that the two malformations most often seen in DiGeorge syndrome are both rare: IAA and persistent TA. When they analyzed their total experience with IAA and TA, they found a strikingly high percentage of DiGeorge syndrome in association: 10 of 28 patients with IAA (68%) and 13 of 39 with TA (33%). A lesson to be learned from this by pediatric cardiologists is that, if we make either of these cardiac diagnoses in a newborn, we should look for the possibility of an associated DiGeorge syndrome.—M.A. Engle, M.D.

Pulmonary Vascular Bed

▶ ↓ Included in this section are abstracts of four articles that pertain to pulmonary vasculature. Two consider the situation of pulmonary atresia and ventricular septal defect with hypoplastic pulmonary arteries fed by collateral arteries. The third concerns the opposite extreme: pulmonary hypertension from pulmonary vascular obstruction in patients with complete atrioventricular canal. The fourth paper considers pulmonary hypertension and the venous bed in the relatively uncommon anomaly of total anomalous pulmonary venous return. All four articles have surgical significance for selection of patients and timing of surgery.—M.A. Engle, M.D.

▶ ↓ This study is relevant for the many children born with tetralogy of Fallot with the extreme variant of atresia rather than stenosis of the right ventricular outflow tract. The question is always raised: Will the intrapulmonary arteries grow and develop normally if the pulmonary blood flow is increased surgically?

What form of palliation should be undertaken? When open-heart repair is planned, will the pulmonary arterial tree be able to accept a full pulmonary blood flow?

These two papers, one from the Mayo Clinic and the other from London and Munich, address the problem.—M.A. Engle, M.D.

Pulmonary Blood Supply in Patients With Pulmonary Atresia and Ventricular Septal Defect

Pui-Kan Liao, William D. Edwards, Paul R. Julsrud, Francisco J. Puga, Gordon K. Danielson, and Robert H. Feldt (Mayo Clinic and Found.)
J. Am. Coll. Cardiol. 6:1343–1350, December 1985   2–10

Pulmonary valve atresia occurring concomitantly with ventricular septal defect and biventricular origin of the aorta is characterized anatomically by the absence of a patent direct connection between the right ventricle and any part of the pulmonary artery tree. In these patients the blood supply to the lungs is derived entirely from the systemic arterial circulation. In pulmonary atresia with ventricular septal defect, the pulmonary blood supply originates from the ductus arteriosus or major systemic to pulmonary collateral arteries, or from both. A third type of blood supply to the lungs comprises numerous small systemic collateral arteries that follow the bronchi or spread over the pleurae. The variety and frequency of natural sources of blood supply to the lungs were investigated in 31 autopsied patients with tetralogy of Fallot and pulmonary valve atresia.

Three types of natural arterial blood supply to the lungs were noted: the ductus arteriosus (12 patients), major collateral arteries (20), and diffuse small pleural arterial plexus coexisting with the ductus arteriosus or major collateral arteries (17). The ductus arteriosus and major collateral arteries did not coexist in the same lung in the latter group. There were confluent central pulmonary arteries in 22 of the 31 patients, including 7 of the 12 with ductus arteriosus, 14 of the 20 with major collateral arteries, and 1 with an aorticopulmonary window. The pulmonary trunk was demonstrated in 24 of the 31 patients. A lung or lungs that connected to a ductus had a complete, unifocal intrapulmonary arterial distribution. The major collateral blood supply was often multifocal and associated with arborization abnormalities. The size of the central pulmonary arteries was not related to the type of arterial blood source, but appeared to be related to the amount of blood flow actually reaching the vessels.

There is a complex arterial system that supplies the lungs in these patients. The size, sources, and relationships among the ductus, the pulmonary artery confluence, the large and small collateral vessels, and the intrapulmonary system are far more varied than has been reported previously. Careful and thorough premortem studies are recommended if surgical intervention is contemplated.

▶ This detailed pathologic study of the central and peripheral pulmonary arteries and ductus arteriosus, as well as the collateral system, led to the same findings and conclusion as the one from London and Munich (Abstract 2–11). Although the central pulmonary arteries were often about as large as would be expected for the size of the patient, the small peripheral arteries were often hypoplastic. They too concluded that "because pulmonary blood flow is the key factor for pulmonary artery growth," early surgical intervention to ensure adequate blood supply to the central, as well as peripheral pulmonary arteries, is often necessary."—M.A. Engle, M.D.

Hypoplasia of the Intrapulmonary Arteries in Children With Right Ventricular Outflow Tract Obstruction, Ventricular Septal Defect, and Major Aortopulmonary Collateral Arteries
Robert J. Johnson, Ursula Sauer, Konrad Bühlmeyer, and Sheila G. Haworth (Inst. of Child Health, London)
Pediatr. Cardiol. 6:137–143, 1985   2–11

In patients with right ventricular outflow tract obstruction (RVOTO), ventricular septal defect (VSD), and major aortopulmonary collateral arteries (MAPCAs), the intrapulmonary arteries often appear hypoplastic on angiographic examination. However, it is easy to underestimate the size of these arteries in this abnormality because it may be difficult to inject sufficient contrast medium into the collateral or hilar pulmonary arteries to produce good definiton of the segmental pulmonary arteries and their branches. Also, contrast medium may be washed out of the injected system by blood from a different uninjected source. Angiography has shown the hypoplastic appearance of the central and lobar pulmonary arteries even after systemic pulmonary anastomosis. However, recent studies suggest that, on occasion, the intrapulmonary vessels may have greater blood flow and therefore develop more normally than indicated previously. The intrapulmonary arterial development was investigated in children with RVOTO., VSD, and MAPCAs and the angiographic appearance of pulmonary vessels in life related to their appearance in postmortem arteriograms.

The study population consisted of four children who died with pulmonary atresia and VSD or severe tetralogy of Fallot with major aortopulmonary collateral arteries; nearly all bronchopulmonary segments had more than one source of blood supply. The intrapulmonary arteries were injected with a barium sulfate-gelatin mixture via the collaterals or hilar pulmonary arteries. Radiographs were obtained and compared with the angiograms. Each specimen was dissected to demonstrate the connections between pulmonary arteries and collaterals. At least ten blocks of tissue were taken for histologic examination and quantitative morphological analysis.

Despite regional variations in the source of blood supply, there was remarkable uniformity of arterial size and number within the respiratory unit in each instance. In addition, all four children had a normal number of arterial pathways, but both preacinar and intra-acinar arteries were

much smaller than normal. Early operative intervention should be undertaken in these patients to ensure the growth of precinar, and particularly
intra-acinar, arteries.

▶ The authors consider that the large, elastic, thin-walled arteries are adapt-
able and should respond by enlarging when the blood flow is increased. It is
more difficult to predict the response of more peripheral intra-acinar arteries,
which have a higher ratio of wall thickness to lumen and are less likely to grow
with more flow. The logical inference is that it would be advantageous to the
child to increase the pulmonary blood flow surgically "as soon as possible after
birth."—M.A. Engle, M.D.

**Pulmonary Vascular Bed in Children With Complete Atrioventricular Sep-
tal Defect: Relation Between Structural and Hemodynamic Abnormalities**
Sheila G. Haworth (Inst. of Child Health, London)
Am. J. Cardiol. 57:833–839, April 1, 1986   2–12

Among children with complete atrioventricular (AV) septal defect, it is
difficult to select those with potentially reversible pulmonary vascular disease for intracardiac repair. In the presence of AV septal defect, some
investigators have found a poor correlation between structural and hemodynamic findings. By applying morphometric techniques, Rabinovitch et
al. improved the correlation between structure and function in patients
with various types of cardiac abnormalities, including 12 with complete
AV septal defect. Recently, however, studies have demonstrated structural
differences in the way in which pulmonary vascular disease develops in
different types of cardiac anomalies. Therefore, pulmonary vascular structure was examined in lung tissue obtained from patients with complete
AV septal defect without significant AV valve regurgitation. These structural abnormalities were then related to age, hemodynamic findings, and
outcome of intracardiac repair.

Lung tissue obtained from open biopsy (27 patients, 71%) or at autopsy
(29%) and the clinical and hemodynamic findings in 38 patients aged 2
weeks to 9 years with complete AV septal defect were analyzed. All 38
children had severe pulmonary hypertension without important left AV
valve regurgitation. Both Heath-Edwards and morphometric criteria were
used. In children older than 5 months, pulmonary artery (PA) systolic,
diastolic, and mean pressure and resistance increased with age, whereas
intra-acinar mean PA arterial medial thickness was inversely related to
age, PA pressure, and resistance. Reduction in intra-acinar PA muscularity
was associated with an increase in severity of obstructive intimal damage
in preacinar PA with age. A PA resistance of less than 6 units per sq mm
was associated with age younger than 3 years and usually younger than
2 years, PA medial thickness of more than 19%, and muscle extension
with or without intimal proliferation. A higher resistance occurred in patients of all ages, but in those younger than 3 years, structural abnormalities

frequently resembled those in patients with lower resistance, whereas older children had a normal or slightly increased PA medial thickness of 14% or less (normal, 7.4%), or classic grade III or IV disease. The four perioperative deaths attributed to pulmonary vascular disease occurred in children who were similar to survivors in age and hemodynamic status, but they had more severe pulmonary vascular abnormalities, i.e., either less muscularity with more severe intimal fibrosis or a much greater increase in muscularity. This finding emphasizes that even potentially reversible abnormalities can prejudice intracardiac repair.

A marked increase in pulmonary vascular smooth muscle probably increases the likelihood of pulmonary hypertensive crises. Any reduction in cross-sectional area of the pulmonary vascular bed by medial hypertrophy, with or without intimal proliferation, increases the right ventricular afterload.

▶ Haworth pooled hemodynamic data and pathologic material (lung biopsy or postmortem examination) from the 14 European centers of Pediatric Cardiology. All patients had severe pulmonary hypertension. The seven children under 2.5 months were extremely ill. Two died before surgery and five after operation. Over the age of 5 months, 16 underwent repair with a 31% mortality and one late death; 3 died unoperated. The known association of Down's syndrome and atrioventricular septal defect was affirmed in this series: Half had this combination.

Not unexpectedly, the severity of pulmonary vascular disease increased with increase in measured pulmonary resistance and also with age. In 75% of children aged 1 year or less, the PAs showed only severe medial hypertrophy; in 77% of those aged 1.1–2.9 years, PAs showed intimal proliferation, whereas in 79% of those older than 3 years the PAs showed either grade III or grade IV pulmonary vascular disease, or else implied severe luminal obstruction when there were no preacinar arteries present in the lung biopsy specimen to show that change.

That observation makes the important point that, when obtaining a lung biopsy, the surgeon should take the specimen sufficiently deep to include small preacinar and terminal bronchial arteries. Intimal proliferation and fibrosis develop initially in small preacinar and terminal bronchiolar arteries. All five patients whose preoperative lung biopsy specimens showed intimal fibrosis died in the hospital soon after repair.

Dr. Haworth concluded that the striking finding in this study of pooled patients with AV septal defect and pulmonary hypertension was the significant inverse relationship between PA muscularity and PA pressure, resistance, and age. Intimal damage increased with age, and patients with the least amount of muscle frequently had the most severe intimal obstruction.—M.A. Engle, M.D.

Restrictive Interatrial Communication in Total Anomalous Pulmonary Venous Connection

Kent E. Ward, Charles E. Mullins, James C. Huhta, Michael R. Nihill, Dan G.

McNamara, and Denton A. Cooley (Baylor Univ., Texas Children's Hosp., and Texas Heart Inst., Houston)
Am. J. Cardiol. 57:1131–1136, May 1, 1986   2–13

The morbidity and mortality associated with early total correction of cardiac defects have decreased because of advances in surgical technique and perioperative care of the neonate with congenital heart disease, including total anomalous pulmonary venous connection (TAPVC) without obstruction. However, early palliation may sometimes be necessary or may enhance the success of a subsequent surgical repair. Short-term palliation and improved hemodynamics were achieved with Rashkind balloon atrial septostomy in some patients with TAPVC without obstruction. The incidence and hemodynamic consequences of a restrictive interatrial communication and the effects of atrial septostomy in the management of patients with TAPVC were examined.

The study population consisted of 21 patients with TAPVC without extra-cardiac obstruction seen at ages 1 day to 10 months. Seventeen (81%) had moderate to severe congestive heart failure, and in the first week after birth, four patients had minimal symptoms of congestive heart failure. Two-dimensional echocardiography or angiography demonstrated a small patent foramen ovale (3 mm or less in diameter) in 19 children (90%). When balloon or blade and balloon atrial septostomy was performed in these 19 patients, significant decreases occurred in the mean right to left atrial pressure gradient (from 2.8 mm Hg to 0.25 mm Hg), systolic pulmonary to femoral artery pressure ratio (from 0.80 to 0.60), and systemic arterial oxygen saturation (from 84% to 79%). One child had nonfatal complications. Surgery was performed in 19 patients from 2 weeks to 29 months after catheterization, with one operative death. Because of persistent heart failure, 4 patients required early total correction; 15 had elective surgical repair. One of two unoperated-on patients died of pneumonia at age 2.5 years.

A restrictive interatrial communication develops after the first month of extrauterine life in most infants with TAPVC. Atrial septostomy leads to improved hemodynamic conditions and clinical palliation. This procedure permits selected patients to undergo elective operative repair in the second year of life and results in a low mortality rate.

▶ Total anomalous pulmonary venous connection is a rare and usually a serious anomaly causing high mortality early in infancy. Surgical methods have reduced the high death rate, but improvement is still sought. The situation that makes the neonate especially at risk is pulmonary hypertension caused by obstruction in the extracardiac course of the anomalous drainage or at the intracardiac level because of an atrial septal defect that is too small. When all the pulmonary venous return eventually enters the right atrium to mix with the systemic venous return, the blood that enters the left atrium and ventricle and the ascending aorta gets there through a patent foramen ovale or native atrial septal defect. If that communication is inadequate, pulmonary venous, as well as arterial, hypertension ensues. These authors found that a balloon-atrial or blade atrial septostomy in 19 infants resulted in satisfactory palliation and converted the situation from one requiring emergency cardiac surgery to one suitable for elective repair at less risk as a toddler.—M.A. Engle, M.D.

Surgical Results

▶ ↓ It is important to know not only what the perioperative morbidity and mortality rates are when patients with congenital heart disease undergo palliative or reparative surgery, but also to have an appreciation of the long-term outcome. Studies such as those presented below enhance our ability to care for postoperative patients with the same attention they received prior to surgery. Most of them benefit from long-term, lifelong follow-up by informed physicians.—M.A. Engle, M.D.

Long-term Follow-up of Valvotomy Before 1986 for Congenital Aortic Stenosis
Kai-Sheng Hsieh, John F. Keane, Alexander S. Nadas, William F. Bernhard, and Aldo R. Castaneda (Children's Hosp., Boston, and Harvard Univ.)
Am. J. Cardiol. 58:338–341, August 1986   2–14

The courses of 59 children who underwent valvotomy for aortic stenosis before 1968 were reviewed. The patients, all older than age 1 year at operation, were followed for a mean of nearly 18 years. The 47 males and 12 females had a median age of 11 years at operation. Indications for operation included symptoms, left ventricular hypertrophy with a strain pattern, and a peak systolic pressure gradient of more than 50 mm Hg. All operations were performed with cardiopulmonary bypass and moderate hypothermia. Fused commissures were incised under direct vision. There were 46 bicuspid and 13 tricuspid valves in the series.

Forty-six patients were alive at review. Actuarial probabilities of survival were 94% at 5 years and 77% at 22 years. Seven of the 13 deaths occurred suddenly, including 4 in patients found 1 to 7 years earlier to have significant obstruction or regurgitation. The two patients with a progressive strain pattern declined operation. Twenty-one patients were reoperated on and three of them died. The likelihood of reoperation rose from 2% at 5 years to 44% at 22 years. Three patients had four episodes of bacterial endocarditis, for a rate of nearly four episodes per 1,000 patient-years. Only 39% of patients were actuarially free from serious events including death, reoperation, and endocarditis at 22 years. Eleven of 29 surviving patients who were not reoperated on were thought to have hemodynamically significant lesions. These findings show the palliative nature of aortic valvotomy and the need for close follow-up of patients undergoing this operation.

▶ The significance of this article is that it documents surgical experience in a cohort of patients operated on before 1968 and followed to the present. It emphasizes that open repair of congenital valvular aortic stenosis is not "total correction" or "cure," but is palliation. The palliation is worthwhile, but by 22 years after the surgery, nearly half needed to be operated on again and 23% were no longer alive. The message is clear: These patients need lifelong cardiologic follow-up and sensitive care if the complications of endocarditis, cardiac deterioration, and sudden death are to be forestalled.—M.A. Engle, M.D.

Experience With Polytetrafluoroethylene Grafts in Children With Cyanotic Congenital Heart Disease

J.C. Opie, L. Traverse, R.I. Hayden, C.Y. Ho, J.A.G. Culham, and P.G. Ashmore (British Columbia Children's Hosp., Vancouver)
Ann. Thorac. Surg. 41:164–168, February 1986   2–15

Expanded polytetrafluoroethylene (PTFE), or Gore-Tex, has been used for shunts in patients with cyanotic congenital heart defects with documented high patency rates and good palliation and postoperative angiographic and hemodynamic findings. The survival and event-free rates of 47 PTFE shunts placed in 42 children during a 2-year period were examined. The mean age at shunt creation was 7.5 months. Modified Blalock-Taussig shunts were used in most instances.

The mean duration of the shunt was 12 months. Five of the 47 grafts had to be replaced, giving an overall 2-year patency rate of 89%. Smaller grafts had a better survival rate. A patent shunt improved the partial pressure of oxygen. The hemoglobin concentration decreased with operation, but increased steadily during follow-up. In eight patients, increased cyanosis and "spells" developed after operation. Two of these underwent a successful second shunt procedure within 6 weeks and two within 15 months. In four patients, progressive cyanosis occurred between 9 and 15 months; three of these died of progressive cyanosis. Congestive heart failure developed in four patients, all of whom had 5-mm grafts. Five patients contracted bronchopneumonia within 6 months of shunting. One patient had early thrombosis, which was finally cleared with intra-arterial streptokinase infusion. Pulmonary artery distortion was observed in three patients. There were no complications associated with 6-mm shunts; the complication rate with the 5-mm shunts was 37%, and was slightly higher (37.5%) with 4-mm shunts. The actuarial patient survival at 2 years was 86%.

Clearly, PTFE shunts are associated with thrombosis, infection, heart failure, repeat shunt operations, shunt reductions, and endarteritis. This suggests that total correction or revision should be performed when the pulmonary vessels have grown sufficiently, or when the patient shows signs of outgrowing the PTFE shunt. Current practice is simply to ligate the graft, which remains in situ. These grafts appear to be an effective form of palliation in patients with cyanotic heart disease and reduced pulmonary flow, but patients must be carefully followed with a strict watch for complications. Inadequate shunts are associated with diminutive pulmonary arteries, and the reverse is also true. The modified Blalock-Taussig anastomosis was the most efficacious prosthetic shunt and was associated with the lowest rate of complications.

▶ One often observes fads in medical and surgical management. This paper reports results after 2 years of palliation of cyanotic congenital heart disease, not by the Blalock-Taussig shunt but by a modification of it that uses a Gore-Tex graft rather than turndown of a divided subclavian artery. The short-term results over 2 years emphasize what had been learned earlier before use of this graft, especially that grafts of 5 mm or larger in young children frequently cause too great an increase in pulmonary blood flow and result in cardiac failure, and that small shunts tend to thrombose. There is a trade-off between the standard and the modified Blalock-Taussig shunt. The former sacrifices an artery to an arm that then relies on collateral circulation for growth and good function, but uses a vessel that is just about the right size for each patient and has the possibility for growth. The Gore-Tex shunt preserves the subclavian artery, but it cannot grow and has only short-term benefits of palliation. When possible, I prefer the classic Blalock-Taussig anastomosis for palliation. If open repair becomes possible, it can simply be ligated.—M.A. Engle, M.D.

Exercise Tolerance and Cardiorespiratory Response to Exercise After the Fontan Operation for Tricuspid Atresia or Functional Single Ventricle
David J. Driscoll, Gordon K. Danielson, Francisco J. Puga, Hartzell V. Schaff, Charles T. Heise, and Bruce A. Staats (Mayo Clinic and Found.)
J. Am. Coll. Cardiol. 7:1087–1094, May 1986   2–16

Surgical repair of tricuspid atresia (Fontan procedure) is an alternative to palliative procedures in patients with a functional single ventricle. Although experience with this operation is too brief to determine its effect on longevity, its impact on exercise tolerance can be evaluated. Investigators who have made this measurement report that exercise tolerance remains subnormal postoperatively. No studies have yet compared preoperative and postoperative exercise tolerance and cardiorespiratory response to exercise, however. Therefore, an attempt was made to determine whether the Fontan procedure improves exercise tolerance and the cardiorespiratory response to exercise by comparing measurements obtained after operation with those obtained before operation.

The study population consisted of 81 patients with tricuspid atresia or a single functional ventricle who underwent maximal exercise study at the Mayo Clinic before the Fontan operation and 29 patients studied after the operation; 7 patients were studied both before and after the operation. The postoperative values for total work performed, duration of exercise, and maximal oxygen uptake were significantly increased. Irrespective of the operative status, the maximal heart rate during exercise was reduced. Cardiac output and the stroke volume response to exercise were subnormal postoperatively. The systemic arterial blood oxygen saturation was reduced markedly preoperatively both at rest and during exercise; postoperatively, it was significantly greater than the preoperative value but it remained slightly abnormal. After operation, the ventilatory response to exercise (respiratory rate, minute ventilation, and ventilatory equivalent for oxygen) decreased toward normal. All indices of exercise tolerance and the cardiorespiratory response to exercise are improved after the Fontan operation although not to normal values.

▶ In 1971 Fontan and Baudet described a more physiologic form of palliation for patients with tricuspid atresia or single ventricle with diminished pulmonary blood flow than had been possible earlier through creation of systemic-to-pulmonary arterial shunts. Right atrial-to-pulmonary arterial connection or right atrial to diminutive right ventricular connection provided a physiologic route for oxygenation of blood while eliminating sites of right-left shunting and avoiding the volume loading of the single ventricle that an artificial ductus imposes. Over the years, criteria for operability have been devised and the mortality rate has declined. When free of postoperative complications (e.g., edema or ascites), patients look well and feel better.

The Mayo Clinic has a large and excellent experience with the Fontan operation. This paper attempts to quantify subjective improvement by studying exercise tolerance and cardiorespiratory response in a group of 81 preoperative patients, another group of 29 postoperative patients, and in 7 who were studied both before and after the operation. Postoperative patients performed better in all respects than did preoperative patients, but they did not do as well as normal controls.

Significantly, they found a negative correlation between age at exercise and exercise tolerance both preoperatively and postoperatively, and between exercise tolerance and age at operation. Patients who had a direct right atrial-to-pulmonary arterial connection had greater exercise tolerance than did those with a right atrial to right ventricular connection. Also ST changes occurred in 21 (27%) of 77 preoperative and in 11 (38%) of 29 postoperative patients. Arrhythmias occurred at rest in 14% and during or after exercise in 28% of the preoperative patients, whereas after the Fontan repair those figures were 21% and 38%, respectively. The authors suggest that postoperative improvement might be better if patients were operated on prior to adolescence.—M.A. Engle, M.D.

Exercise-Induced Hypertension After Repair of Coarctation of the Aorta: Arm Versus Leg Exercise
Howard Markel, Albert P. Rocchini, Robert H. Beekman, Jean Martin, John Palmisano, Catherine Moorehead, and Amnon Rosenthal (C.S. Mott Children's Hosp., Ann Arbor, and Univ. of Michigan)
J. Am. Coll. Cardiol. 8:165–171, July 1986   2–17

Upper limb hypertension on exercise has been documented in children who have undergone repair of coarctation of the aorta. The hypertension is sometimes related to residual or recurrent coarctation, but in other instances blood flow across the repair site may be a major factor in exercise-induced hypertension. Changes in upper limb pressure and the coarctation gradient were compared when arm ergometry and treadmill exercise were performed at equivalent heart rates and peak oxygen consumptions in 28 children with repaired coarctation. The 21 boys and 7 girls had a mean age of 14 years and were studied a mean of 4 years after repair. Seven patients had a resting gradient of less than 15 mm Hg and a treadmill gradient of less than 20 mm Hg; 9 had a higher treadmill gradient, and 12 had a resting gradient of 15 mm Hg or higher.

When patients were exercised to exhaustion, treadmill exercise produced a greater increase in arm systolic pressure and the arm-leg gradient than did arm exercise. Patients with higher gradients had more marked rises in both arm systolic pressure and arm-leg gradient than did controls when treadmill exercise was performed. On arm exercise, patients with the highest gradients had more marked increases in both variables than did controls. These patients had a relatively small ratio of the repair site to the abdominal descending aorta than did patients with a resting gradient of less than 15 mm Hg.

Upper limb hypertension on treadmill exercise in patients with repaired coarctation appears to result from a marked rise in descending aortic blood flow across a mildly to moderately narrowed coarctation repair site. Cardiac catheterization is probably unnecessary in children with a minimal resting arm-leg gradient in whom systolic upper limb hypertension develops on treadmill exercise.

▶ Those of us who study patients long term after surgical repair of coarctation of the aorta have come to expect a hypertensive response to exercise in those healthy, asymptomatic, well-built individuals. This study distinguishes some of the possible reasons for this response and concludes that treadmill exercise increases blood flow to the legs at an increasing pulse rate and exaggerates the pressure difference across the area of coarctation repair. I believe that, in addition, there is probably an abnormality of the aorta and arteries distal to the repair site that renders them less distensible when flow increases.—M.A. Engle, M.D.

Results of Surgical Treatment of Coarctation of the Aorta in the Critically Ill Neonate: Including the Influence of Pulmonary Artery Banding
Scott Goldman, Jacinto Hernandez, and George Pappas (Children's Hosp., Denver)
J. Thorac. Cardiovasc. Surg. 91:732–737, May 1986   2–18

Coarctation of the aorta in neonates is often associated with ventricular septal defect (VSD) or complex cardiac lesions with VSD. The mortality rate is high, but it is improving. The effect of pulmonary banding during operation for coarctation of the aorta was examined in 64 neonates with isolated and complicated VSD. The mean age was 9 days. Thirty-one infants had isolated coarctation or coarctation with minor defects, 18 had coarctation and hemodynamically significant VSD, and 15 had coarctation with VSD and complex cardiac lesions. All of the last were critically ill.

There were no deaths in the operating room, but four patients died within 30 days and seven died in the late postoperative period. Patients with isolated coarctation had a 94% overall survival rate. Eleven of the 18 patients with coarctation plus VSD did not have pulmonary banding. There were no early deaths and only one late death in this group. Among the seven patients who had banding, there was one early death and one late death. On follow-up of the 18 patients in this group, 33% had spontaneous closure of the defect or reduction in size to the extent that the VSD was no longer hemodynamically significant. Among the 15 patients with coarctation, VSD, and complex cardiac lesions, banding was performed in 11. There were no early and two late deaths. Of the four patients who did not have banding, three died in the early postoperative period as a result of cardiac failure. The other died at 3 months of severe cardiac failure. Overall, 12% of the survivors required reoperation for recurrent coarctation within 4 months to 5 years.

Isolated coarctation has a reported mortality of 13% to 21%. When VSD or complex cardiac lesions are also present, mortality rises to 26% to 58%. Use of subclavian flap angioplasty has improved survival and lowered recurrence rates. In this study, 11% of patients so treated required reoperation. Prosthetic patch angioplasty was used infrequently. Although the operation is simple, reports of thrombosis and aneurysm make it a less attractive alternative. However, when resection with end-to-end anastomosis is not feasible, patch angioplasty may be the only choice available for revision of the coarctation. Whether or not to band the pulmonary artery is a question when coarctation is found in association with a large VSD. In this series the large VSD became unmanageable and necessitated repair or banding in two patients during the first 3 months of life. The lack of problems in early life may have resulted from increased pulmonary vascular resistance seen at the high altitude of Denver, in essence, physiologic banding.

Because of the potential adverse effects of banding, the significant rate of spontaneous VSD closure, and the good results obtained in patients with coarctation and a large VSD who had coarctation repair alone, coarctation repair without banding is advocated. However, in patients with coarctation, VSD, and complex defects, banding after completion of coarctation repair decreased mortality.

▶ This study addresses one of the most common problems encountered in the first month of life by pediatric cardiologists and surgeons dealing with critically ill neonates in a Pediatric Cardiac Service. Our approach is similar to that used by these authors: Evaluate the relative severity of the coarctation and the nearby ductus that is usually patent, and the size of the VSD and whether it is simple and perimembranous or muscular or multiple, and determine whether there are other aspects of the malformation, e.g., an abnormal mitral valve.

I believe that the obstruction together with the ductus should be eliminated as soon as medical treatment with digitalis and Lasix has improved the infant's condition. I prefer resection and end-to-end anastomosis over subclavian flap enlargement of the area of coarctation. I prefer to refrain from banding the pulmonary artery for all the reasons cited, but to be prepared to band should the infant fail to improve promptly after relief of the coarctation.—M.A. Engle, M.D.

Subaortic Stenosis, the Univentricular Heart, and Banding of the Pulmonary Artery: An Analysis of the Courses of 43 Patients With Univentricular Heart Palliated by Pulmonary Artery Banding
Robert M. Freedom, Lee N. Benson, Jeffrey F. Smallhorn, William G. Williams, George A. Trusler, and Richard D. Rowe (Univ. of Toronto and Hosp. for Sick Children, Toronto)
Circulation 73:758–764, April 1986   2–19

It is well known that subaortic stenosis may be a major complication after various surgical procedures done to improve blood flow patterns in patients with single-ventricle (univentricular) hearts. It was suggested previously that subaortic stenosis may be caused or accelerated by previous banding of the main pulmonary trunk. A study was conducted to define further the relationship between banding the pulmonary artery in such patients and the subsequent development of subaortic stenosis.

The study group included 29 boys and 14 girls who underwent palliative surgery consiting of pulmonary artery banding. Excluded were patients who had evidence of subaortic stenosis before surgery, those who died within 1 week of the banding procedure, and those who were lost to follow-up.

Subaortic stenosis developed in 31 (72.1%) patients after pulmonary artery banding. The mean age at banding was 0.21 years, and subaortic stenosis was diagnosed at a mean age of 2.52 years. Of the 32 patients who had a main chamber of the left ventricular type that supported the pulmonary artery and a rudimentary right ventricle that supported the transposed aorta, 27 (84.4%) had subaortic stenosis. In patients with univentricular hearts, possibility of subaortic stenosis after pulmonary artery banding is high. Alternative procedures should be investigated.

▶ As simple problems are solved, more complex ones emerge for thoughtful individuals to tackle. The univentricular heart is a problem. These individuals can live a near-normal childhood and adolescence if they have just the right amount of restricted pulmonary blood flow. The more fortunate of these are born with pulmonic stenosis that, if too severe, could be helped by a Blalock-Taussig shunt. Those with no pulmonary stenosis soon experience flooded lungs and cardiac failure, which usually responds to medical measures. What to do next is the problem. The risk of septation operations for a single ventricle is high, and only a few have the right anatomy for this. The risk of a Fontan procedure is still high, even in children over the age of 5 years. It would surely be higher in those under age 2 years.

The best palliation, I believe, is pulmonary artery banding that is done not at a mean age of 0.2 months but around 2 or 3 years, before pulmonary vascular obstructive disease develops. I think that the incidence of development of subaortic stenosis then is not as high as in this series. Furthermore, I know that the band cannot grow and that it does not demand a second palliative operation to increase pulmonary blood flow distal to the band. This second operation can be postponed much longer if the band is placed in a larger child in comparison to a small infant.—M.A. Engle, M.D.

Electrophysiologic Cardiac Function Before and After Surgery in Children With Atrioventricular Canal
Anne Fournier, Ming-Lon Young, Otto L. Garcia, Dolores F. Tamer, and Grace S. Wolff (Univ. of Miami)
Am. J. Cardiol. 57:1137–1141, May 1, 1986   2–20

In the past, surgical repair of atrioventricular (AV) canal defects was associated with a unique vulnerability of the conduction system, which led to the development of surgical techniques aimed at reducing the incidence of subsequent complete heart block. Because few data are available on the electrophysiologic status of the conduction system in this defect, electrophysiologic studies were performed in 32 infants and children with AV canal defects before and after corrective surgery. Ages ranged from 6 months to 16 years.

The patients were divided into two study groups: Group I consisted of 18 preoperative patients, 7 with complete AV canal and 11 with incomplete AV canal; group II had 16 postoperative patients, 11 with complete AV canal and 5 with ostium primum atrial septal defect. Two patients were assessed both preoperatively and postoperatively. All underwent cardiac catheterization and electrophysiologic studies.

First-degree AV block was present in 11 preoperative patients and 12 postoperative patients. Right bundle branch block was confirmed in 6 preoperative patients and in 19 postoperative patients. Only patients in the postoperative group experienced rhythm abnormalities. Atrial and ventricular functions were normal in all preoperative and postoperative patients.

Preoperative patients have few electrophysiologic abnormalities. However, in this study, abnormalities of the conduction system were noted in 38% of all postoperative patients, involving the sinus and AV nodes in 19% and 25%, respectively. If complete heart block can be avoided by modifying surgical techniques, the conduction system will retain good function in almost all postoperative patients.

▶ One of the most challenging anomalies that a surgeon is called upon to repair is the AV septal defect. If the only abnormality is an ostium primum type of atrial septal defect, as it was in eight children in this study, the surgery is less difficult than when there is a complete canal with a single AV valve. These electrophysiologic studies confirm clinical experience, in that symptomatic arrhythmias are rare and that first-degree heart block, though often present, produces little trouble. Postoperatively, however, the intra-atrial surgery, and sometimes intraventricular as well, leaves some sequelae. The good news is that perhaps the most serious of those surgical injuries to the conduction system, complete heart block, is now uncommon (none in these patients) in contrast to the pioneering days 20 years ago when it occurred in 16% of the children.—M.A. Engle, M.D.

Cardiac Arrhythmias in Patients With Surgical Repair of Ebstein's Anomaly

Jae K. Oh, David R. Holmes, Jr., David L. Hayes, Co-Burn J. Porter, and Gordon K. Danielson (Mayo Clinic and Found.)
J. Am. Coll. Cardiol. 6:1351–1357, December 1985   2–21

Ebstein's anomaly is associated with supraventricular and ventricular arrhythmias that may result in high rates of morbidity and mortality, with sudden death reported in up to 20% of these patients. Although surgical techniques aimed at correcting or improving the underlying pathologic characteristics are available, the effect of surgery on subsequent arrhythmia incidence rates has not yet been assessed. A review was made of experience with surgical repair of Ebstein's anomaly, and postoperative arrhythmia rates were assessed.

The study group comprised 52 consecutive patients (25 male and 27 female patients aged 11 months to 64 years) who underwent surgery for Ebstein's anomaly after the diagnosis had been confirmed with cardiac catheterization, echocardiography, or both. There were 34 patients with one or more documented arrhythmias before surgery, including 18 with paroxysmal supraventricular tachycardia, 10 with paroxysmal atrial fibrillation or flutter, 13 with ventricular arrhythmia, and 3 with high-grade atrioventricular block. In seven patients a history consistent with tachyarrhythmia was established, but these patients did not have documented arrhythmias. The remaining 11 patients were asymptomatic at the time of surgery.

During or immediately after surgery, 14 patients experienced atrial tachyarrhythmias and 8 had ventricular tachycardia or ventricular fibrillation. Seven deaths occurred during follow-up for up to 7 months after surgery. Patients without preoperative tachyarrhythmias rarely experienced this complication after surgery; they were younger than the rest of the study population. Of those who had documented supraventricular tachyarrhythmias before surgery, fewer than one third continued to have such symptoms afterward. Patients with perioperative ventricular tachycardia or fibrillation appear to be at increased risk of sudden death.

▶ More than any other congenital cardiac malformation, Ebstein's anomaly predisposes to atrial arrhythmias, perhaps because of the enlarged right atrium and the atrialized right ventricle, but also because of the association in some patients with Wolff-Parkinson-White syndrome. Yet, many patients lead quietly active lives for many years, free of arrhythmias. In a series referred for surgery, the number of symptomatic patients and the number with arrhythmias are, of course, high. The results of open repair in Ebstein's anomaly in 52 patients at the Mayo Clinic show that the repair does not necessarily free the patient from atrial or ventricular arrhythmias or from the risk of sudden death.— M.A. Engle, M.D.

Diagnosis and Natural History of Ebstein's Anomaly
Dorothy J. Radford, R.F. Graff, and G.H. Neilson (The Prince Charles Hosp. Brisbane, Queensland, Australia)
Br. Heart J. 54:517–522, November 1985   2–22

In Ebstein's anomaly, the basic anatomical abnormality consists of downward displacement of the septal and posterior leaflets of the tricuspid valve from the atrioventricular anulus into the body of the right ventricle, resulting in atrialization of a portion of the right ventricle. The anterior leaflet is also abnormal and is usually large and sail-like. In Ebstein's original report in 1866, the specimen also showed absence of the valve to the coronary sinus and a patent foramen ovale. The diagnosis and natural history of Ebstein's anomaly were reviewed in light of currently available diagnostic techniques.

Between 1962 and 1984, Ebstein's anomaly was diagnosed by cardiac catheterization or echocardiography in 35 patients. In 27 the anomaly was an isolated abnormality; the others had additional lesions, chiefly pulmonary stenosis (three patients) or atresia (two). Two had corrected transposition of the great arteries with coarctation. Six patients died, 4 of whom had other cardiac lesions; 13 are currently symptom-free. Twelve patients had cyanosis and heart murmur on the first day of life and eight of these had an associated thrill, an uncommon finding in neonates. When pulmonary vascular resistance fell, clinical improvement occurred; this was assisted by oxygen treatment. Another two children were seen in the first week of life and ten in the first decade, five with a murmur and three with supraventricular tachycardia. Eleven patients were adolescents or adults with a murmur, cardiomegaly, or cardiac symptoms, and three were first seen in the sixth decade. Of the 35 patients, 25 underwent cardiac catheterization. Significant arrhythmias occurred in 12 of these, 2 of whom required cardioversion. It was difficult to enter the pulmonary artery in 11 infants and children. At initial catheter study, the diagnosis was incorrect in four patients. Echocardiography was performed in 29 patients. Earlier M-mode measurements of time delay of tricuspid closure compared with mitral closure did not always lead to the correct diagnosis. However, cross-sectional studies gave good images of tricuspid leaflet displacement, its tethering, and the atrialized portion of the right ventricle. These studies facilitated the diagnosis in more patients in recent years. Echocardiography appears to be the procedure of choice in the diagnosis of Ebstein's anomaly.

▶ I have a long-standing, personal interest in Ebstein's anomaly of the tricuspid valve. When I was a fellow with Dr. Helen Taussig, I first became fascinated with this curious malformation when she asked me to read that chapter of her forthcoming book, Congenital Malformations of the Heart, and to help her correct the galley proof. Then I saw several of these patients in whom we suspected the diagnosis clinically and, unfortunately for them, confirmed it at postmortem examination when they did not survive the palliative surgery of the Blalock-Taussig anastomosis. My first paper with Dr. Taussig on analysis of the clinical syndrome was published in *Circulation* 1:1246–1260, 1950. The beautiful drawings of the specimens by Leon Schlossberg remain the best I have seen on this malformation.

The paper from Queensland confirms the truths that we have learned about this anomaly. Because the series includes infants and adults, it shows the spectrum from the newborn, at risk of dying until pulmonary vascular resistance falls postnatally to the asymptomatic adult. Three adults did not present until they were in their 50s. Six women had 12 children without deterioration in their condition. Eight pregnancies occurred before the cardiologic diagnosis was made. Thirteen patients are now symptom free and 12 have minor symptoms.

Well-known risk factors occurred in this series of 35 patients: obstruction to right ventricular outflow, arrhythmias, and cyanosis related to right-to-left shunt through the patent foramen ovale. Cardiac catheterization was a risk, as 12 of the 25 patients sustained important arrhythmias and 2 required cardioversion. Two-dimensional echocardiography is by far a safer and more informative way to confirm the diagnosis.—M.A. Engle, M.D.

Pulsed Doppler Echocardiographic Assessment of the Pulmonary Venous Pathway After the Mustard or Senning Procedure for Transposition of the Great Arteries
J.F. Smallhorn, R. Gow, R.M. Freedom, G.A. Trusler, P. Olley, M. Pacquet, J. Gibbons, and P. Vlad (Hosp. for Sick Children, Toronto, Montreal Children's Hosp., and Ottawa Children's Hosp., Canada)
Circulation 73:765–774, April 1986   2–23

The Mustard procedure and the Senning procedure are the operations most commonly used for interatrial rerouting of pulmonary and systemic venous blood in patients with simple transposition of the great arteries. However, systemic venous obstruction or pulmonary venous obstruction (PVO) may complicate both procedures. Cardiac catheterization and cross-sectional echocardiography have been used to identify this complication, but both techniques have disadvantages. Pulsed Doppler echocardiography was used to compare pressure and flow profiles in patients who had undergone the Mustard or Senning procedure with profiles in normal persons and in patients with PVO.

The study comprised three groups of children: group I consisted of 59 patients who had undergone the Mustard operation; group II, 12 who had undergone the Senning procedure; and group III, patients with midbaffle obstruction of the pulmonary venous atrium or isolated stenosis of the pulmonary vein, 2 of whom had had a Mustard repair and 6 of whom had undergone a Senning procedure. All patients underwent pulsed Dopp-

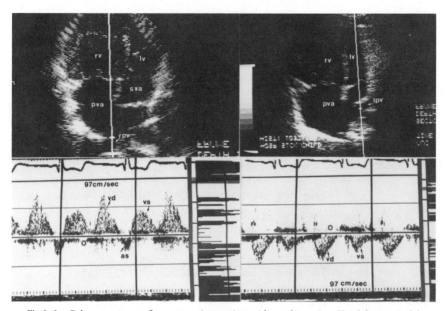

Fig 2–3.—Pulmonary venous flow pattern in a patient without obstruction. **Top left,** an apical four-chamber cut from a patient who underwent the Mustard procedure. The sample volume is placed where the right pulmonary veins enter the pulmonary venous atrium. **Bottom left,** the spectral trace from the same patient. Note the three phases of flow, one reversed peak during atrial systole followed by one forward during the x descent and a second peak during the y descent. **Top right,** an apical four-chamber view demonstrating the sample volume in a left pulmonary vein. **Bottom right,** the spectral trace demonstrating a biphasic flow pattern. The velocity of flow is lower than from the right pulmonary veins because of the increased angle between the Doppler sample volume and the direction of pulmonary venous flow. Abbreviations: *as,* atrial systole; *lpv,* left pulmonary vein; *lv,* left ventricle; *pva,* pulmonary venous atrium; *rv,* right ventricle; *sva,* systemic venous atrium; *rpv,* right pulmonary ventricle; *vd,* flow during y descent; *vs,* flow during the x descent. (Courtesy of Smallhorn J.F., et al: Circulation 73:765–774, April 1986. By permission of the American Heart Association, Inc.)

ler echocardiography, and flow patterns were compared with those obtained from normal persons.

The pulmonary venous flow pattern in patients without obstruction mirrored the left atrial pressure trace (Fig 2–3), whereas obstruction produced a specific high-velocity turbulent pattern (Fig 2–4). Pulsed Doppler echocardiography is a reliable, noninvasive diagnostic technique for monitoring pulmonary venous atrial pressure flow changes after a Mustard or Senning procedure and for detecting the presence of midbaffle obstruction and isolated stenosis of the pulmonary vein before and after either procedure.

▶ A venous switch operation by the Mustard or Senning technique for transposition of the great arteries carries a lower mortality rate at the present time than the arterial switch operation of Jatene. Obstruction to superior vena caval flow is often noted after the Mustard operation, but its effects can usually be compensated for by development of collateral circulation via the azygous system. Such a compensatory scheme does not exist in the case of pulmonary

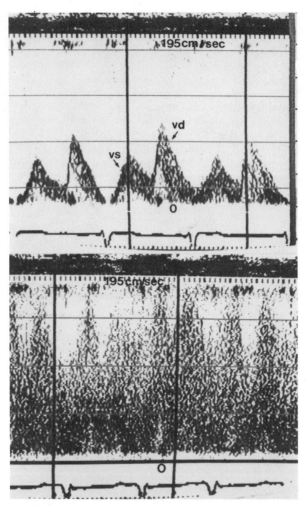

Fig 2–4.—Pulmonary venous flow pattern in a patient with obstruction. **Top,** the Doppler spectral trace from the right pulmonary veins demonstrates normal biphasic pulmonary venous flow. **Bottom,** the sample volume is placed in the vicinity of the left pulmonary veins. Note the high-velocity turbulent flow characteristic of pulmonary venous obstruction. Abbreviations: *vs,* flow during the x descent; *vd,* flow during the y descent. (Courtesy of Smallhorn, J.F., et al.: Circulation 73:765–774, April 1986. By permission of the American Heart Association, Inc.)

venous obstruction. Therefore, it is good to know that a noninvasive technique can be used with confidence to assess this possible complication over long-term follow-up.—M.A. Engle, M.D.

The Midterm and Long-Term Results of the Mustard Operation in Patients With Transposition of the Great Vessels and Dynamic Left Ventricular Outflow Tract Obstruction

Scott Stewart, Peter J. Harris, and James Manning (Univ. of Rochester, N.Y.)
Ann. Thorac. Surg. 41:272–275, March 1986   2–24

Left ventricular (LV) outflow tract obstruction may be present in a third of patients with transposition. It may result from supravalvular or valvular narrowing or from subvalvular obstruction. Forty-three consecutive patients with transposition and an intact ventricular septum or only a very small septal defect were studied for outflow tract obstruction.

Eight patients (19%) had dynamic LV outflow tract obstruction. The mean age was 1 year. All had elevated LV systolic pressure and no evidence of pulmonary vascular disease. Left ventricular–pulmonary artery pressure gradients ranged from 14 mm Hg to 60 mm Hg in the five evaluable patients. The outflow tract obstruction was clearly dynamic in six cases. The upper ventricular septum bulged posteriorly into the outflow tract, and the anterior mitral leaflet moved forward in systole, compressing the outflow tract to an inverted cone of contrast medium. Study of the outflow tract at the time of the Mustard operation was unrewarding. The gradient was unchanged or increased in all patients but one at follow-up, and all patients continued to have a murmur of LV outflow tract obstruction. However, all have been asymptomatic during follow-up for 1–11 years.

Dynamic LV outflow tract obstruction persists after the Mustard operation, but is not inconsistent with an excellent clinical outcome. The LV outflow tract presently is not explored in patients with dynamic obstruction.

▶ Although the right ventricle and the ventricular septum are hypertrophied to support systemic pressure when the great arteries are transposed and the patient survives because of a venous switch operation that accomplishes physiologic repair, the possibility of encroachment on the outflow tract of the left ventricle is more a theoretical than a real handicap. That has been our experience, and it is the experience of these authors as well. We support their conclusions.—M.A. Engle, M.D.

Wall Thickness, Cavity Dimensions, and Myocardial Contractility of the Left Ventricle in Patients With Simple Transposition of the Great Arteries: A Multicenter Study of Patients From 10 to 20 Years of Age
Ana-Maria Carceller, Jean-Claude Fouron, Jeffrey F. Smallhorn, Jean-Louis Cloez, Nicolaas H. van Doesburg, Pierre Mauran, Gilles Ducharme, Claude Pernot, and André Davignon (l'Hôpital Sainte-Justine, Montreal, The Hosp. for Sick Children, Toronto, l'Hôpital d'Enfants de Brabois, CHU de Nancy, France, and Univ. of Montreal)
Circulation 73:622–627, April 1986   2–25

Surgical rerouting of the venous return is the standard operative procedure for correction of simple transposition of the great arteries (TGA) in patients with normal pulmonary pressure. One consequence of this procedure is that the left ventricle maintains its anatomical relationship

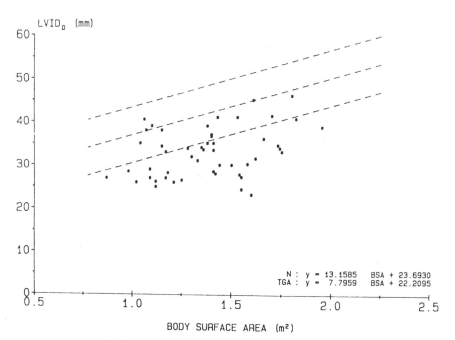

Fig 2–5.—Individual values for left ventricular internal dimensions at end-diastole (LVID$_d$) in patients with uncomplicated transposition of the great arteries (TGA) in relation to body surface area (BSA). The *dotted lines* correspond to the regression line *(middle)* and 95% tolerance limits for the same variables in a normal, age-matched population (N). (Courtesy of Carceller, A.-M., et al.: Circulation 73:622–627, April 1986. By permission of the American Heart Association, Inc.)

with the pulmonary circulation, thus influencing the muscular growth and general dynamics of the ventricular walls. Wall thickness and cavity dimensions of the left ventricles in patients with corrected uncomplicated TGA were compared with those measurements in normal children.

The study group comprised 51 patients aged 10–20 who had undergone correction of uncomplicated TGA by either the Mustard procedure or the Senning procedure. The control group consisted of 69 normal individuals. Echocardiographic studies were performed to measure left ventricular posterior wall (LVPW) thickness and cavity dimensions at end-systole (LVID$_s$) and at end-diastole (LVID$_d$).

There was a positive correlation between body surface area and LVID$_s$ and LVID$_d$ within the group of TGA patients (Fig 2–5); in comparison with normal persons, however, the LVID was significantly smaller than that measured in controls. A positive correlation between body surface area and LVPW thickness was also found in the TGA patients (Fig 2–6). The LVPW thickness in the TGA patients was always thinner than in the control group. In addition, a progressive increase in LVPW thickness was noted as the patients grew older. These findings should aid in future interpretation of echocardiographic findings in patients with TGA.

▶ In individuals who survive with completely transposed great arteries, the left

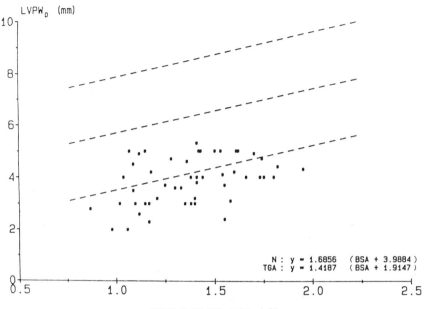

LVPW$_D$ (mm)

N : y = 1.6856 (BSA + 3.9884)
TGA : y = 1.4187 (BSA + 1.9147)

BODY SURFACE AREA (m²)

Fig 2–6.—Dimensions of left ventricular posterior wall at end-diastole (LVPW$_d$) in patients with transposition of the great arteries (TGA) in relation to body surface area (BSA). The *dotted lines* represent the regression line *(middle)* and the 95% tolerance limits for the same variables in a normal, age-matched population (N). (Courtesy of Carceller, A.-M., et al.: Circulation 73:622–627, April 1986. By permission of the American Heart Association, Inc.)

ventricle is required to act as a low-pressure pump to the pulmonary circuit, and the right ventricle acts as a high-pressure pump to the systemic circulation. The adaptations of these two chambers over many years have been the subject of speculation. This multicenter report focuses on the left ventricle in patients now aged 10–20 years who survived for that long, thanks to an operation (Mustard or Senning) that rerouted venous blood at the atrial level to match the transposed arteries. Not unexpectedly, they found that the thickened ventricular septum bowed back into the thin-walled left ventricle, making its cavity size smaller than in a left ventricle that gives rise to the aorta. Changes in left ventricular geometry probably accounted for the high indices of myocardial contractility and shortening fraction that were found in these patients.—M.A. Engle, M.D.

Hemodynamic and Electrophysiologic Results of the Senning Procedure for Transposition of the Great Arteries

Craig J. Byrum, Edward L. Bove, Henry M. Sondheimer, Rae-Ellen W. Kavey, and Marie S. Blackman (UNY, Upstate Med. Ctr.)
Am. J. Cardiol. 58:138–142, July 1, 1986   2–26

A review was made of the results with the modified Senning procedure, a surgical technique used in the physiologic repair of congenital transposition of the great arteries. During a 3-year period, 24 children between the ages of 6 days and 24 months underwent a modified Senning procedure. Two children died perioperatively, and one who survived the operation died of sepsis 17 days afterward. Of the 21 surviving children, 20 underwent elective postoperative catheterization for hemodynamic and electrophysiologic assessment about 13 months after surgery.

All survivors were clinically well at the time of follow-up and had normal weight gain. Systemic arterial blood showed normal oxygen saturation. Left ventricular function and pulmonary artery pressures also were normal. No pulmonary venous obstruction was noted. Four patients had narrowing at the junction of the superior vena cava and the systemic venous atrium, but only one had clinical manifestations that necessitated corrective surgery. Atrioventricular conduction in response to programmed electric stimulation was normal in all children. However, sinus node dysfunction was noted in six. The Senning procedure led to an excellent hemodynamic and electrophysiologic status in all survivors.

▶ Venous rerouting of the circulation to correct physiologically for completely transposed great arteries has been performed for about 20 years with a low operative mortality of about 5%. After the Mustard operation in long-term follow-up was found to be associated with atrial arrhythmias that seemed to become more common as the years added up after surgery, and because obstruction of the superior vena cava was common, some surgeons changed to the Senning operation for this kind of physiologic repair.

These authors reported on 21 survivors of the Senning operation performed about 1 year previously. They found a similar incidence of sinus node dysfunction and of superior vena caval obstruction as associated with the Mustard operation.—M.A. Engle, M.D.

Laboratory Investigations

General Guidelines

Recommendations for Use of Laboratory Studies for Pediatric Patients With Suspected or Proven Heart Disease: A Statement of the Committee on Congenital Cardiac Defects of the Council on Cardiovascular Disease in the Young of the American Heart Association
Thomas P. Graham, Ira H. Gessner, William F. Friedman, Welton M. Gersony, Howard Gutesell, Arno R. Hohn, Jay M. Jarmakani, Barry J. Maron, Amnon Rosenthal, Karen Uzark, Victoria Vetter, Roberta G. Williams, and Steven Yabek (American Heart Assoc., Dallas)
Am. J. Cardiol. 58:443A–450A, August 1986   2–27

In this special report, the American Heart Association sets forth its recommendations for the use of laboratory studies in pediatric patients in whom a congenital or acquired cardiac problem is suspected. These recommendations are issued not only for the purpose of promoting the proper use of diagnostic tests, but also to encourage avoidance of unnecessary tests. These recommendations are not applicable to research protocols for which informed consent and institutional approval have been obtained.

Indications are provided for appropriate use of roentgenologic examinations of the chest, ECG, vectorcardiography, cardiac ultrasound examinations, phonocardiography, continuous ambulatory ECG monitoring, stress testing, nuclear cardiac studies, electrophysiologic studies, and cardiac catheterization. General and special indications are given, as well as recommended frequency limitations and special comments. Physicians are encouraged to evaluate both risk-benefit and cost-benefit ratios for each procedure in each patient.

▶ As modalities for use in diagnosis have multiplied, the physician has more to choose *from,* not just to *choose.* Nothing supplants the clinical acumen of the good cardiologist who listens to what the parents and the child tell him on questioning and who carefully examines his patient. By this time he has already made a presumptive diagnosis and he chooses the few tests that will most help him to confirm or to reject that diagnosis and to manage the patient.

The studies used most frequently are noninvasive: ECG and initial x-ray examination (to be repeated only when necessary), supplemented most often by echocardiography. One needs a specific indication to carry out the other studies listed in this report. Recommendations for choosing each study are offered here to help the cardiologist to be selective rather than all inclusive.—M.A. Engle, M.D.

Cardiac Catheterization

Complications and Mortality Associated With Cardiac Catheterization in Infants Under One Year: A Prospective Study
Herbert E. Cohn, Michael D. Freed, William F. Hellenbrand, and Donald C. Fyler (Harvard Univ. and Children's Hosp. Med. Ctr., Boston, and Yale Univ.)
Pediatr. Cardiol. 6:123–131, 1985   2–28

Since the Cooperative Study on Cardiac Catheterization was conducted 20 years ago, there have been many advances in the techniques of cardiac catheterization of young infants. In addition, cardiovascular surgery is now being carried out on an increasing number of infants, and knowledge of more details of cardiovascular anatomy and physiology is necessary for success. Although the Cooperative Study reported a high incidence of complications and deaths in early infancy, a more recent evaluation wit hin the New England Regional Infant Cardiac Program (NERICP) found a mortality rate of approximately 8%, including catheterizations of patients who died of inoperable congenital heart lesions or died after surgery. Because the NERICP data collection suggested a mortality rate so different from that previously reported, a multicenter study was designed to assess the incidence of complications and deaths directly attributable to cardiac catheterization.

To evaluate complications and mortality in children younger than 1 year of age, findings were reviewed in 273 patients who had undergone 312 catheterizations. Among those performed on infants less than 4 months of age, the incidence of complications requiring treatment was 12%, and for those aged 4–12 months it was 1.5%. It was determined by precardiac catheterization risk assessment that 13% of these procedures were high risk, 21% were medium risk, and 66% were low risk. As expected, the incidence of complications was much greater in the high-risk group (30%) than in the medium-risk group (14%) or the low-risk group (4%). The overall mortality rates at 24 hours, 48 hours, and 1 week after cardiac catheterization were 3.8%, 8.3%, and 13.5%, respectively, including patients with inoperable lesions and those having cardiac surgery. On the other hand, deaths directly attributable to cardiac catheterization complications were 0,0.3% and 0.3%, respectively.

Prior to cardiac catheterization, patients at high risk in whom major complications and death are most likely to occur can be predicted. The incidence of death from cardiac catheterization-related complications is low in patients younger than 1 year of age, compared with the incidence of death from the underlying lesion or after cardiac surgery.

▶ This important prospective study was conducted among six hospitals cooperating within the New England Region to diagnose and treat infants with critical congenital heart disease. Half of the 273 patients were less than 1 month of age, and a third of the studies were performed in the first week of life.

The incidence of death from cardiac catheterization-related complications was extremely low: 2.5%. Arrhythmia was the most common major complication: supraventricular tachyarrhythmias during catheter manipulation in four infants aged 3 weeks to 3 months. Sinus bradycardia occurred in four catheterizations of infants up to 6 weeks. Profound hypotension occurred in two infants and a major arterial complication in one, a day-old child who required embolectomy for a femoral arterial thrombosis after percutaneous arterial catheterization. Cardiac perforation occurred three times but did not cause death. Catheter problems were associated in two instances with CO_2-filled balloons, and embolism was noted twice.

The use of noninvasive techniques may render cardiac catheterization unnecessary in some instances. Prostaglandin infusion in infants with ductus-dependent lesions makes these infants more safe for needed cardiac catheterization.

I agree with the authors' statement that, "Since the incidence of catheterization-related morbidity and mortality in this study is very low . . . we believe catheterization should not be withheld from a moribund infant if there is any possibility of finding a correctable cardiac lesion."—M.A. Engle, M.D.

Variability of Right-Sided Cardiac Oxygen Saturations in Adults With and Without Left-To-Right Intracardiac Shunting
L. David Hillis, Brian G. Firth, and Michael D. Winniford (Univ. of Texas at Dallas and Parkland Mem. Hosp., Dallas)
Am. J. Cardiol. 58:129–132, July 1, 1986   2–29

In many cardiac catheterization laboratories, left-to-right shunting is evaluated by first taking single blood samples from the superior vena cava, right atrium, and pulmonary artery during right-sided catheterization and measuring the oxygen saturation of these single blood samples. Based on the findings, it is then decided whether to pursue further detailed oximetric studies, which are costly and time consuming. However, the variability of single samples in adults with and without intracardiac left-to-right shunting has not yet been assessed. Evaluation was made of oxygen saturation in single samples from adults without intracardiac shunting to establish normal standards of variability.

During a period of about 5 years, 524 male and 507 female aged 14–82 years underwent cardiac catheterization. In 980 patients, no shunting was present, and the differences in oxygen saturation of blood samples between the superior vena cava and right atrium, right atrium and pulmonary artery, and superior vena cava and pulmonary artery from these patients were measured for setting standards.

The normal limits of variability for these saturation differences were found to be 8.7%, 5.7%, and 9.0%, respectively. When these norms were applied to 51 patients with diagnosed left-to-right shunting, it was found that 46 patients (90%) could be identified correctly just from oxygen saturation measurements in their single blood samples. Assessment of oxygen saturation from single blood specimens has a high predictive accuracy (more than 94%) and excellent sensitivity (more than 90%) and specificity (94% to 95%) in the identification of patients with and without intracardiac left-to-right shunting. In patients with large shunts (Qp/Qs ratio of 2 or more), the sensitivity of these measurements is especially high.

▶ The limited number of samples for analysis of oxygen saturation has economic benefits in a cost-containment environment, but is it cost effective for the patient if his condition is not diagnosed correctly? The authors found that large shunts could be detected with accuracy, sensitivity, and specificity, but that smaller shunts with Qp/Qs ratio of 1.9 or less were sometimes missed. Fortunately, the authors used indocyanine green dye studies to exclude or quantitate a left-to-right shunt. It is this kind of backup that can permit limitation of samples for oxygen saturation in adults undergoing cardiac catheterization, 98% of whom have no intracardiac shunting (980 of 1,031 patients).

The authors extended their study to 541 patients in the intensive care units. There, customarily detailed oximetric analysis is undertaken only when pulmonary artery saturation exceeds that in the inferior vena cava. They found that a difference between superior vena cava and pulmonary artery saturation of at least 9% occurred in 90% of patients with shunting and in only 6% of those without shunting, a predictive accuracy of 94%.—M.A. Engle, M.D.

Magnetic Resonance Imaging

▶ ↓ Just as two-dimensional echocardiography with Doppler studies brought a new dimension to accurate anatomical definition of congenital cardiac anomalies noninvasively and without radiation, so too has magnetic resonance imaging (MRI) emerged as a technique for visualization of cardiovascular structures through which blood flows, without radiation or injection of contrast medium.

The first of the three papers abstracted below describes the methodology and general applications of MRI in congenital heart disease. The other two describe use of the method in two specific common forms of congenital heart disease, ventricular septal defect and coarctation of the aorta.

My impressions of this technique are that it is dramatic in its revelations, but that it is quite costly and it is difficult to use in infants and small children with high heart rates and the inability to lie still for the relatively long time required to obtain the cuts.—M.A. Engle, M.D.

Congenital Heart Disease: Gated MR Imaging in 72 Patients
Dominique Didier, Charles B. Higgins, Madeleine R. Fisher, Luci Osaki, Norman H. Silverman, and Melvin D. Cheitlin (Univ. of California at San Francisco and San Francisco Gen. Hosp.)
Radiology 158:227–235, January 1986   2–30

Recent studies have described the effectiveness of gated magnetic resonance imaging (MRI) in demonstrating cardiovascular lesions in a small group of patients. Rapidly flowing blood produces no MRI signal, thus a good natural contrast is provided between blood and cardiovascular structures. As opposed to x-ray imaging techniques, intravenous injection of contrast medium is not necessary, making MRI a completely noninvasive method. The clinical valve of gated MRI was assessed for making the definitive diagnosis of segmental anatomy and for detection of cardiac abnormalities in a large series of patients with congenital heart disease. In most instances the ability of MRI to demonstrate various lesions was compared with angiography. Seventy-two patients with a variety of congenital anomalies of the heart and great vessels underwent gated MRI using the multisectional spin-echo technique. Transverse, sagittal, and coronal images were obtained. The MRI were graded as excellent, diagnostic, or nondiagnostic, and the MRI findings were corroborated by angiography or two-dimensional echocardiography.

In 96% of the studies MRI was excellent (20) or diagnostic (49). Visceroatrial situs, the type of ventricular loop, and the relationship of the great vessels were identified in all patients with studies encompassing the entire heart. Also, 44 of 47 abnormalities at the level of the great vessels were identified with MRI including coarctation of the aorta and vascular rings. Of 35 ventricular abnormalities, MRI showed 32. However, two small ventricular septal defects and one Ebstein anomaly were missed. All of the abnormalities at the atrial level and those of systemic and pulmonary venous return were observed on MRI. Complex cardiac anomalies (e.g., single ventricles) and the status of the pulmonary arteries were shown clearly, and good assessment of total and palliative postoperative anatomy was possible.

Results in this large series of patients with congenital heart disease

demonstrate the clinical efficacy of MRI in detecting congenital abnormalities of the heart and great vessels. Considering its accuracy, MRI might
replace angiography in the diagnosis of septal defects and great vessel
abnormalities. The combination of two-dimensional echocardiography
and MRI could be the safest and most cost-effective approach to the
preoperative and postoperative assessment of both simple and complex
congenital cardiovascular disease.

▶ This report presents the principles of and the rationale for using MRI. The
age range of the patients studied was wide, from 2 months to 78 years. The
number of infants and small children studied was nine between the ages of 2
months to 3.5 years. Because most serious malformations produce their bad
effects early in infancy, this is the age group in which one would like most of
all to have safe, brief, informative diagnostic studies that are noninvasive and
that do not require anesthesia for sedation. These nine young patients received
pentabarbital sodium intramuscularly. The authors, in fairness, point out limitations of the method. An important one is the inability to evaluate valvular
abnormalities, especially of semilunar valves. Another is the low signal intensity provided by the thin structures in the atrial septum or membranous ventricular septum.—M.A. Engle, M.D.

**Identification and Localization of Ventricular Septal Defect by Gated Mag-
netic Resonance Imaging**
Dominique Didier and Charles B. Higgins (Univ. of California at San Francisco
and Univ. Hosp. Saint Jacques, Besançon, France)
Am. J. Cardiol. 57:1363–1368, June 1, 1986   2–31

Imaging of the ventricular septum has traditionally been accomplished
by angiography. Newer noninvasive techniques, including two-dimensional echocardiography (2-D echo) and echo Doppler and color flow
imaging with 2-D echo, have recently been added as valuable tools for
diagnosis. Gated magnetic resonance imaging (MRI) is a still-newer technique that has already been tested in the diagnosis of congenital cardiac
abnormalities. Its potential for visualization of abnormalities associated
with the most common form of congenital heart disease was evaluated in
11 male and 11 female patients, aged 2 months to 51 years, in whom
various types of ventricular septal defects (VSDs) had been diagnosed
previously, by cardiac catheterization and angiography in 19 and by 2-D
echo in 3. As a control, 17 normal volunteers were examined to define
the normal morphologic characteristics of the ventricular septum.

The four portions of the ventricular septum were easily identified with
MRI, especially on the transverse images. In 20 of the 22 patients, the
VSD was visualized. In the other two patients, failure occurred as a result
of excessive movement by the patient or, in one infant, because there was
a 3-mm gap between sections in the VSD. The VSD was perimembranous
in ten patients and of the inlet type in four, the complete atrioventricular
canal type in three, and the outlet type in six others. This imaging technique

has great potential as an alternative to angiography for confirmation of the diagnosis and localization of a VSD before surgery.

▶ Despite the limitations of imaging abnormalities in the area of the thin membranous ventricular septum noted above, the authors pooled experience from the University of California in San Francisco and from Besançon, France, to report their observations in patients with this most common of congenital heart defects. The age span was wide, from 2 months to 51 years, in their 22 patients. The studies successfully identified the defect and its location in all but two, one of whom was an infant. Although perimembranous VSD is the most common type, it was underrepresented in these 20 successful studies. It was imaged in ten patients. Defects in other locations were more often the subject of study; outlet VSD, for example, was studied in six. The smallest defect imaged was 0.3 cm. They recommend transverse images as the most useful in demonstration of the VSD.—M.A. Engle, M.D.

Nuclear Magnetic Resonance Imaging in Evaluation and Follow-Up of Children Treated for Coarctation of the Aorta
Robert A. Boxer, Michael A. LaCorte, Sharanjeet Singh, Rubin Cooper, Marcia C. Fishman, Mitchell Goldman, and Harry L. Stein (North Shore Univ. Hosp. and Cornell Univ., Manhasset, N.Y., and Brookdale Hosp. Med. Ctr., Brooklyn)
J. Am. Coll. Cardiol. 7:1095–1098, May 1986   2–32

Traditionally, coarctation of the aorta has been visualized by cardiac catheterization and angiography. More recently, digital subtraction angiography and two-dimensional ultrasonography have been used for diagnosis. However, ECG-gated nuclear magnetic resonance (NMR) imaging is a newer, noninvasive technique used to visualize many congenital cardiac malformations. This technique was evaluated in patients with coarctation of the aorta and in the follow-up of such patients after surgery or balloon dilation angioplasty.

The study group comprised ten patients aged 2.5–18 years with coarctation of the aorta who underwent NMR imaging studies. In seven patients the diagnosis was confirmed by cardiac catheterization and angiography, and the other three had clear clinical evidence of the disorder. One patient underwent surgical repair of the coarctation and six underwent balloon dilation angioplasty. In addition to the ten diagnostic NMR studies, NMR studies were done in three children after they had been treated.

In all pretreatment studies, the sagittal and 60-degree left anterior oblique imaging planes visualized the coarctation most adequately, but the coronal view did not adequately visualize it. In all cases, NMR imaging done after treatment confirmed effective relief of the coarctation. The technique offers several advantages over conventional methods in evaluation of coarctation of the aorta in that it is noninvasive, does not require the use of contrast agents intravenously, and provides excellent resolutuion of vascular wall structures.

▶ This study reports the application of magnetic resonance imaging to another specific congenital anomaly, namely, coarctation of the aorta in ten children. Three were not operated on, one was treated surgically, and six by balloon dilation angioplasty. The area of discrete narrowing, and even the shelf in one illustrative case, was seen, and there was an area of aneurysm formation distal to the coarctation in one paitent studied 16 months after balloon dilation. Although one image identified a large collateral artery, this technique in my experience does not show the extent of collateral circulation as well as aortography does. To learn about collateral vessels is one of the chief reasons for preoperative diagnostic studies in patients with this malformation.—M.A. Engle, M.D.

Radionuclide Measurement of Right Ventricular Function in Atrial Septal Defect, Ventricular Septal Defect, and Complete Transposition of the Great Arteries
Edward J. Baker, Chen Shubao, Susan E. M. Clarke, Ignac Fogelman, Michael N. Maisey, and Michael Tynan (Guy's Hosp., London)
Am. J. Cardiol. 57:1142–1146, May 1, 1986   2–33

Nuclide assessments of right ventricular function were compared in 30 patients having ventricular septal defect (VSD), 30 with a secundum atrial septal defect, and 20 with surgically corrected complete transposition of the great arteries. The overall mean age was 9 years. First-pass and gated equilibrium nuclide angiographic studies were performed.

The mean right ventricular ejection fraction in patients with VSD was 64%, compared with 61% for the group with atrial septal defect. The mean value of 49% in patients with transposition was significantly lower than in the VSD group. Measurements of right ventricular ejection fraction were reproducible, with a correlation coefficient between two data sets of 0.93. The ratio of pulmonary to systemic flow correlated significantly with the phase difference in patients with VSD. Age did not correlate with ejection fraction or phase difference in this group.

First-pass gated nuclide angiography is a valid means of estimating the right ventricular ejection fraction. Delayed right ventricular contraction on phase analysis may be a sensitive index of early right ventricular dysfunction. The method is not applicable to measurement of right ventricular ejection fraction if intracardiac right-to-left shunting is present.

▶ The technique of first-pass and gated equilibrium cineangiography has had wide acceptance in medical cardiology, where it is used especially to evaluate left ventricular function in adults with acquired heart disease. This study, in contrast, is an attempt to evaluate right ventricular function in 80 patients, mostly children, with an atrial defect (30) or with VSD (30) who had not been operated on, and in 20 patients with a physiologic repair by intra-atrial rerouting for transposition of the great arteries (TGA).

They found right ventricular function to be within normal limits in all. The mean ejection fraction was lower in the TGA group (49%) than in the other two groups with left-to-right shunting lesions. Two obvious differences that pertain in the TGA patients is that their right ventricle supports a systemic systolic pressure and therefore hypertrophies, and that it functions with a normal volume load, whereas the other two conditions have a volume-loaded right ventricle because of the left-to-right shunt.—M.A. Engle, M.D.

Echocardiography and Doppler Studies

▶ ↓ Two-dimensional echocardiography has become the single most informative noninvasive means of defining cardiac anatomy and function. Doppler methodology, in the form of pulsed-wave and continuous-wave ultrasound, has added physiologic parameters of flow through defects and across stenotic or regurgitant valves. Color Doppler increases the sensitivity of these measurements. The rapid progress in this field is truly impressive, and the good keeps getting better. In many situations, cardiac catheterization is no longer necessary in preoperative evaluation and follow-up.

Here are several examples of studies of this methodology and of applications to some problems in heart disease in childhood.—M.A. Engle, M.D.

Use of Doppler Techniques (Continuous-Wave, Pulsed-Wave, and Color Flow Imaging) in the Noninvasive Hemodynamic Assessment of Congenital Heart Disease

Guy S. Reeder, Philip J. Currie, Donald J. Hagler, A. Jamil Tajik, and James B. Seward (Mayo Clinic and Found.)
Mayo Clin. Proc. 61:725–744, September 1986   2–34

Because Doppler echocardiography is a relatively new technique, a review was made of its principles and application to date in the diagnosis of congenital cardiac abnormalities. Doppler ultrasound makes use of a change in sound frequency that occurs when ultrasound is reflected from a moving target. With continuous-wave Doppler ultrasound, the crystals function continuously. This technique allows for accurate measurement of high velocities, but spatial localization of abnormal velocities is lacking. With pulsed-wave Doppler ultrasound echocardiography, short bursts of ultrasound are emitted; this technique has depth acuity. The two Doppler modes complement each other and are frequently used in combination. Two-dimensional color Doppler echocardiography has depth acuity, but it lacks the ability to quantitate high velocities.

Doppler echocardiography is used to detect intracardiac shunts because the decrease in pressure across the defect can be quantitated. The size of an atrial septal defect is measured with pulsed-wave Doppler and color flow imaging techniques because flow velocities across this defect are relatively low. Small ventricular septal defects are measured with pulsed-wave Doppler, whereas large ventricular septal defects are usually imaged by two-dimensional echocardiography. Uncomplicated patent ductus arteriosus can be assessed by either pulsed-wave or continuous-wave Doppler examination. Stenotic lesions may best be examined by continuous-wave

Doppler study, but pulsed-wave Doppler may facilitate spatial localization of peak velocities.

Doppler echocardiography in combination with two-dimensional echocardiography provides comprehensive data in a noninvasive setting. This new technique facilitates the diagnosis of congenital heart disease significantly, and in some patients its use may even avoid cardiac catheterization.

▶ The authors of this informative review article on Doppler techniques are at the Mayo Clinic and are experts in this field. They share their extensive experience of the past few years and illustrate their observations liberally in black and white and in color as they discuss the approach to diagnosis of congenital cardiac lesions and postoperative congenital heart disease. It was many years from the time Doppler in Prague described the Doppler shift to the application of pulsed-wave Doppler to echocardiography (around 1980) and then of continuous-wave Doppler (around 1983), but once the idea and the instrumentation caught on, the methodology advanced rapidly and it has now become an essential tool in pediatric cardiology centers.—M.A. Engle, M.D.

Comparison of High Pulse Repetition Frequency and Continuous Wave Doppler Echocardiography for Velocity Measurement and Gradient Prediction in Children With Valvular and Congenital Heart Disease
A. Rebecca Snider, J. Geoffrey Stevenson, James W. French, Albert P. Rocchini, MacDonald Dick, II, Amnon Rosenthal, Dennis C. Crowley, Robert H. Beekman, and Jane Peters (Univ. of Michigan and Univ. of Washington)
J. Am. Coll. Cardiol. 7:873–879, April 1986   2–35

Doppler echocardiography has been used extensively to quantitate the pressure drop across stenotic and regurgitant valves and across septal defects. For severely stenotic valves and for most regurgitant lesions, the peak flow velocity is high. Two techniques have been described to detect and display these high velocities clearly, namely, continuous-wave Doppler echocardiography and high pulse repetition frequency Doppler echocardiography. The ability of these two techniques to detect the peak velocity of a jet flow disturbance and to predict pressure gradients accurately was compared.

The study was carried out in two groups of children with valvular or congenital heart disease. The first study group included 84 children or adolescents who underwent examination in the echocardiography laboratory with both Doppler techniques in randomized sequence. In these experiments the peak velocity recorded with high pulse repetition frequency Doppler echocardiography was compared with the peak velocity recorded with the continuous-wave technique. The second study group to determine accuracy included 41 children or adolescents who were examined with both Doppler techniques at the time of cardiac catheterization. The first study showed a high correlation between peak velocities detected by high pulse repetition frequency and continuous-wave Doppler echocardiography. The accuracy study showed a close correlation between measured peak-to-peak pressure gradients and pressure gradients calculated from continuous-wave and high pulse repetition frequency Doppler echocardiography. Close correlations were also observed between measured peak instantaneous gradients and pressure gradients calculated from continuous-wave and high pulse repetition frequency Doppler echocardiography.

In children and adolescents, no difference was determined in the ability of the two Doppler techniques to detect the peak velocity of a jet flow disturbance. Further, both Doppler techniques were equally accurate in their ability to predict pressure gradients measured at cardiac catheterization.

▶ Dr. Snider and colleagues studied 84 children by two Doppler techniques and 41 by the two Doppler methods when they had cardiac catheterization for their predominantly obstructive cardiac lesions. Their results showed remarkably similar results by the two methods and great accuracy of both when compared with pressures measured at cardiac catheterization, the "gold standard."—M.A. Engle, M.D.

The Role of Cross Sectional Echocardiography and Pulsed Doppler Ultrasound in the Management of Neonates in Whom Congenital Heart Disease Is Suspected: A Prospective Study
Maurice P. Leung, C.K. Mok, K.C. Lau, Roxy Lo, and C.Y. Yeung (Univ. of Hong Kong)
Br. Heart J. 56:73–82, July 1986   2–36

The value of combined cross-sectional echocardiography and pulsed Doppler ultrasound in the management of symptomatic neonates suspected of having congenital heart disease was examined in 96 consecutive infants whose mean age was 11 days; all had cardiorespiratory symptoms. Cardiac catheterization was performed in all except for seven who were moribund when admitted.

Of 536 cardiovascular anomalies identified at cardiac catheterization and autopsy, 95.5% were correctly diagnosed by echocardiography. Seven false positive echocardiographic diagnoses were made, for a specificity of 99%. Nearly all missing diagnoses and all false positive findings represented extracardiac vascular anomalies. Normal cardiovascular anatomy was consistently identified as such. Eight of 84 proposed management plans were found after catheterization to be inappropriate. Nearly 80% of neonates in this study could have been managed correctly without cardiac catheterization.

The availability of high-resolution cross-sectional echocardiography and pulsed Doppler ultrasound, with competent interpretation, can lower the number of cardiac catheterizations needed in the management of neonates suspected of having congenital heart disease. In most cases, sound clinical decisions on management may be made from the echocardiographic findings.

▶ When a diagnostic technique is evaluated and validated, it is logical that applications should be extended to a wider range of conditions and to a wider age range. This study in symptomatic infants with suspected congenital heart disease both validates this application for specificity and sensitivity and provides justification to use in these, the sickest and the highest at risk of any age group with congenital heart disease, this noninvasive and informative diagnostic tool to plan management.—M.A. Engle, M.D.

Noninvasive Assessment of Pulmonary Valve Stenosis, Aortic Valve Stenosis, and Coarctation of the Aorta in Critically Ill Neonates
Donald J. Hagler, A. Jamil Tajik, James B. Seward, and Donald G. Ritter (Mayo Clinic and Found.)
Am. J. Cardiol. 57:369–372, Feb. 1, 1986   2–37

Despite improved diagnosis, two-dimensional (2-D) echocardiography often does not allow accurate noninvasive assessment of the severity of pulmonary valve stenosis, aortic valve stenosis, or coarctation of the aorta. However, continuous-wave Doppler examination, when combined with 2-D echocardiography, enhances the management of these stenotic lesions without confirmatory cardiac catheterization. During a 2-year period, 14 consecutive neonates, aged 3 months or younger and having obstructive lesions, underwent combined 2-D echocardiography and continuous-wave Doppler examinations. Four neonates had pulmonary valve stenosis, five had aortic valve stenosis, and five had coarctation. Thirteen were critically ill and required emergency evaluation.

All 14 infants underwent 2-D echocardiography with a 7.5-MHz imaging transducer. Continuous-wave Doppler examinations were performed with a 2-MHz non-imaging transducer. Fine adjustments in transducer position and angulation allowed for measurement of a Doppler signal of highest audible frequency, maximal velocity, and clear spectral velocity envelope at the parasternal, apical, subcostal, and suprasternal positions. With the modified Bernoulli equation, the resultant valve pressure gradient equaling $4V^2$ related gradient to four times the square of the maximal velocity.

The 2-D echocardiographic examination allowed accurate anatomical prediction of all defects as confirmed on surgery. However, continuous-wave Doppler showed confirmatory evidence of the severity of valve gradient, providing additional information for either surgical or medical management. No infant required cardiac catheterization prior to treatment. However, one with severe coarctation of the aorta subsequently underwent therapeutic cardiac catheterization and balloon angioplasty. Another child with an estimated gradient of 30 mm Hg confirmed at surgery or catheterization subsequently underwent pulmonary valvotomy elsewhere. Studies with 2-D echocardiography also provided additional information about chamber dimension and ventricular function assessed by ejection fraction by the method of Quinnes, et al.

Combined 2-D echocardiography and continuous-wave Doppler examination allows noninvasive evaluation of both anatomical and hemo-dynamic variables in the diagnosis and management of critical stenotic lesions in the neonates. The combined approach is the preferred to cardiac catheterization and avoids the risk, trauma, and osmotic load associated with cardiac catheterization.

▶ The Mayo Clinic team applied their technique of 2-D echocardiography and continuous-wave Doppler to study 14 neonates, 13 of them critically ill. They derived sufficiently accurate information from these studies to forego cardiac catheterization as they planned surgical and/or medical management.

These are the patients most in need of prompt recognition and accurate, noninvasive assessment, which should include not just these Doppler and echocardiographic studies but a history, well-performed physical examination, ECG, and chest x-ray examination. Analysis of these features guides the observer in performing echocardiography and in molding all of the data logically into diagnosis and a plan of management.—M.A. Engle, M.D.

Doppler Ultrasound in the Estimation of the Severity of Pulmonary Infundibular Stenosis in Infants and Children

A.B. Houston, I.A. Simpson, C.D. Sheldon, W.B. Doig, and E.N. Coleman (Royal Hosp. for Sick Children, Glasgow)
Br. Heart J. 55:381–384, April 1986   2–38

The pressure gradient in obstructive cardiac lesions can be calculated with Doppler echocardiography by measuring maximal velocity of blood flow across an obstruction and applying the modified Bernoulli equation. However, there is a potential for error in patients with infundibular pulmonary stenosis, because obstruction can occur on more than one level. The validity of the modified Bernoulli formula was assessed by measuring the pressure gradient in 31 children aged 7 days to 16 years with infundibular pulmonary stenosis, including 16 with tetralogy of Fallot.

All children underwent Doppler echocardiography, and pressure gradients were measured from various parasternal and subcostal positions. In 21 children who underwent cardiac catheterization, pressure gradients were measured from separate right ventricular and pulmonary arterial recordings while the catheter was advanced, and measurements were then compared with those obtained on catheter withdrawal. Measurements from both procedures were correlated and interpreted.

The Doppler recordings obtained were satisfactory in all cases. Good correlation was found between gradients measured at catheterization and those calculated from Doppler measurements. Doppler ultrasound provides accurate, noninvasive assessment of the severity of pulmonary infundibular stenosis.

▶ Houston and colleagues from Glasgow showed convincingly that Doppler ultrasound with two-dimensional echocardiography can provide an accurate estimate of the severity of infundibular stenosis, often an elongated obstruction, just as it has been shown by others that the method is valid for discrete valvular stenosis.—M.A. Engle, M.D.

Accuracy and Pitfalls of Doppler Evaluation of the Pressure Gradient in Aortic Coarctation
Gerald R. Marx and Hugh D. Allen (Univ. of Arizona, Tucson)
J. Am. Coll. Cardiol. 7:1379–1385, June 1986   2–39

The pressure gradient in aortic coarctation can usually be obtained by comparison of upper and lower extremity blood pressures measured by sphygmomanometry. However, some patients may have upper or lower extremity compromise because of prior procedures or anomalous origin of the subclavian arteries, which may preclude accurate measurement of the gradient. At cardiac catheterization, Doppler echocardiography can estimate pressure drops across discrete obstructions. Because the obstruction in coarctation also is discrete, it was hypothesized that Doppler echocardiography should predict the pressure drop. This hypothesis was tested in 31 patients with the diagnosis of aortic coarctation who underwent cardiac catheterization. Ages ranged from 6 days to 20 years. The mean Doppler-estimated gradient, calculated using only jet velocities distal to the obstruction, was 44 ± 17 mm Hg, and the mean catheterization gradient was 36 ± 21 mm Hg. Using both the precoarctation and postcoarctation velocities, the mean Doppler-estimated gradient was 36 ± 20 mm Hg and the mean catheterization gradient was 36 ± 21 mm Hg.

Doppler echocardiography closely estimated the pressure gradient in aortic coarctation, and estimation improved when the velocities proximal as well as distal to the obstruction were included in the calculation.

▶ Yet another useful application of Doppler technology is reported: estimation of the pressure gradient across discrete coarctation of the aorta. The investigators were unable to obtain jet velocities in three neonates with severe coarctation and patent ductus arteriosus, but they were well satisfied with the accuracy of the method in the others, especially when they included velocities both proximal and distal to the coarctation.—M.A. Engle, M.D.

Continuous-Wave Doppler in Children With Ventricular Septal Defect: Noninvasive Estimation of Interventricular Pressure Gradient
Daniel J. Murphy, Jr., Achi Ludomirsky, and James C. Huhta (Baylor Univ. and Texas Children's Hosp., Houston)
Am. J. Cardiol. 57:428–432, Feb. 15, 1986   2–40

Pulsed Doppler echocardiography has been used extensively to detect the presence of flow disturbances within the heart caused by ventricular septal defect (VSD). Currently, continuous-wave Doppler is being used to estimate transvalvular pressure gradients in a variety of cardiac lesions, including aortic, pulmonary and mitral stenosis. In addition, limited suc-

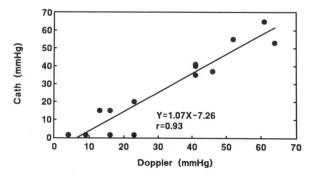

Fig 2–7.—Comparison of the ventricular septal defect (VSD) gradient by Doppler echocardiography and cardiac catheterization in 14 children with isolated perimembranous VSD. (Courtesy of Murphy, D.J., et al.: Am. J. Cardiol. 57:428–432, Feb. 15, 1986.)

cess has been reported in predicting systolic pressure differences between the left and right ventricle in patients with VSD. To evaluate infants and children with VSD for medical or surgical care, right ventricular and pulmonary artery pressures have been measured by cardiac catheterization. A noninvasive method would be valuable in selecting patients for cardiac catheterization or surgical intervention. An attempt was made to determine the accuracy of continuous-wave Doppler estimates of left-to-right ventricular pressure gradients in 28 children with VSD as the only lesion or as part of more complex congenital heart disease.

Doppler measurement of maximal velocity was carried out during catheterization and the Doppler-predicted gradient was compared with the peak-to-peak gradient measured simultaneously by catheter (Fig 2–7). The Doppler gradients ranged from 10 mm to 71 mm Hg and correlated well with the measured gradient. Fourteen children were discovered to have isolated VSD, and in these patients Doppler measurements of gradient allowed accurate estimation of right ventricular pressure. An inverse correlation was noted between the ratio of pulmonary to systemic resistance and maximal velocity.

Continuous-wave Doppler is an accurate means of measuring the instantaneous VSD pressure gradient in children with congenital heart disease and can be used to estimate the right ventricular and pulmonary artery pressure in those with isolated VSD. Further, this noninvasive method can be used to distinguish restrictive from nonrestrictive VSD.

▶ In the foregoing articles we have read about the value of Doppler methodology in evaluating infants and children with congenital heart disease, chiefly that caused by discrete valvular pulmonic or aortic stenosis or coarctation, and even with more diffuse subpulmonic stenosis. Now we find that Murphy and colleagues have validated the method in a common left-to-right shunting lesion, namely, VSD.

In this study of 28 children, the defect was isolated in 14, but in the rest it was associated with other lesions (e.g., transposition of the great arteries) or with severe pulmonic stenosis as part of tetralogy of Fallot. Doppler estimates correlated well with the studies at cardiac catheterization, thereby extending the utility of this terrific tool and also justifying the elimination in some patients of cardiac catheterization done simply for measurement of the size of the defect and the shunt of blood across it.—M.A. Engle, M.D.

Anatomical-Echocardiographic Correlations in Pulmonary Atresia With Intact Ventricular Septum: Use of Subcostal Cross-Sectional Views
B. Marino, E. Franceschini, L. Ballerini, C. Marcelletti, and G. Thiene (Ospedale "Bambino Gesù," Rome, and Univ. of Padova, Italy)
Int. J. Cardiol. 11:103–109, April 1986   2–41

Pulmonary atresia and an intact ventricular septum in neonates must be promptly diagnosed and treated. Cross-sectional echocardiography is an important technique for the evaluation and expeditious treatment of these infants. The efficacy of echocardiography was evaluated in the diagnosis and classification of these patients, and anatomical cuts were correlated with subcostal cross-sectional echocardiographic images.

Cross-sectional echocardiographic images obtained in 26 infants with pulmonary atresia and intact ventricular septum were compared with anatomical findings in specimens having the same anomaly. The echocardiographic study was based on a subcostal approach using oblique projections; specimens were cut using the same approach. The infants could be classified into three groups. In the first group of 12, the morphologically right ventricle was represented by all of its three component parts including the inlet, trabecular, and outlet. In the second group, all six infants had overgrowth of the apical component; consequently, the right ventricle had only two effective component parts, namely, the inlet and outlet. In the third group of eight infants, muscular overgrowth of both outlet and apical portions meant that the right ventricle was represented by only an inlet portion. Good morphological assessment and correlation with anatomical cuts, obtained in particular by using the "right oblique equivalent" view, can avoid invasive study in this malformation prior to palliative surgery.

► When cyanotic neonates present with pulmonary atresia and an intact ventricular septum, their heart size can range from an enormously dilated right atrium and ventricle, or a "wall-to-wall" heart, to one of near-average size with only a diminutive right ventricle. Most of these children have a poor prognosis, because their anatomy limits a skillful cardiac surgeon's ability to help them. If one could simplify their diagnosis and avoid cardiac catheterization, this might spare these infants from one stress while they are supported medically and while cardiologists and surgeons discuss palliation. This echocardiographic anatomical correlation provides a basis for translating echo-depicted anatomy into what we have become accustomed to interpret on angiocardiography.—M.A. Engle, M.D.

Specific Lesions

Arrhythmias

Modes of Onset ("Initiating Events") for Paroxysmal Atrial Tachycardia in Infants and Children

Ann Dunnigan, David G. Benditt, and D. Woodrow Benson, Jr. (Univ. of Minnesota)

Am. J. Cardiol. 57:1280–1287, June 1, 1986   2–42

Electrocardiographic documentation of spontaneous episodes of paroxysmal atrial tachycardia (PAT) has been reported only infrequently. Consequently, although PAT is relatively common in young patients, the initiating events are not well understood. A group of young patients with a history of spontaneous onset of PAT were investigated to gain insight into the precipitating events.

Thirty young patients with ECG-documented spontaneous-onset PAT were divided into two groups: Group 1 consisted of 22 infants between the ages of 1 day and 7 months who were monitored during continuous ECG recording as inpatients; group 2 consisted of 8 children between the ages of 2 and 14 years with an average of one PAT episode per week who were monitored during continuous ECG recording on an outpatient basis. All were monitored for at least 24 hours, and all underwent transesophageal study to evaluate PAT characteristics.

All 30 patients experienced at least one spontaneous episode of PAT during continuous ECG monitoring. In group 1, from one to more than ten episodes of PAT were recorded, whereas one or two episodes occurred in group 2. Four types of initiating events were observed: atrial extrasystole, ventricular extrasystole, sinus acceleration, and sinus pause with junctional escape. Whereas atrial extrasystole was an initiating event of PAT in both infants and children, sinus acceleration was observed exclusively in infants. Ventricular extrasystole and sinus pause with junctional escape were observed exclusively in the older children. Multiple onsets of PAT were observed exclusively in infants with sinus acceleration. Antiarrhythmic drug therapy may be facilitated if the initiating event of PAT is known in each patient.

▶ The 30 infants and children studied were representative of more general experience in PAT in that most were young infants and almost all had structurally normal hearts. The risk to a small infant of a sustained rapid rate was also borne out in this study, because nine infants were in congestive heart failure. We would have digitalized these infants to control the cardiac failure, and prevent its return by maintenance therapy with digitalis to minimize or prevent recurrence of tachyrhythmia. These investigators stopped medication to carry out this study, designed to capture the onset and offset of tachycardia. The arrhythmia did return, and they did learn about four types of initiating events. They quite sensibly conclude that this knowledge may help in management of children with arrhythmias. The data support the experienced clinician's impression that young infants especially should be maintained with digitalis therapy through their first year to try to prevent recurrences.—M.A. Engle, M.D.

Intravenous and Oral Amiodarone for Arrhythmias in Children
Clifford A. Bucknall, Barry R. Keeton, Paul V.L. Curry, Michael J. Tynan, George R. Sutherland, and David W. Holt (Guy's Hosp., London, and Southampton Gen. Hosp., England)
Br. Heart J. 56:278–284, September 1986   2–43

Amiodarone reportedly is effective in children with cardiac arrhythmias. Adverse effects may be less frequent than in adults. Thirty children with a mean age of 7 years received amiodarone therapy between 1979 and 1984. Other drugs had been ineffective in 29. Nineteen had supraventricular tachycardia, four had atrial flutter, and seven had ventricular tachycardia. Eight patients had congenital structural heart disorders. Five children initially received amiodarone intravenously, but all were treated orally.

Amiodarone given intravenously controlled arrhythmia in all five children treated, two of whom had ventricular tachycardia. Oral treatment suppressed arrhythmia in 28 of the 30 children. It was the only antiarrhythmia agent used in 19 of them, whereas 8 children required digoxin in addition to amiodarone. The mean oral dosage of amiodarone associated with initial suppression of arrhythmia was 10 mg/kg daily, and the mean maintenance dosage was 6 mg/kg daily. Young infants required higher dosages to control arrhythmia. Adverse effects were frequent, particularly photosensitivity. In one child complete heart block developed. Sleep disorder and corneal deposits were also observed. Treatment was withdrawn from five patients because of side effects.

Amiodarone is an effective antiarrhythmia drug for use in children, but only those with resistant, life-threatening arrhythmias should receive it. The oral dosage should be calculated by surface area estimation; more data on plasma concentrations are needed. Particular care is necessary in infants because they require a higher weight-related oral dosage of amiodarone for suppression of arrhythmia.

► Most arrhythmias respond to the common antiarrhythmic agents, but when they do not, one seeks alternative drugs. Amiodarone is one of these. Experience in children is limited, so it is helpful to have this analysis of wanted and unwanted effects in 30 children with atrial or ventricular arrhythmia refractory to therapy. Just as in adults, there is good news and bad news. The good news is that in 19 children the drug as the sole agent effectively controlled the arrhythmia and did so in 9 others in combination with other drugs. Just as is true for infants treated with the familiar drug digoxin, the dose needed on a per kilogram basis was higher for infants than for older children. The bad news is that untoward effects were common and were unrelated to size of dose, blood level, or duration of therapy. Whereas amiodarone offers some promise for children with refractory arrhythmias, we have not yet found the best drug or the best management.—M.A. Engle, M.D.

Doppler Echocardiography in the Diagnosis and Management of Persistent Fetal Arrhythmias

Janette F. Strasburger, James C. Huhta, Robert J. Carpenter, Jr., Arthur Garson, Jr., and Dan G. McNamara (Baylor Univ., Texas Children's Hosp., and St. Luke's Episcopal Hosp., Houston)
J. Am. Coll. Cardiol. 7:1386–1391, June 1986   2–44

Persistent fetal arrhythmias are rare. Although they are life-threatening, they are potentially treatable. Doppler echocardiography was evaluated as a diagnostic aid in the management of 27 fetuses with persistent arrhythmias. Gestational age at the time of diagnosis ranged from 18 weeks to 39 weeks.

All 27 had persistent fetal arrhythmias, defined as an abnormality in cardiac rhythm with a ventricular rate of more than 180/minute or less than 100/minute, or an irregular ventricular rate. Thirteen fetuses were studied by combined noninvasive echocardiography consisting of M-mode, two-dimensional, and pulsed Doppler studies. Data from this group were compared with data obtained from only M-mode and two-dimensional echocardiography in the other 14 fetuses.

Eleven of the 27 fetuses had atrioventricular block, and 6 of these had congenital heart disease; 10 had tachycardia and 6 had atrial premature contractions. These prenatal diagnoses were later confirmed by ECG in 18 surviving infants who had postnatal tachycardia. Although Doppler echocardiography provided correct antenatal diagnostic data in all 13 fetuses in which it was performed, it was not more sensitive than M-mode recording. However, interpretation was much easier to obtain. It also provided additional information about valvular incompetence and the functional state of the fetal heart. Experience with quantitation of Doppler recordings in the fetus is still limited and the technique requires further evaluation.

▶ During a 7-year period, 27 fetal arrhythmias were detected and investigated by echocardiography. Fetal hydrops was a serious consequence of the arrhythmia, because it represented late cardiac failure. Four of five fetuses in the second trimester had fetal hydrops and all four died. Overall, only 18 of the 27 with persistent arrhythmia survived. Clearly, detection of fetal arrhythmia, especially early in the midtrimester, is a serious matter. It is possible to digitalize some mothers and thereby treat fetal atrial tachycardia. If the fetus has complete heart block, however, intrauterine management is limited. This fetus needs frequent monitoring of ventricular rate and function so that the perinatologists can decide on the risks and rewards of premature delivery and treatment of the newborn.—M.A. Engle, M.D.

Maternal Antibodies Against Fetal Cardiac Antigens in Congenital Complete Heart Block

Pamela V. Taylor, James S. Scott, Leon M. Gerlis, Eva Esscher, and Olive Scott (Univ. of Leeds, England, and Univ. Hosp., Uppsala, Sweden)
N. Engl. J. Med. 315:667–672, Sept. 11, 1986   2–45

Previous studies have suggested that there is a strong association between maternal connective tissue disease and congenital complete heart block as a consequence of transplacental passage of antibodies to soluble tissue ribonucleoprotein antigens. A search was made for antibodies directed against fetal cardiac conducting tissue by examining serum samples obtained from women who had given birth to an infant with heart block, as well as samples from normal controls.

Samples were obtained from 41 mothers of infants with congenital complete heart block, 44 mothers of infants with cardiac anomalies other than complete heart block, and 50 mothers of normal infants. In addition, serum samples were collected within 3 months after birth from 8 infants with congenital complete heart block and from 50 normal infants. Fetal heart, liver, kidney, and skin tissue from various sources was also available for examination.

Of the 41 mothers of infants with heart block, 17 had symptoms of connective tissue disease. Twenty-one (51%) had IgG antibody that was reactive with fetal heart tissue, whereas this was the finding in only 9 (10%) of the 94 control mothers. Of the eight samples available from infants with complete heart block, three were positive for the antibody; all control serum samples were negative. In addition, a higher occurrence of antibodies to cytomegalovirus, but not to Epstein-Barr virus, was found in the 41 mothers than in the controls. These data support the concept that maternally derived antibody may often, but not always, be involved in the pathogenesis of congenital complete heart block.

▶ This well-designed study follows a long-standing interest in Uppsala in the natural history of congenital complete heart block. When an unusually high association of maternal lupus and complete heart block in the offspring was recognized first in Virginia and then in other states and in other countries, it was logical to look for maternal antibodies against fetal cardiac antigens. They found a 50% incidence of anti-IgG in the 41 mothers whose infants had heart block, in contrast to 10% in the others. They also found an unexpected elevation of antibody against cytomegalovirus in these mothers that was not present in controls. This suggests to me the possibility of a neoantigen, virus-infected fetal cell against which an antibody develops.—M.A. Engle, M.D.

Hypertrophic Cardiomyopathy

Left Ventricular Diastolic Filling in Children With Hypertrophic Cardiomyopathy: Assessment With Pulsed Doppler Echocardiography
Samuel S. Gidding, A. Rebecca Snider, Albert P. Rocchini, Jane Peters, and Rebecca Farnsworth (C.S. Mott Children's Hosp., Ann Arbor, and Univ. of Michigan)
J. Am. Coll. Cardiol. 8:310–316, August 1986   2–46

Noninvasive studies have suggested abnormal left ventricular (LV) diastolic filling in patients with hypertrophic cardiomyopathy. Doppler pulsed ultrasound studies of LV inflow were performed with simultaneous

M-mode echocardiography and phonocardiography in 17 children and young adults, 10 of whom had hypertrophic cardiomyopathy and 7, a normal heart. None of the study patients had an outflow gradient at rest of more than 16 mm Hg on Doppler study. All had evidence of trivial or mild mitral insufficiency.

Left ventricular systolic and diastolic dimensions were significantly smaller in the patients with cardiomyopathy, and LV posterior wall and septal thickness were significantly greater. Significant prolongation of the isovolumic relaxation time was observed in the patient group. Peak flow velocity during the rapid filling phase was lower in the patient group. Mitral valve Doppler area measurements showed the percent total area in the first third of diastole to be lower in the patients than in the controls.

Diastolic filling is abnormal in these children and young adults with hypertrophic cardiomyopathy who underwent mitral valve Doppler study. This technique is an alternative to M-mode echocardiography for serial assessment of ventricular diastolic function in this setting. The Doppler method is well suited to detecting changes in function with drug treatment.

▶ If a visitor from Mars saw what is being learned from Doppler technology and he chose an unusual condition (e.g., hypertrophic cardiomyopathy) to investigate, he might be a "quick study" and postulate the results that this study found. M-mode echocardiography has since its infancy played a dominant role in diagnosis and in following results of therapy for this condition. The authors suggest that two-dimensional echocardiography with pulsed Doppler ideally fills the need as a method of serial evaluation in patients with hypertrophic cardiomyopathy.—M.A. Engle, M.D.

Development and Progression of Left Ventricular Hypertrophy in Children With Hypertrophic Cardiomyopathy
Barry J. Maron, Paolo Spirito, Yvonne Wesley, and Javier Arce (Natl. Heart, Lung, and Blood Inst., Bethesda)
N. Engl. J. Med. 315:610–614, Sept. 4, 1986   2–47

It is not known whether the magnitude and distribution of left ventricular (LV) hypertrophy in patients with hypertrophic cardiomyopathy are evident at the time of birth or shortly after, or whether hypertrophy develops during the first years of life. An echocardiographic study was conducted in an effort to gain insight into this phenomenon in 39 children aged 4–15 years who had a personal history of hypertrophic cardiomyopathy or a family history of the disorder. Only patients who were followed for at least 2.5 years were included; the mean length of follow-up was 4 years. Two-dimensional echocardiograms were obtained at onset of the study and during follow-up.

Sixteen patients had normal wall thicknesses in all LV segments at initial evaluation, whereas the other 23 patients had increased wall thickness in one to four segments. At the most recent follow-up, 17 patients had no significant change in wall thickness in any LV segment in comparison with the values at their initial evaluation, whereas 22 had a substantial increase in LV wall thickness between evaluations. In the latter group, the anterior ventricular septum was involved in 19 patients, the posterior septum in 10, the anterior free wall in 11, and the posterior free wall in 1. The increases in wall thickness, which exceeded those expected as a consequence of normal growth to a significant degree, were not associated with symptomatic deterioration or subaortic obstruction. Echocardiographic screening should be repeated during adolescence in asymptomatic children who have a family history of hypertrophic cardiomyopathy.

▶ This is the most recent of many studies by Maron and his group on hypertrophic cardiomyopathy. Because there is a strong familial occurrence, his group studied echocardiographically children aged 4 years and older with such a history to see whether and when the hypertrophy begins. They found that 16 of the 39 children were normal on initial examination, but found hypertrophy in some segments in the others and that in all but 1 of these, hypertrophy advanced strikingly between examinations, yet the patients continued asymptomatic. He did not study any children younger than 4 years, so he has not yet answered to his satisfaction the question of whether this process is present at birth.—M.A. Engle, M.D.

Hypertension

Changes in Ponderosity and Blood Pressure in Childhood: The Muscatine Study
William R. Clarke, Robert F. Woolson, and Ronald M. Lauer (Univ. of Iowa)
Am. J. Epidemiol. 124:195–206, August 1986   2–48

Previous studies have shown that blood pressure increases from birth through adolescence, and that there is great variability between children of the same age and sex. Also, ponderosity, an index computed from height and weight, and body size are related to systolic and diastolic blood pressures. A study was conducted in schoolchildren in Muscatine, Iowa, to assess the association between changes in longitudinal blood pressure and ponderosity measurements.

The data were collected during an 11-year period and comprised measurements of 2,925 students (1,530 girls, 1,395 boys) obtained between the ages of 15 and 18 years. All participants were measured at least once in a previous school survey when they were between ages 6 and 15 years. Measurements included height, weight, triceps skinfold thickness, and systolic and diastolic blood pressure.

There was a direct correlation between changes in ponderosity and changes in blood pressure: children whose ponderosity decreased in relation to that of other children of the same age and sex experienced a drop in systolic and diastolic blood pressure, whereas an increase in ponderosity was associated with a similar increase in blood pressure. These changes were independent of a child's initial blood pressure, but were totally related to the degree of ponderosity gain or loss in the child. When lean children are seen with high blood pressure, further investigation is always indicated, because this finding may be a symptom of secondary hypertension.

▶ Two towns came to be household words among pediatricians as the result of research projects directed toward understanding hypertension in the community. These were Bogalusa, Louisiana, and Muscatine, Iowa. This report is one of a series by the Iowa group seeking risk factors, associations, and meaningful indices for prediction of hypertension. Their series of adolescent boys and girls was large and their work was done over an 11-year period. They found a direct correlation between height, weight (ponderosity index), and blood pressure.—M.A. Engle, M.D.

Left Ventricular Structure and Function in Normotensive Adolescents With a Genetic Predisposition to Hypertension
Maria Radice, Claudio Alli, Fausto Avanzini, Marco Di Tullio, Giancarlo Mariotti, Emanuela Taioli, Alessandro Aussino, and Giuseppe Folli (Università di Milano, Italy)
Am. Heart J. 111:115–120, January 1986   2–49

Although the hemodynamic changes that lead to the development of arterial hypertension remain unclear, the heart is believed to play an active role. Support for this suggestion is provided by evidence that strains of rats prone to the development of hypertension have a greater myocardial mass than do control rats before hypertensive levels are recorded. In these rats the early stage of hypertension is represented by a hyperkinetic state consisting of an elevation in cardiac output with normal peripheral vascular resistance. Some studies suggest that similar changes occur in man. To determine whether cardiac involvement precedes or follows the development of hypertension, it is necessary to study normotensive individuals in whom hypertension probably will develop later in life. Differences in cardiac morphology or function were assessed in three groups: normotensive adolescent boys with hypertensive parents, who thereby carry a high risk of becoming hypertensive later in life; normotensive adolescent boys with normotensive parents; and adolescent boys with borderline hypertension.

The study population consisted of 131 males aged 14–19 years; 106 were normotensive and 25 were borderline hypertensive. Among the 106 normotensive males, 51 had at least one hypertensive parent and 55 had parents who were both normotensive. The following morphological parameters were significantly greater in the group with at least one hypertensive parent: interventricular septum (0.54 cm/sq mm vs. 0.49 cm/sq mm; posterior wall thickness (0.54 cm/sq mm vs. 0.50 cm/sq mm); left ventricular mass (125.0 gm/sq mm vs. 109.2 gm/sq mm); and cross-sectional area (9.9 sq cm/sq mm vs. 8.9 sq cm/sq mm). There were no significant differences betwen boys with at least one hypertensive parent and those with borderline hypertension. Excursion of the left ventricular posterior wall was markedly higher in the borderline hypertensive group. However, there were no differences between the males with at least one hypertensive parent and those with normotensive parents.

It seems that the same kinds of change in cardiac morphology are present in normotensive individuals with a family history of hypertension and in those with borderline hypertension. These findings suggest that cardiac involvement may precede elevation in blood pressure.

▶ In order to answer the "chicken and the egg" question of which came first, left ventricular hypertrophy or hypertension, the authors used two-dimensional echocardiography to study sets of adolescent boys with and without borderline hypertension. One group of normotensive boys was considered at risk for the development of hypertension because a parent had high blood pressure. The last group had subtle changes that suggested the answer: cardiac structural changes precede hypertension.—M.A. Engle, M.D.

Hypercholesterolemia

Safety and Efficacy of Long-term Diet and Diet Plus Bile Acid-Binding Resin Cholesterol-Lowering Therapy in 73 Children Heterozygous for Familial Hypercholesterolemia
Charles J. Glueck, Margot J. Mellies, Mark Dine, Tammy Perry, and Peter Laskarzewski (Univ. of Cincinnati)
Pediatrics 78:338–348, August 1986   2–50

Reduction of the plasma cholesterol concentration by diet alone or diet in combination with cholestyramine resin can prevent coronary heart disease. Because there is also evidence that atherosclerosis starts to develop in childhood, the safety and efficacy of a long-term diet with or without bile acid-binding therapy were examined in a group of 73 children who were heterozygous for familial hypercholesterolemia (FH). Thirty-nine normal children not restricted in their diets were followed prospectively as controls.

The 35 boys and 38 girls (69 of them white and 4 black) were aged 3 months to 18 years. Forty were maintained on a low-cholesterol diet alone for an average of 5.8 years; the other 33 were first treated with a low-fat diet alone for about 1 year, after which low doses of bile acid-binding resins were added to the regimen for an average of 4.3 years. All children were tracked for height and weight percentiles throughout the study.

No significant differences in height and weight over time were found during 6 years of follow-up in the 73 FH children when compared with normal controls, or in a comparison of the 40 FH children receiving the diet alone with the 33 FH children receiving the diet plus resin therapy. Whereas 35 of the FH children treated with diet alone had a reduction in total plasma cholesterol level of 9.6% ± 2%, the children receiving the diet plus resin therapy had a mean reduction in total plasma cholesterol concentration of 12.5% ± 2% beyond the effects of diet alone. Although the combination of long-term diet and bile acid-binding resin therapy did not affect normal growth, it did significantly effect a reduction in the total plasma cholesterol level.

▶ The long-term benefits to humankind from this long-term (11 years) study of

73 children with heterozygous inheritance of the rare lipid disorder, hypercholesterolemia, could be that the epidemic of atherosclerosis and coronary artery disease might be terminated. Dr. Glueck is a noted investigator in the field of disorders of lipid metabolism. He reasoned that "the anatomic genesis of atherosclerosis is in childhood." In early life the major risk factors can be identified and perhaps be modified: lipid and lipoprotein abnormalities, obesity, hypertension, and starting to smoke cigarettes. If it could be demonstrated that with proper diet alone, or with diet and a cholesterol-lowering drug, the elevated cholesterol levels in children with FH could be lowered without affecting normal growth and development, that would be a significant first step. This paper shows that this is possible. The second step is to make the diet palatable and the drugs tasteless and affordable. The third step is to make our health-conscious public want to do something to protect their coronaries enough to adopt new feeding habits and to comply with the new lean and active life-style.— M.A. Engle, M.D.

Kawasaki Syndrome

▶ ↓ Kawasaki syndrome is like the new guy on the block for many pediatric cardiologists. Those of us in the States read with interest about this new mucocutaneous lymph node syndrome that Dr. Kawasaki described about 20 years ago, but we didn't really expect to see a case. That attitude has certainly changed. Although in the United States we do not see the thousands of affected children that Japanese physicians do, especially in epidemic years, nonetheless, we are seeing more children with Kawasaki syndrome now than the number of children with rheumatic fever seen at this medical center in the late 1940s and early 1950s when that kind of myocarditis was prevalent. This was also before penicillin treatment of acute β-hemolytic streptococcal pharyngitis became prevalent and the benefit of ongoing penicillin prophylaxis was established. Kawasaki syndrome today is a bit like rheumatic fever in earlier times—a dreaded pancarditis of unknown etiology, uncertain treatment, and as yet impossible prevention. Because the most severe cardiac complication of the syndrome concerns coronary aneurysms, they are the focus of the abstracts that follow.—M.A. Engle, M.D.

Comparison of Macroscopic, Postmortem, Angiographic and Two-Dimensional Echocardiographic Findings of Coronary Aneurysms in Children With Kawasaki Disease

Takako Fujiwara, Hisayoshi Fujiwara, Tadashi Ueda, Kenya Nishioka, and Yoshihiro Hamashima (Kyoto Women's Univ. and Kyoto Univ., Japan)
Am. J. Cardiol. 57:761–764, Apr. 1, 1986   2–51

Kawasaki disease is an acute systemic inflammatory disease with acute angiitis, especially of the coronary arteries. It most commonly affects infants and young children. Usually, 20% of patients with Kawasaki disease have coronary aneurysms. The main cause of death is coronary artery disease as a result of thrombi or organization in the coronary aneurysm.

The two methods that have been used to detect coronary aneurysm in patients with Kawasaki disease are two-dimensional echocardiography (2-D echo) and coronary cineangiography. However, the results of these two studies may differ. A comparison was made of the macroscopic, post-mortem, angiographic, and 2-D echo findings of coronary aneurysm in Kawasaki disease using the hearts of eight affected infants and children obtained at autopsy. Ages ranged from 5 months to 11 years.

Postmortem angiography and 2-D echo yielded similar results in aneurysms in which there was no thrombus, organization, or marked thickening of the arterial wall. However, in aneurysms with complete or incomplete occlusion of the dilated cavity caused by thrombi, organization, or marked thickening of the arterial wall, angiography showed only the free cavity of the coronary aneurysm and not the original aneurysm. On the other hand, 2-D echo revealed an echo-free space representing the original aneurysm in which material suggestive of thrombi or organization was found, but did not disclose whether the aneurysm was occlusive.

The discrepancies between the results of cineangiography and 2-D echo are attributable to the formation of large thrombi, organization, or marked thickening of the arterial wall in the aneurysmal cavity. It is important to recognize these limitations of angiography and 2-D echo.

▶ Coronary arterial abnormality is the chief threat to life in children with Kawasaki syndrome. In addition to aneurysmal dilatation of the origins of the coronary arteries, there may be one or more areas of dilatation more peripherally, as well as areas of stenosis. The advent of two-dimensional echocardiography simplified the detection of proximal aneurysms but, of course, it cannot image more distal involvement. Nonetheless, it has pretty much replaced angiocardiographic studies as a means of identifying the changes in the vessels and in following their course. This article points out the anatomical reasons for discrepancies in echocardiographic and angiocardiographic views and pictures.— M.A. Engle, M.D.

Repeated Quantitative Angiograms in Coronary Arterial Aneurysm in Kawasaki Disease
Hiroyuki Nakano, Ken Ueda, Akihiro Saito, and Keiko Nojima (Shizuoka Children's Hosp., Japan)
Am. J. Cardiol. 56:846–851, Nov. 15, 1985   2–52

Kawasaki disease is an acute febrile illness that predominately affects infants and young children. During the acute stage of illness it produces coronary aneurysms, and sudden death may result from occlusion of the coronary artery. Although more than half of the coronary aneurysms may regress within 1 year after onset, some progress into completely obstructive or markedly stenotic coronary lesions. It is important to assess the condition of the coronary lesions accurately and to observe their natural course carefully, because the morbidity and mortality of Kawasaki disease depend on the extent of associated coronary artery disease. The severity of coronary aneurysms caused by Kawasaki disease was classified using quantitative coronary cineangiography and retrospective follow-up observations.

In all, 138 patients with Kawasaki disease underwent coronary angiography between January 1980 and December 1984 in evaluation of coronary artery involvement. There were 188 angiographic studies available for assessment. Based on these angiograms and retrospective follow-up findings, the coronary aneurysms were quantitatively graded as 0 (normal), with no significant enlargement in any portion of the coronary artery; I (mild), with aneurysmal dilatation of the coronary artery evident but localized, with a maximal diameter of less than 4.0 mm; II (moderate), with a maximal diameter of coronary aneurysms between 4.0 mm and 8.0 mm, regardless of body size; and III (severe), a giant aneurysm with a maximal diameter of more than 8.0 mm. Mild coronary aneurysms usually regressed to normal within a short time and the patient's prognosis was good. However, the course of grade II aneurysms varied, depending on initial angiographic coronary diameter, but all were eventually reduced in size. Conversely, grade III aneurysms usually progressed to become obstructive or stenotic, or the large aneurysm persisted. Follow-up observations demonstrated that the course of coronary artery disease depended on the size and distribution of aneurysms at initial angiography.

This grading of the severity of coronary lesions may provide useful criteria for predicting the prognosis of patients with Kawasaki disease. It is of clinical importance to prevent coronary artery disease; if coronary aneurysms should occur, however, every effort should be make to preclude the development of very large aneurysms.

▶ In a large group of 138 Japanese children with Kawasaki syndrome, angiocardiography was carried out usually within 3 months of onset, but in some the first study was much later and in one instance, 9 years later. Fifty patients who were found to have coronary abnormalities underwent a second study between 3 and 22 months later.

The authors stated that the single most important determinant of the child's prognosis is the size of the aneurysm on initial study, small ones tending to regress. They say that "every effort should be made to preclude the development of very large aneurysms." We all agree, but we do not know for sure how to do this.—M.A. Engle, M.D.

Sensitivity, Specificity, and Predictive Value of Two-Dimensional Echocardiography in Detecting Coronary Artery Aneurysms in Patients With Kawasaki Disease
Thomas E. Capannari, Stephen R. Daniels, Richard A. Meyer, David C. Schwartz, and Samuel Kaplan (Children's Hosp. Med. Ctr., Cincinnati)
J. Am. Coll. Cardiol. 7:355–360, February 1986   2–53

Kawasaki disease is an inflammatory illness of unknown etiology that affects infants and children. It is accompanied by persistent fever, mucocutaneous involvement, and cervical adenopathy. However, the most serious consequence is the formation of coronary artery aneurysms, which may led to coronary thrombosis, stenosis, and eventually myocardial infarction. It has been suggested that aneurysms can be detected noninvasively with two-dimensional echocardiography, but there are few data to support this. Therefore, a prospective study was undertaken to test the sensitivity, specificity, and predictive value of two-dimensional echocardiography in detecting coronary artery aneurysms.

Seventy patients with Kawasaki disease underwent selective coronary arteriography. The study was divided into two periods because of increased experience and the use of a systematic approach with two-dimensional echocardiography in the second period. Aneurysms were observed in 9 of the 70 patients (13%). The coronary artery system was broken up into six regions: the proximal third of the main right coronary artery, distal right coronary artery, left main coronary artery, left anterior descending coronary artery, circumflex coronary artery, and distal left coronary artery. Sensitivity and specificity were high when imaging the proximal regions and improved from the first to the second period. However, both sensitivity and specificity were lower for the more distal regions of the right and left coronary arteries. Overall, the sensitivity of two-dimensional echocardiography was 100% because there were no patients who had isolated distal coronary artery aneurysms. Two-dimensional echocardiography is a sensitive and specific test for detecting aneurysms in the proximal portions of both the right and left coronary arteries and is useful in selecting patients for invasive investigation with selective coronary arteriography.

▶ This excellent study correlates in the same patient the angiocardiographic and echocardiographic images of the coronary arterial abnormalities of this syndrome. It provides a sound basis for the current practice in most pediatric cardiologic centers of following their patients with this syndrome by two-dimensional echocardiography.—M.A. Engle, M.D.

The Treatment of Kawasaki Syndrome With Intravenous Gamma Globulin
Jane W. Newburger, Masato Takahashi, Jane C. Burns, Alexa S. Beiser, Kyung Ja Chung, C. Elise Duffy, Mary P. Glode, Wilbert H. Mason, Venudhar Reddy, Stephen P. Sanders, Stanford T. Shulman, James W. Wiggins, Raquel V. Hicks, David R. Fulton, Alan B. Lewis, Donald Y. M. Leung, Theodore Colton, Fred S. Rosen, and Marian E. Melish (Harvard Univ. and other U.S. universities)
N. Engl. J. Med. 315:341–347, Aug. 7, 1986   2–54

Kawasaki syndrome is an acute childhood illness of unknown origin. In about 15% to 25% of all patients it is associated with the development of coronary artery aneurysms or ectasia, often leading to myocardial infarction, sudden death, or chronic coronary artery insufficiency. To date, conventional treatment has consisted of aspirin administration, but a reduction in incidence of coronary artery abnormalities has not been observed. Findings from a recent Japanese study suggest that gamma globulin, given in high doses intravenously, may prevent coronary abnormalities associated with this syndrome. A multicenter, randomized clinical trial was conducted to compare the efficacy of concomitant gamma globulin and aspirin administration intravenously with the efficacy of aspirin administration alone.

The series included 168 children with Kawasaki syndrome, who were divided into two groups of 84 children each. The first group was given aspirin alone, whereas the second group received gamma globulin, 400 mg/kg intravenously, for 4 days, plus aspirin. All patients were followed with two-dimensional echocardiography.

Two weeks after enrollment, 18 (23%) of 78 children in the aspirin group and 6 (8%) of 75 children in the gamma globulin group had coronary artery abnormalities. After 7 weeks, abnormalities were present in 14 (18%) of 79 children in the aspirin group, but in only 3 (4%) of 79 children in the gamma globulin group. No serious side effects were noted with gamma globulin administration. High-dose gamma globulin administration appears to be safe and effective in the reduction of coronary artery abnormalities associated with Kawasaki syndrome.

▶ Kawasaki syndrome is a condition of unknown etiology, a spontaneous tendency to heal, uncertain management, and impossible prevention. The greatest risk to life is involvement of coronary arteries. This group of collaborative investigators followed the suggestion of a Japanese investigator that gamma globulin in high doses intravenously might reduce the incidence of coronary artery abnormalities. Six centers cooperated in a controlled study, which showed a statistically significant decrease in the number of patients treated with intravenous gamma globulin who had aneurysms in the acute stage, and more regression of aneurysms or ectasia in the subacute stage. If this study is confirmed, it offers the first hope not of preventing the disease, but of preventing the serious component of the illness—abnormality of the coronary arteries.—M.A. Engle, M.D.

3 Heart Disease in Adults

Introduction

In this section of the YEAR BOOK OF CARDIOLOGY, selected articles are reviewed in a variety of areas. In the subsection on valvular disease, a simple new bedside technique for the evaluation of heart murmurs is described; an attempt is made to establish major and minor criteria for the diagnosis of mitral valve prolapse; recent advances in Doppler echocardiography in the evaluation of patients with valve disease are presented; the criteria for surgery in endocarditis of the aortic and tricuspid valves is reviewed; the difficult management of patients with prosthetic valves during pregnancy is discussed; and the status of balloon valvuloplasty of the aortic and mitral valve is updated.

In the subsection on myocardial and pericardial diseases, experimental data are presented that emphasize the potential hazards of treating viral myocarditis with cyclosporine; the history of several patients who had both acquired immunodeficiency syndrome and acute myocarditis is presented; the current status of peripartum heart disease, involvement of the heart in Lyme disease, Chagas disease, and Friedrich's ataxia are each updated in fine papers; the potential reversibility of cardiomyopathy in conditions associated with excess iron storage is further documented; evidence is presented implying that prolonged tachycardia by itself may produce myocardial dysfunction in rare patients; an excellent study documents the benefits of captopril, but not of nifedipine, in patients with heart failure from dilated cardiomyopathy; the ventricular function and natural history of an intriguing group of patients who appear to have localized hypertrophic cardiomyopathy is reviewed; and the natural history and difficult management of recurrent, chronic pericarditis are reviewed.

In the subsection on disturbances of cardiac rhythm and conduction, the very important potential adverse reactions to antiarrhythmic agents are emphasized; the findings of 24-hour ambulatory ECG recordings are presented to establish a baseline of normality; the natural history of lone atrial fibrillation and right bundle branch block is reviewed; the clinically important relationship between hypokalemia and a prolonged QT interval is discussed; the value of electrophysiologic testing in patients at high risk of ventricular arrhythmias is reviewed; the antiarrhythmic value of β-blockers and flecainide are discussed; the hazards of amiodarone are appropriately emphasized; the continued development and usefulness of the implantable defibrillator in selected patients is reviewed; and the promise of the relatively simple technique of signal averaging of late QRS potentials to detect individuals at high risk of ventricular arrhythmias is updated.

In the subsection of miscellaneous papers the influence of varous dietary lipids on serum lipids is reviewed, with the suggestion made that certain monosaturated fats may be as beneficial as polyunsaturated fatty acids; the potential beneficial effects of activated charcoal on serum lipids is discussed; the beneficial effects of plasmapheresis in familial hypercholesterolemia is illustrated; the importance of platelets and the endothelial surface in clinical coronary artery syndromes is demonstrated; the potentials of small amounts of cocaine to produce severe myocardial ischemia, and of radiation to produce myocardial and coronary artery disease many years later, are reviewed; and from Seattle come words of caution regarding strenuous exercise in patients with severe coronary artery disease. The final paper further documents the benefits of weight reduction in overweight patients with hypertension in helping to control the blood pressure and to produce regression of left ventricular hypertrophy.

Robert C. Schlant, M.D.

Valvular Heart Disease

Diagnosis of Left-Sided Regurgitant Murmurs by Transient Arterial Occlusion: A New Maneuver Using Blood Pressure Cuffs

Nicholas J. Lembo, Louis J. Dell'Italia, Michael H. Crawford, and Robert A. O'Rourke (Univ. of Texas at San Antonio and VA Hosp., San Antonio)
Ann. Intern. Med. 105:368–370, September 1986   3–1

The results of transient arterial occlusion were compared with those of isometric handgrip exercise, squatting, and amyl nitrite inhalation in the diagnosis or exclusion of left-sided regurgitant murmurs in 60 patients aged 6–85 years (mean, 47 years). Left-sided regurgitant murmurs were present in 50%. For transient arterial occlusion, a sphygmomanometer was placed around each upper arm with change in murmur recorded. To assess hemodynamic changes, seven additional patients with right and left heart catheterization were evaluated. For the isometric handgrip exercise, a hand dynamometer was used. For the squatting procedure patients were instructed to squat rapidly from a standing position. The amyl nitrite inhalation procedure consisted of breathing 0.3 ml of the gas three times rapidly.

Transient arterial occlusion augmented the intensity of left-sided regurgitant murmurs. This maneuver was more effective than squatting and equalled that of the handgrip exercise and amyl nitrite inhalation (Fig 3–1). Transient arterial occlusion did not intensify any murmurs not caused by left-sided regurgitation. Thus a false positive diagnosis was less likely with this technique. No changes were observed in aortic pressure, right atrial pressure, heart rate, cardiac output, or systemic vascular resistance. The effect of a single hemodynamic alteration, i.e., an acute change in arterial compliance, may explain its success.

Isometric handgrip exercise caused multiple hemodynamic effects and increased afterload. It appeared less useful in changing the intensity of the

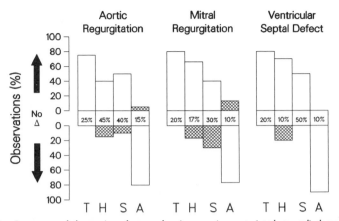

Fig 3–1.—Percentage of observations that noted an increase *(arrow pointed upward)*, decrease *(arrow pointed downward)*, or no change *(no delta)* in murmur intensity of aortic regurgitation, mitral regurgitation, and ventricular septal defect using transient arterial occlusion (T), handgrip exercise (H), squatting (S), and amyl nitrite inhalation (A). *Open bars* indicate expected correct observations; *cross-hatched bars* indicate observations that were opposite to those expected, or incorrect. (Courtesy of Lembo, N.J., et al.: Ann. Intern. Med. 105:368–370, September 1986.)

aortic regurgitation murmur, and by increasing murmur intensity in aortic sclerosis could give a false diagnosis of left-sided regurgitant murmur. The multiple hemodynamic events that take place with squatting appeared to lessen its usefulness in the diagnosis or exclusion of left-sided regurgitant murmurs. It was also observed that many flow murmurs, in addition to left-sided regurgitant murmurs, increased during squatting. Amyl nitrite, which caused a decrease in systemic arterial pressure within 15 seconds, was as effective as arterial occlusion in identifying or excluding left-sided regurgitant murmurs. The advantages of transient arterial occlusion include its ease and speed in diagnosis, with no need for patient participation or vasoactive drug administration.

▶ This simple bedside test appears to be very promising in the safe assessment of heart murmurs. I hope that the technique will be studied extensively under standardized conditions to further document its diagnostic accuracy, perhaps with simultaneous color Doppler studies.—R.C. Schlant, M.D.

New Guidelines for the Clinical Diagnosis of Mitral Valve Prolapse
Joseph K. Perloff, John S. Child, and Jesse E. Edwards (Univ. of California at Los Angeles and United Hosp., St. Paul)
Am. J. Cardiol. 57:1124–1129, May 1986   3–2

Mitral valve prolapse (MVP) usually denotes a connective tissue abnormality of leaflets, anulus, and chordae tendineae. Agreement on standards of definition remain elusive. This is partly because superior displacement of mitral leaflets, generally referred to as mitral valve prolapse, is not necessarily abnormal. An attempt was made to provide information

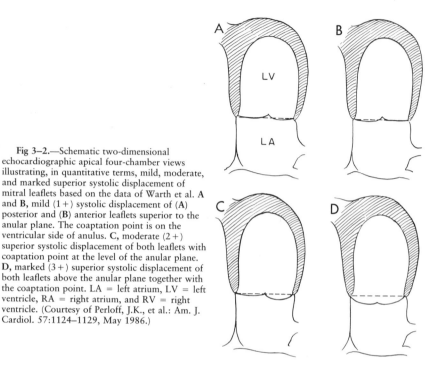

Fig 3–2.—Schematic two-dimensional echocardiographic apical four-chamber views illustrating, in quantitative terms, mild, moderate, and marked superior systolic displacement of mitral leaflets based on the data of Warth et al. **A** and **B,** mild (1 +) systolic displacement of (**A**) posterior and (**B**) anterior leaflets superior to the anular plane. The coaptation point is on the ventricular side of anulus. **C,** moderate (2 +) superior systolic displacement of both leaflets with coaptation point at the level of the anular plane. **D,** marked (3 +) superior systolic displacement of both leaflets above the anular plane together with the coaptation point. LA = left atrium, LV = left ventricle, RA = right atrium, and RV = right ventricle. (Courtesy of Perloff, J.K., et al.: Am. J. Cardiol. 57:1124–1129, May 1986.)

to resolve the dilemma posed by the gray zone between normal and abnormal and to establish new guidelines for the clinical diagnosis of pathologic MVP.

The normal mitral valve leaflets bow or arch upward in systole within the gaussian curve of normal distribution. Displacement becomes abnor-

TABLE 1.—Nonspecific Findings

Symptoms
  "Atypical" chest pain, dyspnea, fatigue, lassitude
    giddiness, dizziness, syncope
  Psychological disturbances
Physical appearance
  Thoracic bony abnormalities
  Hypomastia
Electrocardiogram
  T-wave inversions in inferior limb leads or lateral
    precordial leads
  Premature ventricular beats at rest, on exercise or
    on ambulatory ECG
  Supraventricular tachycardia
X-ray
  Scoliosis, pectus excavatum or carinatum, or loss of
    thoracic kyphosis
Two-dimensional echocardiogram
  Mild superior systolic displacement of anterior or anterior
    and posterior mitral leaflets

(Courtesy of Perloff, J.K., et al.: Am. J. Cardiol. 57:1124–1129, May 1986.)

TABLE 2.—MINOR CRITERIA

Auscultation
    Loud first heart sound with an apical holosystolic murmur
Two-dimensional echocardiogram
    Isolated mild to moderate superior systolic displacement of
        the posterior mitral leaflet
    Moderate superior systolic displacement of both mitral
        leaflets
Echocardiogram plus history
    Mild to moderate superior systolic displacement of mitral
        leaflets with
        Focal neurologic attacks or amaurosis fugax in the young
        First-degree relatives with major criteria

(Courtesy of Perloff, J.K., et al.: Am. J. Cardiol. 57:1124–1129,
May 1986.)

TABLE 3.—MAJOR CRITERIA

Auscultation
    Mid- to late systolic clicks and late systolic murmur
        or whoop alone or in combination at the cardiac apex
Two-dimensional echocardiogram
    Marked superior systolic displacement of mitral leaflets
        with coaptation point at or superior to anular plane
    Mild to moderate supérior systolic displacement of mitral
        leaflets with
        Chordal rupture
        Doppler mitral regurgitation
        Anular dilatation
Echocardiogram plus auscultation
    Mild to moderate superior systolic displacement of mitral
        leaflets with
        Prominent mid to late systolic clicks at the cardiac apex
        Apical late systolic or holosystolic murmur in the young
        Late systolic "whoop"

(Courtesy of Perloff, J.K., et al.: Am. J. Cardiol. 57:1124–1129,
May 1986.)

---

mal or pathologic when it is caused by primary connective tissue disease of the leaflets, chordae tendineae, and anulus, or when it is present in connection with certain developmental diseases of connective tissue or by a secondary response to disorders, e.g., papillary muscle dysfunction or altered left ventricular geometry or cavity size. The fundamental process involved in abnormal leaflet displacement is weakening caused by interruption of the fibrosa because of intrusion of excess elements of the spongiosa layer of the valve. Four morphological features argue for a pathologic process: (1) obviously excessive degrees of prolapse associated with a gelatinous appearance of valve tissue; (2) degrees of MVP that vary distinctly from one segment of the leaflet to the other; (3) fibrosis additive to existing leaflet structure that does not obscure identification of leaflet layers; and (4) the gross secondary extravalvular features and complications of MVP that sometimes occur, especially focal fibrous lesions of the left ventricular mural endocardium caused by friction from the chordae tendineae.

Nonspecific symptoms associated with MVP are listed in Table 1; minor and major criteria are outlined in Tables 2 and 3, respectively. Most of the ECG signs are nonspecific, but they take on new meaning when the diagnosis of MVP is established independently. Chest radiographic signs are also nonspecific. The angiocardiogram can be a major source of diagnostic information, but has given way to the two-dimensional echocardiogram. Gradations from normal to abnormal must be established. Because displacement of the pathologic MVP is superior and systolic, all leaflets that prolapse abnormally must have superior systolic motion. The converse is not the case, however. The gradations of mitral valve displacement, depicted in Figure 3–2, are quantitatively defined in the apical four-chamber view.

Echocardiography has become the reference standard for diagnosing MVP. An abnormal pattern is clear when a mitral leaflet is flail, or when the bellies of either or both leaflets are markedly superior to their anular plane together with the coaptation point. When displacement is only mild or moderate, an unqualified assumption of abnormality cannot be made. Doppler echocardiography can identify mitral valve regurgitation accompanying disruption of leaflet edge coaptation where echocardiography is less sensitive. Arguments applied to the mitral valve apply also to the tricuspid valve. Pathologic anular dilatation, seen in some MVP patients, is defined as more than 2 SD larger than mean normal. Ruptured chordae tendineae are uniformly pathologic. An apical holosystolic murmur with or without a loud first heart sound establishes the diagnosis of mitral regurgitation, whereas the echocardiogram identifies the origin as pathologic MVP.

One or more of the major criteria listed establish the probability of pathologic MVP. Prophylaxis for endocarditis is warranted. Nonspecific features do not provide a basis for the diagnosis of pathologic MVP.

▶ This is a valuable paper. The authors' stated objective is to set the stage for increasing the probability of accurately diagnosing pathologic mitral valve prolapse by consideration of both clinical and echocardiographic criteria, which they divide into nonspecific findings and minor and major criteria. They properly state that such formulations, which increase diagnostic probability, cannot be expected to encompass all observable variations or to eliminate all doubt. It is hoped that the more widespread use of these and other criteria will decrease the too-frequent overdiagnosis of MVP, with all of the attendant hazards of establishing iatrogenic heart disease in patients with minor, "normal" variations. The detrimental effects of a false diagnosis of heart disease in children was shown by Bergman and Stamm (*N. Engl. J. Med.* 276:1008, 1967), and Haynes et al. (*N. Engl. J. Med.* 299:741, 1978) found an increased absenteeism in steelworkers after they were found to have hypertension in a screening program. Retchin et al. (*Arch. Intern. Med.* 146:1081, 1986) recently observed that the finding of MVP in patients referred for echocardiography because of the clinical suspicion of MVP was not associated with greater symptoms or functional disability. They found a surprisingly high rate of functional disability in such patients, whether or not MVP was confirmed by echocardiography. Interestingly, a high rate of functional disability developed during the follow-up period of 1–3 years in both the 75 patients with MVP (43%) and the 83 non-MVP patients (46%). Alpert et al. (*Am. Heart J.* 111:1123, 1986) found that both M-mode and two-dimensional echography had moderately high diagnostic accuracy for the diagnosis of MVP, but concluded that this accuracy was not high enough to support the use of either echo modality as the diagnostic standard for MVP.

Panidis et al. (*J. Am. Coll. Cardiol.* 7:768, 1986) evaluated Doppler echocardiography in 80 patients with MVP and found that mitral regurgitation was common (69%); 20 (36%) of the 55 patients with mitral regurgitation had no detectable systolic murmurs, and all 20 had mild regurgitation by Doppler.—R.C. Schlant, M.D.

Determination of the Stenotic Aortic Valve Area in Adults Using Doppler Echocardiography
Catherine M. Otto, Alan S. Pearlman, Keith A. Comess, Robyn P. Reamer, Carolyn L. Janko, and Lee L. Huntsman (Univ. of Washington)
J. Am. Coll. Cardiol. 7:509–517, March 1986   3–3

It is important to be able clinically to diagnose hemodynamically significant aortic stenosis. Although the results of physical examination may be misleading, aortic stenosis can be excluded with two-dimensional (2-D) echocardiography, which demonstrates normal separation of leaflets. However, patients with severe stenosis cannot be distinguished from those with milder obstruction when separation of leaflets is diminished. Doppler ultrasound permits noninvasive measurement of the velocity of blood flow; in the stenotic valve a laminar high-velocity jet of flow occurs. Four methods of determining the severity of aortic stenosis in adults were evaluated using results at cardiac catheterization as a reference standard. These methods involved the Doppler pressure gradient, aortic valve area as calculated from Doppler and catheterization data, aortic valve area as calculated from Doppler and 2-D echocardiographic data, and a dimensionless index using Doppler data alone.

The severity of aortic stenosis was evaluated by Doppler echocardiography in 48 adults with a mean age of 67 years undergoing cardiac catheterization. The maximal Doppler systolic gradient correlated with the peak-to-peak pressure gradient, and the mean Doppler gradient correlated with the mean pressure gradient by manometry. However, the transvalvular pressure gradient was flow dependent and an association with left ventricular (LV) dysfunction was observed in 33% of these patients. Thus, among 32 patients with an aortic valve area of no more than 1.0 sq cm at catheterization, 6 (19%) had a peak Doppler gradient of less than 50 mm Hg.

To account for the influence of volume flow, the aortic valve area was calculated as stroke volume, measured simultaneously by thermodilution, divided by the Doppler systolic velocity integral in the aortic jet. When aortic valve areas calculated by this method were compared with results at catheterization, it was found that in the subgroup without significant coexisting aortic insufficiency, there was closer agreement of valve area with that found at catheterization.

Transaortic stroke volume can be determined noninvasively by Doppler echocardiographic measures in the LV outflow tract just proximal to the stenotic valve. The aortic valve area can then be calculated as the cross-sectional area of the LV outflow tract times the systolic velocity integral to the flow of the outflow tract, divided by the systolic velocity integral in the aortic jet. When aortic valve areas calculated by this method were compared with results at catheterization, it was found that the noninvasive valve area compared well with valve areas calculated at catheterization. In fact, a simple index, derived as the ratio of the systolic velocity integral in the LV outflow tract to that in the aortic jet, gave better identification of patients with severe stenosis than did the Doppler pressure gradient alone.

These results show that noninvasive calculation of the aortic valve area using Doppler echocardiography is feasible. The simple Doppler ratio may be useful clinically for identifying patients with severe stenosis, particularly when low transaortic flow is suspected.

▶ This study, in which four Doppler echo methods for determining the severity of aortic stenosis were compared, logically demonstrates the superior usefulness of newer Doppler techniques that eliminate the need for an independent examination of cardiac output. The author demonstrates the clinical usefulness of calculations using the continuity equation to estimate aortic valve area and the dimensionless ratio of the systolic velocity integral of flow in the aortic outflow tract to the systolic integral of the aortic jet. Of 32 patients with a valve area of less than 1.0 sq cm, 31 had a dimensionless Doppler ratio of no more than 0.3, including 5 or 6 patients with severe stenosis but a Doppler maximal pressure gardient of less than 50 mm Hg. These newer techniques, in experienced hands, will probably prove to be of great clinical usefulness after they have been more adequately evaluated in larger numbers of patients. Other recent studies of the value of Doppler echocardiography in aortic stenosis have also used the continuity equation (Skjaerpe et al.: *Circulation* 72:810, 1985; Richards et al.: *Circulation* 1986; 73:964) as well as earlier Doppler techniques (Currie et al.: *Circulation* 71:1162, 1985; Smith et al.: *Am. Heart J.* 111:245, 1986; Zoghbi et al.: *Circulation* 73:452, 1986; Ohlsson and Wranne, *J. Am. Coll. Cardiol.* 7:501, 1986; Yeager et al.: *Am. J. Cardiol* 57:644, 1986; and Panidis et al.: *Am. Heart J.* 112:150, 1986).—R.C. Schlant, M.D.

Comparative Accuracy of Two-Dimensional Echocardiography and Doppler Pressure Half-Time Methods in Assessing Severity of Mitral Stenosis in Patients With and Without Prior Commissurotomy
Mikel D. Smith, Rodney Handshoe, Sharon Handshoe, Oi Ling Kwan, and Anthony N. DeMaria (Univ. of Kentucky and VA Med. Ctr., Lexington)
Circulation 73:100–107, January 1986   3–4

It is well established that M-mode echocardiography is useful in detecting mitral stenosis, but this technique is neither sensitive nor specific in estimating actual mitral valve area. On the other hand, two-dimensional (2-D) echocardiography can provide measurements of mitral valve area that correlate well with those obtained by cardiac catheterization and direct surgical examination. An alternative noninvasive approach for estimating mitral valve area is based on Doppler echocardiographic measurement of blood flow velocity across the orifice. This method involves measurement of the interval required for the Doppler-estimated transmitral gradient to fall to half its maximal diastolic value; this is called the pressure half-time. The relative accuracy of these two noninvasive techniques was compared with the accuracy of measurements obtained from cardiac catheterization in 4 consecutive patients with mitral stenosis.

All had 2-D echocardiography before catheterization. In addition, continuous-wave Doppler echocardiographic examinations were carried out in 45 patients. Thirty-seven of the patients had undergone mitral commissurotomy about 11 years previously. The mean valve area as determined at catheterization for the total group of patients ranged from 0.37 to 2.30 sq cm (mean, 1.08 sq cm). Linear regression analysis of data from the 33 patients who had not been operated on previously demonstrated good correlation between the results of 2-D echocardiographic measurements of the mitral valve area at catheterization. Correlation was also good between Doppler measurements of mitral valve area and measurements at catheterization. However, in the 35 patients who had undergone commissurotomy, measurements of Doppler pressure half-time correlated much better with measurements at catheterization than with 2-D echocardiographic estimates. Reproducibility was similar for the two noninvasive methods, with a mean error of 0.14 sq cm for 2-D echocardiographic planimetry and of 0.15 sq cm for Doppler pressure half-time.

Both the 2-D echocardiographic and Doppler pressure half-time methods provide accurate noninvasive estimates of mitral valve area in patients who have not undergone surgery. However, the Doppler pressure half-time is superior to 2-D echocardiography in estimating mitral valve area in those patients with prior commissurotomy.

▶ The superiority of the continuous-wave Doppler technique compared with 2-D echocardiography in patients with mitral stenosis who have undergone prior commissurotomy is probably the result of severe distortion of the mitral orifice caused by fibrosis and calcification, both of which may limit the ability of the echocardiogram to image the valve orifice. Smith et al. (*JAMA* 255:3145, 1986) also reviewed the value and limitations of continuous-wave Doppler echocardiography in estimating the severity of stenosis of each of the cardiac valves.—R.C. Schlant, M.D.

Semiquantitative Grading of Severity of Mitral Regurgitation by Real-Time Two-Dimensional Doppler Flow Imaging Technique
Kunio Miyatake, Shiro Izumi, Mitsunori Okamoto, Naokazu Kinoshita, Hirohiko Asonuma, Hiroshi Nakagawa, Katsuhiro Yamamoto, Makoto Takamiya, Hiroshi Sakakibara, and Yasuharu Nimura (Natl. Cardiovascular Ctr., Suita, Osaka, Japan)
J. Am. Coll. Cardiol. 7:82–88, January 1986   3–5

It is now possible to observe and record the two-dimensional (2-D) aspects of intracardiac blood flow topography in real time using the newly developed real-time 2-D Doppler flow imaging technique. This technique is expected to yield information about valve regurgitation unobtainable using other techniques. An attempt was made to estimate the severity of mitral regurgitation using this new Doppler technique in 109 patients who underwent left ventriculography.

Using Doppler (color-coded) flow imaging techniques, signals caused by blood flow in the cardiac chambers were processed using a high-speed autocorrelation method so that the direction, velocity, and turbulence of the intracardiac blood flow were displayed in the color-coded mode on the monochrome B-mode echocardiogram in real time. The mitral regurgitant flow was imaged as a jet spurting from the mitral valve orifice into the left atrial cavity. The regurgitant jet in the left atrial cavity was seen to have a variety of orientation and dynamic features. The sensitivity of the technique in detection of mitral regurgitation was 86% compared with the sensitivity of left ventriculography. The mitral regurgitation in the false negative cases was usually mild. The severity of regurgitation was graded on a four-point scale on the basis of the farthest distance reached by the regurgitant flow signal from the mitral valve orifice. When these results were compared with those of angiography, a significant correlation ($r = .87$) was found between the two methods in evaluation of the severity of mitral regurgitation. A comparable result was found for the evaluation based on the area covered by regurgitant signals in the left atrial cavity. Noninvasive semiquantitative evaluation by real-time 2-D Doppler (color-coded) flow imaging appears to be a promising clinical technique.

▶ Real-time, 2-D Doppler (color-coded) flow imaging is one of the more promising imaging techniques developed in the past decade. This paper describes methods for semiquantifying Doppler flow imaging by using planimetry to measure the entire depth and breadth of the recipient flow. In experienced hands the technique should prove faster and perhaps be more accurate than other Doppler or nuclear cardiology techniques in the estimation of valvular regurgitation. The technique is also of great value in the assessment of patients with intracardiac shunts. Its application requires greater skill than routine Doppler echocardiography, and the amount of regurgitation can be overestimated or underestimated by subtle gain-setting changes. Unfortunately, it is also very expensive; however, this technique undoubtedly represents a major advance in noninvasive diagnostic imaging.—R.C. Schlant, M.D.

Contribution of Echocardiography and Immediate Surgery to the Management of Severe Aortic Regurgitation From Active Infective Endocarditis

Pinhas Sareli, Herman O. Klein, Colin L. Schamroth, Anthony P. Goldman, Manuel J. Antunes, Wendy A. Pocock, and John B. Barlow (Univ. of The Witwatersrand and Baragwanath Hosp., Johannesburg)
Am. J. Cardiol. 57:413–418, Feb. 15, 1986   3–6

Severe aortic regurgitation associated with left ventricular (LV) failure and infective endocarditis presents a challenge to physicians. Although results of medical therapy are unsatisfactory, surgeons are sometimes reluctant to operate early because of the presence of infected friable tissues and an unstable hemodynamic state. Echocardiography contributes significantly to identification of those patients with severe aortic regurgitation who are at high risk. A systematic approach was developed that comprises immediate echocardiographic evaluation of all patients with a clinical diagnosis of severe aortic regurgitation and LV failure followed by surgery within 24 hours if vegetations are observed on the aortic valve or diastolic closure of the mitral valve is seen.

Thirty-four patients aged 15–60 years with severe aortic regurgitation underwent immediate (within 24 hours of diagnosis) aortic valve surgery. All were in New York Heart Association class IV for LV failure, and 18 had right-sided heart failure. The decision for immediate surgery was based on the echocardiographic demonstration of diastolic closure of the mitral valve or vegetations on the aortic valve. Seventeen patients had premature closure of the mitral valve, and 13 of these have diastolic crossover of LV and left atrial pressure tracings recorded at surgery. Surgery confirmed infective endocarditis of the aortic valve in 29 patients, 27 of whom had vegetations on echocardiography. Both the aortic and mitral valves were replaced in seven patients. Antibiotic therapy was begun immediately after blood was obtained for culture and was continued for 4–6 weeks postoperatively. The mortality rate within 30 days of surgery was 6% overall and 7% for patients with infective endocarditis. The mean follow-up period was about 11 months, and two late deaths occurred. None of the patients had periprosthetic regurgitation or persistence of endocarditis. Procrastination in referral for surgery of these extremely ill patients is not justified and is likely to be associated with higher risks of morbidity and mortality.

▶ It should be emphasized that all of the 34 patients recommended for prompt surgery were in New York Heart Association functional class IV, and that interstitial or frank pulmonary edema was observed in all on chest radiography despite diuretics. The authors believe that aortic valve endocarditis is more benign if no vegetations are detected by echocardiography. This finding, however, can vary significantly with the experience of the echocardiographer as well as the particular instrument and technique used. Unfortunately, it will probably never be possible to conduct a proper study to compare with the author's aggressive approach, in which surgery was performed within 24 hours. I am not convinced that all such patients require surgery so urgently.— R.C. Schlant, M.D.

Right-Sided Valvular Endocarditis: Etiology, Diagnosis, and an Approach to Therapy

Michael J. Robbins, Ruy Soeiro, William H. Frishman, and Joel A. Strom (Albert Einstein College of Medicine, Bronx)
Am. Heart J. 111:128–135, January 1986   3–7

Right-sided valvular endocarditis often develops in intravenous drug abusers. Recently, there has been an increase in the prevalence of isolated right-sided involvement among patients with endocarditis. Among 351 intravenous drug abusers with endocarditis, 54% had disease limited to the tricuspid and pulmonic valves. A review was made of the etiologic and clinical features of the disease, and certain aspects of the treatment of right-sided endocarditis.

Right-sided and left-sided endocarditis are different clinical and experimental entities and they require different clinical approaches. A diagnosis of right-sided endocarditis can be based on a high index of suspicion that is often raised when an intravenous drug abuser is seen with fever, especially when pulmonary infiltrates are detected. In approximately 80% of these patients the disease was confirmed with two-dimensional (2-D) echocardiography. Both prognostic and therapeutic information can be obtained by measuring the echocardiographically visualized vegetation. When growth is less than 1.0 cm in diameter, antibiotic therapy is likely to cure the infection. However, if it is 1.0 cm or more in diameter, there is a frequent lack of response to medical management, perhaps because of the slower metabolic rate of bacterial colonies within these large vegetations. Surgical intervention should be contemplated if fever persists after 3 weeks of antibiotic therapy in a patient in whom 2-D echocardiography reveals a vegetation of 1.0 cm or larger in size. The physician should carefully document adequate levels of antibiotics, and other sources of fever must be excluded prior to surgical intervention.

It is speculated that there may be a role for anticoagulation in these patients to potentiate the effects of antibiotic therapy. However, because left-sided disease clearly contraindicates anticoagulant therapy, left-sided disease must be excluded before anticoagulant therapy is instituted. Persistent pyrexia necessitates surgical intervention in approximately one third of the patients with vegetation that is 1.0 cm or greater in diameter. When initial surgery is performed, the authors currently insert a prosthetic valve and have had no difficulties with recurrent infection or valve dysfunction.

▶ This is a very pertinent review of a condition that has tragically become a frequent occurrence in many hospitals in the United States. The authors properly emphasize that there is no justification at this time, for the use of anticoagulant therapy in this setting in an attempt to minimize vegetation size, although future studies may prove its usefulness. The recommendation for valve replacement in patients with both a vegetation 10 mm or larger in diameter and a persistent fever for at least 3 weeks is in accord with that of most clinicians dealing with these problems.—R.C. Schlant, M.D.

Pregnancy in Patients With Mechanical Prosthetic Heart Valves: Our Experience Regarding 98 Pregnancies in 57 Patients

E. Vitali, F. Donatelli, E. Quaini, G. Groppelli, and A. Pellegrini (Ente Ospedaliero Niguarda Ca'Granda, Milan, Italy)

J. Cardiovasc. Surg. 27:221–227, March–April 1986   3–8

Pregnancy in women with prosthetic heart valves poses several medical and ethical problems. Ninety-eight pregnancies occurred in 57 patients who underwent valve replacement with ball or tilting disk prostheses. All of the patients were in New York Heart Association functional class I or II at conception. No significant changes in functional status were noted during pregnancy. Atrial fibrillation was present in 48 patients. All of the patients were treated with anticoagulant therapy orally at conception. Although different antithromboembolic prophylactic regimens were used, the recommended regimen included coumarin at the time when pregnancy was diagnosed and heparin intravenously 3 weeks before delivery; coumarin therapy was resumed and supplemented with heparin 2 days after delivery.

There were 13 voluntary interruptions of pregnancy and 37 spontaneous abortions. In the 47 live births, two congenital malformations (warfarin syndrome and cleft palate) and four hemorrhagic complications without sequelae were observed. Maternal thromboembolic complications included fatal mitral prosthesis thrombosis in two women and systemic embolization in seven. There was a high risk of complications in the absence of antithromboembolic prophylaxis and the use of subcutaneous heparin alone throughout pregnancy and after delivery or spontaneous abortion. In addition, there was a risk of failure in prophylaxis with intravenous heparin. The use of coumarin was associated with a lower risk of complications. No maternal hemorrhagic complications were observed.

Pregnancy after mechanical valve replacement exposes the mother and the fetus to a high risk of complications. Contraceptive prophylaxis should be strongly advised to these patients during the fertile years. Should pregnancy be desired, coumarin appears to be the most reliable antithromboembolic prophylactic agent.

▶ Overall, a very sobering retrospective review of the consequences of 98 pregnancies in 57 patients with mechanical prosthetic heart valves. In patients with mechanical valves who desire to become pregnant, the authors recommend planned conception and heparin therapy for the first 3 months of pregnancy. In general, the disappointing results in this report further support the use of bioprostheses in such patients and/or contraceptive prophylaxis. Interestingly, 48 of the 57 patients had atrial fibrillation and may have required anticoagulant therapy even if they had a bioprosthesis.—R.C. Schlant, M.D.

Percutaneous Transluminal Valvuloplasty of Acquired Aortic Stenosis in Elderly Patients: An Alternative to Valve Replacement?
Alain Cribier, Nadir Saoudi, Jacques Berland, Thierry Savin, Paulo Rocha, and Brice Letac (Centre Hospitalier et Universitaire and Hôpital Charles Nicolle, Rouen, France)
Lancet 1:63–67, Jan. 11, 1986   3–9

Percutaneous transluminal balloon catheter aortic valvuloplasty (PTAV) was performed in three adults with isolated severe calcific aortic stenosis. All were elderly (aged 68–79 years) and in addition had progressive angina

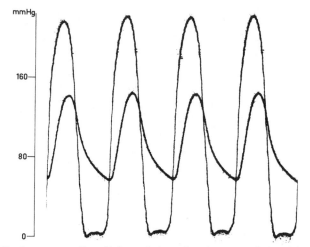

Fig 3–3.—Simultaneous recording of left ventricular and aortic pressures before (left) and at the end of PTAV (right) in a patient with a residual gradient of 40 mm Hg. Transvalvular systolic gradient decreased from 90 to 40 mm Hg. (Courtesy of Cribier, A., et al.: Lancet 1:63–67, Jan. 11, 1986.)

or exertional dyspnea. In one patient PTAV was done as an alternative to surgical valve replacement. The second patient refused surgery and instead accepted PTAV. The third patient also had an acute episode of pulmonary edema and had multiple vessel lesions; PTAV was decided upon as a less risky procedure than surgery.

For the PTAV procedure, 9F balloon catheters designed for dilatation of congenital valve stenosis were used. Three inflations with three balloons 8 mm, 10 mm, and 12 mm in diameter, respectively, were carried out by 10 ml injections of a 50/50 mixture of saline solution and contrast medium.

The immediate results were encouraging because dilatation resulted in a change from severe to moderate aortic stenosis. By the time of completion of the third series of inflations, a pronounced decrease was noted in the ventriculo-aortic systolic pressure gradient; one patient had a residual gradient of 40 mm Hg (Fig 3–3), with 30 mm Hg in the other two. Improvement in the gradient, confirmed by angiography and echocardiography, was the result of better systolic valve opening. The balloon inflations probably resulted in a partial tear of the stenosed valve. Patient tolerance during the inflations was excellent. The inflated balloon was not totally occlusive, perhaps because of the irregular shape of the aortic orifice as the aortic pressure remained satisfactory during the procedure. Findings on follow-up examinations for 9–15 weeks were unremarkable. Additional studies need to be done, but results in these three patients illustrate the feasibility of PTAV as a simple therapeutic alternative to valve replacement when surgery is too risky or impossible.

Percutaneous Mitral Valvuloplasty in an Adult Patient With Calcific Rheumatic Mitral Stenosis

Raymond G. McKay, James E. Lock, John F. Keane, Robert D. Safian, Julian M. Aroesty, and William Grossman (Beth Israel Hosp., Harvard Univ., and Children's Hosp., Boston)
J. Am. Coll. Cardiol. 7:1410–1415, June 1986   3–10

Balloon valvuloplasty has found many uses in younger patients, but its efficacy in older adults with long-standing calcific valve obstruction is uncertain. The method was evaluated in an elderly patient with long-standing rheumatic mitral stenosis.

Man, 75, had right and left heart failure and severe chronic obstructive lung disease. The mean diastolic gradient across the mitral valve was 20 mm Hg, and the calculated mitral valve area was 0.6 sq cm. The Fick cardiac index was 1.6 L/minute/sq m. After transseptal catheterization and balloon dilation of the interatrial septum, a 25-mm valvuloplasty balloon was advanced over a guidewire across the septum and placed across the mitral anulus; inflation at 3 atmospheres of pressure reduced the mean mitral gradient to 12 mm Hg, increasing the cardiac index to 2.5 L. The mitral valve area increased to 1.4 sq cm. Mitral regurgitation increased from 1+ to 2+. Dyspnea decreased postoperatively and exercise tolerance increased. Catheterization 2 months after operation showed reductions in filling pressures and pulmonary vascular resistance and no evidence of restenosis. The pulmonary-systemic flow ratio was 1.8.

The findings indicate that percutaneous valvuloplasty is feasible in the adult with rheumatic mitral stenosis and may lead to significantly improved valve function without producing serious complications. The procedure is not indicated in patients with moderate to severe mitral regurgitation or in those with left atrial thrombus.

Percutaneous Transvenous Balloon Valvotomy in a Patient With Severe Calcific Mitral Stenosis

Igor F. Palacios, James E. Lock, John F. Keane and Peter C. Block (Massachusetts Gen. Hosp., Children's Hosp., and Harvard Univ., Boston)
J. Am. Coll. Cardiol. 7:1416–1419, June 1986   3–11

Percutaneous transvenous balloon mitral valvotomy was performed successfully in a man who had refractory congestive heart failure caused by calcific mitral stenosis.

Man, 57, who had acute rheumatic fever as a child, experienced dyspnea on exertion in 1978. Because of additional major medical problems, cardiac surgery was not considered. Using the transseptal technique, balloon mitral valvotomy was performed. To permit the passage of larger balloon valvotomy catheters to the mitral anulus, dilation of the interatrial septum was done, using an 8-mm balloon catheter. The procedure was completed in 2 hours, and the patient tolerated it well with minimal discomfort. No significant mitral regurgitation resulted. Within 48 hours the patient was transferred from the intensive care unit to a ward bed.

Hemodynamic measurements improved after this procedure. The prevalvotomy left atrial diastolic mean pressure of 38 mm Hg decreased to 19 mm Hg, and the corresponding left ventricular diastolic mean pressure decreased from 18 mm Hg to 15 mm Hg. The mean diastolic gradient across the mitral valve decreased from 20 mm Hg to 4 mm Hg. Cardiac output increased to 5.7 L/minute from 3.4 L/minute. The mitral valve area increased from 0.7 sq cm to 2.5 sq cm. The mean pulmonary artery pressure dropped to 40 mm Hg.

This procedure may be preferred or may even represent the only alternative for patients with incapacitating symptoms caused by a stenotic, calcified, mitral valve who cannot undergo cardiac surgery. Advantages of this technique include the possibility of decreasing morbidity, shortening hospital stay, and reducing costs. If safety and effectiveness are established, this technique may have particular importance for application in those countries in which rheumatic heart disease is common.

▶ These three papers (3–9 to 3–11) are important landmarks in the further experimental application of balloon valvuloplasty to the treatment of selected patients with aortic and mitral stenosis. To date, the results are better than might have been predicted from earlier attempts at digital or instrumental dilatation at surgery. Not only have the pressure differences across the stenotic valves been decreased, but there has been an unexpectedly low incidence of valvular regurgitation and peripheral embolus. Previous reports have indicated the value of the technique in the treatment of patients with congenital pulmonary valve stenosis (Kan, J. S., et al.: *N. Engl. J. Med.* 370:540, 1982; Pepine, C. J., et al.: *Am. J. Cardiol.* 50:1442, 1982); patients with coarctation of the aorta (Singer, M. I., et al.: *Am. Heart J.* 103:131, 1982); in 23 patients aged 2–17 years with valvular aortic stenosis (Lababidi, Z., et al.: *Am. J. Cardiol.* 53:194, 1984); and in patients with mitral stenosis (Babic, U. U., et al.: *Am. J. Cardiol.* 57:1101, 1986).

We must await additional studies that will determine the subsets of patients most likely to benefit from the procedure with the fewest adverse effects. One wonders whether or not it might be more successful in patients without extensive calcification.—R.C. Schlant, M.D.

Myocardial Disease

The Effects of Cyclosporine on Acute Murine Coxsackie B3 Myocarditis
John B. O'Connell, Elizabeth A. Reap, and John A. Robinson (Loyola Univ., Maywood, Ill.)
Circulation 73:353–359, February 1986   3–12

Cyclosporine adequately controls rejection in allotransplantation by suppressing T helper lymphocyte interleukin-2 production. In viral infections, the timing of immunosuppression is critical; any inflammatory reaction is to be modified without production of overwhelming viral dissemination. It is thought that immunopathologic mechanisms that culminate in a chronic dilated cardiomyopathy are set in motion during acute viral myocarditis. Coxsackievirus B3 is cardiotropic, leading to cell mediated toxicity toward myocardial cells. Initially, there is minimal inflammation and necrosis. After viral clearance, a smoldering inflammatory reaction, myocyte necrosis, and clinical emergence of congestive heart failure occurs. The effects of cyclosporine given at various times after viral infection with coxsackievirus B3 were studied in mice.

Seven days after infection, untreated mice had survived with sporadic clinical evidence of viral infection, e.g., coat ruffling. Mild-to-moderate mononuclear cell infiltration and necrosis occurred. Infected mice treated with cyclosporine from the day of infection had a 75% mortality at day 7. All had gross evidence of viral infection, and histologic examination revealed myocyte necrosis but no inflammation. Fourteen days after infection, untreated mice had necrosis and inflammation similar to that seen at 7 days. Of 16 mice in which cyclosporine was begun 7 days after infection, 55% were dead by day 14; most deaths occurred within 72 hours of the start of the drug. Inflammation in these mice was similar to that in mice in which treatment was started on day 0, but the necrosis score was higher. When the same experiments were performed on another strain of mice, mortality rates were not as high, but necrosis was more severe in cyclosporine-treated animals. Cultures showed virus in all cyclosporine-treated mice, but not in infected, untreated mice at 7 days or 14 days.

Systemic viral infections can commonly lead to myocarditis, especially those with coxsackievirus B3. It is possible that dilated cardiomyopathy is an immunologic sequel to such viral infection. The prognosis in dilated cardiomyopathy is poor, with a 50% mortality within 2 years. This animal model shows progression from viral infection to myocardial hypertrophy and fibrosis with coxsackievirus B3 infection. After the virus is cleared from the body, a chronic inflammatory reaction ensues, resulting in progressive myocyte damage, hypertrophy, ventricular dilatation, and heart failure within 1–2 years after infection in mice. Administration of cyclosporine in this study appeared to interfere with normal virus clearance after infection, and to increase mortality and necrosis while inhibiting the inflammatory response. The use of cyclosporine may also promote antigen persistence or interfere with antigen clearance, enhancing myocardial destruction. The precise timing of cyclosporine administration may be critical. Further studies are needed to examine the effects of the drug when given in the established chronic phase, when all virus had disappeared from the body. Clearly, the drug is hazardous if given during the acute viral phase.

▶ This paper is important because it demonstrates that cyclosporine, given to mice either concurrently with coxsackievirus B3 or 1 week later, results in an increase in myocardial mortality and necrosis, possibly secondary to enhanced viral survival. Monrad et al. (*Circulation* 73:1058, 1986) reported similar findings in mice infected with encephalomyocarditis (EMC) virus and treated with cyclosporine. They also found greater myocardial failure when cyclosporine was administered during the early recovery period. It would appear to be very important that all trials of cyclosporine or other immunosuppressive therapy for viral myocarditis are conducted with great caution and only as part of a well-designed and controlled clinical trial.—R.C. Schlant, M.D.

Congestive Cardiomyopathy in Association With the Acquired Immuno-deficiency Syndrome

Ira S. Cohen, David W. Anderson, Renu Virmani, Bernard M. Reen, Abe M. Macher, Joel Sennesh, Paul DiLorenzo, and Robert R. Redfield (Walter Reed Army Med. Ctr., Armed Forces Inst. of Pathology, Walter Reed Army Inst. of Res., Washington, D.C., Fairfax Hosp., Falls Church, Va., and Uniformed Services Univ. of the Health Sciences, Bethesda)
N. Engl. J. Med. 315:628–630, Sept. 4, 1986   3–13

Fatal acquired immunodeficiency syndrome (AIDS) occurred in three patients with clinical, echocardiographic, and morphological findings of dilated cardiomyopathy in the absence of Kaposi's sarcoma. In each case, recurrent opportunistic infection was present for more than 6 months prior to the fatal acute cardiac illness that became evident clinically 4–8 weeks before death.

Pronounced four-chamber dilatation was present at postmortem ex-

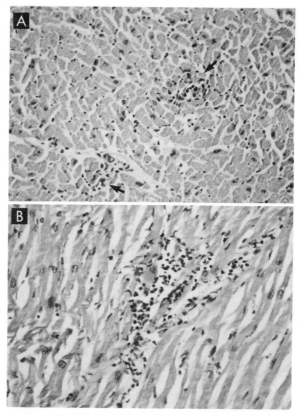

Fig 3–4.—Focal myocarditis (**A**), *(arrows* ×86) and focal lymphocytic infiltrate with myocyte necrosis (**B**) (x180) in patient 1. (Hematoxylin and eosin.) (Courtesy of Cohen, I.S., et al.: N. Engl. J. Med. 315:628–630, Sept. 4, 1986. Reprinted by permission of The New England Journal of Medicine.)

amination in two patients. Focal myocarditis and focal inflammatory infiltrates consisting mostly of lymphocytes and histiocytes with myocyte necrosis were observed as isolated findings in three of four histologic sections obtained from one patient (Fig 3–4). Each patient had a negative history regarding cardiotoxin exposure. All were cachectic at death. Even though multivitamin therapy was administered orally throughout the clinical course, vitamin deficiency could not be excluded entirely as an etiologic factor.

Autopsy findings in two patients of generalized cardiomyopathy with focal lymphocytic myocarditis in the absence of evidence of bacterial or parasitic infection suggested a viral pathogenesis. Cytomegalovirus and Epstein-Barr virus may cause myocardial damage in AIDS patients. Also, the possibility of primary human immunodeficiency virus-induced myocardial damage cannot be ruled out. In view of the severe T and B cell deficiency associated with AIDS, the myocarditis and dilated cardiomyopathy present in two patients raises the possibility that appreciable myocyte damage and myocardial dysfunction may occur as a result of a primary, nonimmune process as well. As a complication of AIDS, clinical and subclinical cardiac dysfunction should be considered in patient evaluation.

▶ It was almost bound to occur: Infection with human immunodeficiency virus (or human T cell lymphotropic virus type III/lymphadenopathy virus), which results in global immune dysfunction, appears to have been a major predisposing condition for rapidly fatal cardiac illness in the three patients described in this report. Although not completely documented, the clinical course and microscopic findings in the two patients who were autopsied make it likely that these patients died of viral myocarditis. Unfortunately, more will probably follow.—R.C. Schlant, M.D.

Peripartum Cardiomyopathy: Clinical, Hemodynamic, Histologic and Prognostic Characteristics
John B. O'Connell, Maria Rosa Costanzo-Nordin, Ramiah Subramanian, John A. Robinson, Diane E. Wallis, Patrick J. Scanlon, and Rolf M. Gunnar (Loyola Univ., Maywood, Ill.)
J. Am. Coll. Cardiol. 8:52–56, July 1986   3–14

Peripartum cardiomyopathy is defined as the onset of left ventricular dilation and congestive heart failure occurring either during the third trimester of pregnancy or in the first 6 postpartum months. This relatively rare syndrome had been thought to be more common in patients older than age 30 years, in multiparous or eclamptic patients, and in twin gestations. Hypertension, myocarditis, and nutritional or dietary deficiencies are factors that have been implicated as possible causes, but the etiology remains controversial. Is the condition a specific disease of heart muscle, or is the presentation of congestive heart failure in the peripartal period simply the initial presentation of latent idiopathic dilated cardiomyopathy?

To clarify these points and further characterize the syndrome, peripartum cardiomyopathy was examined in a middle class population of 14 patients and findings compared with those in a nonselected group of patients with idiopathic dilated cardiomyopathy.

In the 14 study patients the risk factors for development of coronary or myocardial disease was unusual. One was a cigarette smoker, two were diabetic, and none admitted to regular alcohol use. Gestational hypertension was found in four of the women, and a viral prodrome before onset of heart failure was noted in two. Eight women sustained heart failure with their first pregnancy, but three had one or more previous pregnancies without problems. Three infants were premature, and six women (43%) required cesarean section. Heart failure occurred in two in connection with twin gestation. In eight patients the initial presentation of cardiac disease occurred before delivery; in three patients it was seen in the first postpartum week. In the remaining three patients heart failure developed within 2–8 weeks post partum. All infants were normal. Six of the patients (43%) with the peripartum cardiomyopathy group were younger than age 30 years, compared with only five patients (9%) with idiopathic dilated cardiomyopathy. The duration of symptoms was shorter in the study group. Complex ventricular arrhythmias and wall motion abnormalities were common in both groups. Endomyocardial biopsy specimens showed myocyte hypertrophy, nuclear hyperchromaticity, and interstitial fibrosis in both groups. Active myocarditis was noted in 29% of study patients but in only 9% of those with idiopathic dilated cardiomyopathy.

Treatment for the study group was standard medical therapy for congestive heart failure, restriction of activity, and treatment with anticoagulants. Only one patient with myocarditis received immunosuppressive therapy. Six study patients died during follow-up, but seven improved dramatically with resolution of clinical symptoms, discontinuation of cardiotonic medication, and normalization of cardiac function. Two patients with active myocarditis died. Survivors had higher ejection fractions and smaller left ventricular end-diastolic dimensions.

The incidence of myocarditis was more frequent in the study patients. Myocarditis may play an early role in the development of peripartum cardiomyopathy and may be missed if biopsy is not performed until later. The prognosis for peripartum cardiomyopathy is different from that of idiopathic dilated cardiomyopathy in that patients either improved dramatically within 6 weeks or died. Because dietary and nutritional factors were probably not involved, other factors must be considered. Pregnancy may predispose women to a more severe form of viral myocarditis when they are infected by a cardiotropic virus. After delivery, immunologic function begins to normalize, which may enhance viral clearance and account for the rapid lessening of symptoms and hemodynamic abnormalities. Although this study has not defined peripartum cardiomyopathy as an entity distinct from idiopathic dilated cardiomyopathy, there are features specific to both syndromes. The previously reported risk factors may no longer be valid. After early institution of medical management, if further clinical deterioration is evident, early cardiac transplantation should be considered.

► In this study of peripartum heart disease, 4 of 14 patients (29%) had histologic evidence of myocarditis. Sanderson et al. (*Br. Heart J.* 56:285, 1986) also found evidence of myocarditis in 5 of 11 African women in Nairobi. It is possible that the patients in both series were infected with a cardiotropic virus during their pregnancy, although this was not documented, nor has our knowledge about the relationships between pregnancy and the immune system suggested whether or not the association is likely to be more than coincidental.—R.C. Schlant, M.D.

Cardiac Involvement in Lyme Disease: Manifestations and Management
Lyle J. Olson, Emmanuel C. Okafor, and Ian P. Clements (Mayo Clinic and Found.)
Mayo Clin. Proc. 61:745–749, September 1986   3–15

Lyme disease is caused by a *Treponema*-like spirochete, *Borrelia burgdorferi*, carried by the tick *Ixodes dammini*. The condition was originally described in residents of Lyme, Connecticut, but it is now known to occur nationwide. Lyme disease with cardiac involvement was diagnosed in a woman referred because of complete heart block.

Woman, 28, with no previous history of heart diseases, was seen for complete heart block. Four days earlier she noticed a pruritic, erythematous, vesicular rash behind the left knee. The joint became painful and stiff within days. Fever, malaise, myalgia, headache, stiff neck, photophobia, and paresthesia of the right arm also developed. In a local emergency room a 10-day oral course of erythromycin was prescribed, and the symptoms resolved within days. Two weeks later the patient had aching pain in the right parasternal region and severe dyspnea on exertion. When she was seen, her heart rate was 55 beats per minute, blood pressure was 80/50, and an ECG showed complete heart block. A palpable, nontender cervical lymph node was found, and a 20-cm, erythematous lesion with central clearing was seen behind the left knee. A chest x-ray film showed no cardiac enlargement, and clear lungs. Phenoxymethyl penicillin was started for presumed Lyme carditis. Within 24 hours the rash on the leg disappeared, and within 48 hours the patient felt completely well. Serial ECGs showed 2:1 atrioventricular block, followed by first-degree atrioventricular conduction delay, and then normal rhythm by hospital day 6. Serum antibodies to *B. burgdorferi* were found, which were considered to be diagnostic of Lyme disease. The patient was dismissed on the sixth hospital day taking a course of penicillin. At follow-up, she was asymptomatic and had a normal ECG.

Remissions and different clinical manifestations occur at each of the three stages of Lyme disease. Stage 1 is characterized by erythema chronicum migrans and nonspecific constitutional symptoms. Stage 2 can occur weeks or months later and includes cardiac and neurologic abnormalities. Stage 3, typified by arthritis, occurs in about 60% of the patients and may occur weeks to years after stage 1. The incidence of cardiac involvement in patients with Lyme disease is estimated at 8%. Fluctuating degrees of atrioventricular block have been described previously, with narrow QRS complexes suggesting a block proximal to the bundle of His. The patients in this series were treated with prednisone and aspirin. However, prednisone required 3–4 months of therapy because of recurrent neurologic or joint involvement when the dosage was tapered. Although antibiotic therapy was given to several patients, it did not appear significantly to shorten the duration of cardiac involvement. Electrocardiograms return to normal in days to weeks after appropriate treatment.

Reversible ECG and radionuclide abnormalities are attributed to myopericarditis. Cardiac involvement in Lyme disease can be clinically occult and fatal. Erythema chronicum migrans is the best clinical marker for Lyme disease, but it is not seen in every case. Acute rheumatic fever, Rocky Mountain spotted fever, and *Yersinia enterocolitica* infection may be confused with Lyme disease with cardiac involvement. However, complete heart block is unusual in these other diseases. Serologic testing may be helpful in the diagnosis of Lyme disease. Antibiotic therapy is recommended for all patients with Lyme disease to reduce the incidence and decrease the duration of neurologic or joint involvement. Tetracycline, penicillin, or erythromycin is appropriate. Parenteral administration of penicillin is most effective for active neurologic or joint involvement. Corticosteroids and salicylates can also be used in Lyme carditis when high-degree atrioventricular block, P-R prolongation of more than 0.30 second, or cardiomegaly develops.

▶ This disease, which was first described in 1977 in the city of Lyme, Connecticut, is now thought to be endemic to Minnesota and Wisconsin, as well as the coastal northeastern and northwestern United States. The responsible spirochete is usually spread by tick bite between May and October. The heart block can be severe and may require temporary transvenous cardiac pacing. In addition to heart block, others have reported pericarditis and severe, even fatal, myocarditis. Interestingly, the cardiac valves appear to be spared.—R.C. Schlant, M.D.

Abnormal Left Ventricular Diastolic Function in Chronic Chagas' Disease: An Echocardiographic Study
Tomás Caeiro, Luis M. Amuchastegui, Eduardo Moreyra, and Derek G. Gibson (Hosp. Privado, Cordoba, Argentina, and Brompton Hosp., London)
Int. J. Cardiol. 9:417–424, December 1985   3–16

A major feature of chronic Chagas' disease is left ventricular (LV) involvement. At an early stage, contrast angiography reveals anteroapical involvement, often followed by generalized cavity dilatation. It is possible that the overall effect on LV function might be similar to that of chronic coronary artery disease. However, it was noted that incoordinate relaxation, so characteristic of the latter condition, was absent in patients with Chagas' disease despite the obvious segmental abnormalities of function. Because incoordinate relaxation can also be detected echocardiographically, an attempt was made to use this method to investigate diastolic LV function in detail in patients with Chagas' disease.

To investigate systolic and diastolic LV function, simultaneous M-mode echocardiograms and phonocardiograms were recorded in 19 patients with chronic Chagas' disease; these were then digitized and compared with normal. Five patients were in New York Heart Association class I, nine in class II, and five in class III. The LV cavity dimensions were increased in three patients and the shortening fraction was reduced in one. The peak velocity of circumferential fiber shortening was below the 95% confidence limit of normal in nine. In contrast to previous echocardiographic studies, diastolic abnormalities were common, with prolongation of isovolumic relaxation time in 9 patients and a reduced rate of dimension increase in 11. Nevertheless, despite regional disease, documented angiographically in five of six patients, there was no evidence of asynchronous wall motion during relaxation as noted in patients with coronary artery disease and comparable segmental abnormalities of wall motion. The relative timing of aortic valve closure and minimum cavity dimension was normal in all but three patients, and a significant dimension change occurred during isovolumic relaxation in only one. Diastolic disturbances are common at all stages of Chagas' disease and may represent a fundamental aspect of the pathologic process as it affects the left ventricle.

▶ The findings that patients with Chagas' disease have a striking reduction in the peak rate of LV dimension filling and prolongation of the early diastolic period of rapid filling suggest that Chagas' disease may produce early changes in LV diastolic function. These diastolic abnormalities may contribute significantly to the functional disability of patients with this condition. This is another recent example of the current special interest in diastole. Brecher would be pleased.—R.C. Schlant, M.D.

Cardiac Involvement in Friedreich's Ataxia: A Clinical Study of 75 Patients
John S. Child, Joseph K. Perloff, Philip M. Bach, Allan D. Wolfe, Susan Perlman, and R. A. Pieter Kark (Ataxia Ctr., Reed Neurologic Res. Ctr. and Jerry Lewis Neuromuscular Inst., and Univ. of Calif. at Los Angeles)
J. Am. Coll. Cardiol. 7:1370–1378, June 1986   3–17

To establish the prevalence and to characterize the types of involvement of the heart, 39 males and 36 females aged 10–66 years (mean, 24 years) with classic Friedreich's ataxia were studied prospectively. Electrocardiograms were performed in all 75 patients, vectorcardiograms in 34, and echocardiograms in 58.

Both ECG and vectorcardiographic abnormalities were observed in 69 patients (92%). The ECGs revealed ST-T wave abnormalities in 79%, right axis deviation in 40%, short PR interval in 24%, abnormal R waves in lead V_1 in 20%, abnormal inferolateral Q waves in 14%, and left ventricular (LV) hypertrophy in 16%. The M-mode echocardiograms were reviewed in 57 (77%) patients, 47 of whom were also studied by two-dimensional echocardiography. Concentric LV hypertrophy was revealed in 11%, asymmetric septal hypertrophy in 9%, and globally decreased LV function in 7%. The ECG and echocardiographic findings in LV hypertrophy were compared. Five of six patients with concentric LV hypertrophy on echocardiography had ECG-observed hypertrophy. All patients with hypertrophy seen on echocardiography had ST-T wave abnormalities seen on ECG.

Overall, 95% of the patients had at least one cardiac abnormality. Two patients died, and necropsy revealed a minimally dilated but flabby left ventricle in both.

In general, there appeared to be two fundamentally different types of cardiac disease: a common "dystrophic" form manifested by ECG initial force deformities without detectable echographic wall motion abnormalities, but occasionally extension throughout the left ventricle with global hypokinesia and reduced QRS voltage; and a hypertrophic form represented by symmetric or asymmetric LV hypertrophy with normal cavity size and ventricular function. That Friedreich's ataxia, a phenotypically homogeneous neuropathic disorder, expressed itself as two basically different types of cardiac disease, and that a nonmyopathic systemic disorder afflicted the myocardium, are puzzling observations.

▶ Virtually all patients with Friedreich's ataxia have occult, asymptomatic involvement of the heart that produces ECG abnormalities. Ultimately, it may progress and become the cause of death. In the authors' patient series, which is one of the largest studied systematically and nonselectively, hypertrophic cardiomyopathy was less frequent than in other series, some of which may have been more selective. The 7% of patients with "dystrophic" cardiomyopathy did not meet criteria for dilated cardiomyopathy and were not thought to be the end result of hypertrophic cardiomyopathy, but rather a fundamentally different type of cardiac involvement. This study raises the possibility of ultimately subclassifying patients with Friedreich's ataxia on the basis of their cardiac abnormalities and ultimately, different genetic biochemical abnormalities. Alboliras et al. (*Am. J. Cardiol.* 58:518, 1986) also found a wide spectrum of cardiac abnormalities in 22 patients with Friedreich's ataxia studied at the Mayo Clinic. Casazza et al. (*Br. Heart J.* 55:400, 1986) reported no beneficial effects of verapamil therapy for a mean of 8 months in nine patients with ventricular hypertrophy in Friedreich's ataxia.—R.C. Schlant, M.D.

Tachycardia-Induced Cardiomyopathy: A Reversible Form of Left Ventricular Dysfunction
Douglas L. Packer, Gust H. Bardy, Seth J. Worley, Mark S. Smith, Frederick R. Cobb, R. Edward Coleman, John J. Gallagher, and Lawrence D. German (Duke Univ.)
Am. J. Cardiol. 57:563–570, March 1, 1986   3–18

The effect of acute tachycardia on left ventricular (LV) function in patients with paroxysmal supraventricular arrhythmias has been well documented. With the abrupt increase in heart rate, the right and left atrial pressures increase and end-diastolic volume and stroke volume decrease. The cardiac output may either increase or decrease depending on the degree to which the decrease in stroke volume is offset by the increase in heart rate. When tachycardia is terminated, stroke and end-diastolic volumes quickly return to normal, atrial pressures return to baseline, and a post-tachycardia diuresis may ensue. In contrast, the effect of chronic tachycardia on otherwise normal myocardium is not well established. An attempt was made to determine if there is a relationship between chronic supraventricular tachycardia and LV dysfunction.

The study population consisted of eight patients aged 5–57 years. Uncontrolled symptomatic tachycardia had been present for 2.5–41 years as well as significant LV dysfunction in the absence of other apparent underlying cardiac disease. Seven patients had incessant tachycardia for 0.5–6.0 years; one had ectopic atrial tachycardia, and seven had an accessory atrioventricular pathway that participated in reciprocating tachycardia. Surgery was carried out on six patients; the ectopic focus was ablated in one, and an accessory pathway was divided in five. In addition, one patient underwent open ablation of the His bundle, and one underwent closed chest ablation of the atrioventricular conduction system. Although myocardial biopsy specimens were obtained from five patients, none suggested a specific diagnosis. Pretreatment radionuclide angiography revealed a mean ejection fraction (EF) of 19%. After tachycardia control substantial improvement in LV function was observed in six of eight patients at rest and in one additional patient during exercise. The mean EF increased to 33% within an average of 8 days after treatment and was 45% at late follow-up 17 months later. Seven patients remained asymptomatic 11–40 months after the corrective procedure was carried out. Chronic uncontrolled tachycardia may result in significant LV dysfunction that is reversible in some cases after control of the arrhythmia.

▶ This report found that only 3% of patients referred with supraventricular tachycardia refractory to conventional medical therapy had ventricular dysfunction without apparent underlying heart disease. The pathophysiology of the decreased function, which the authors note has also been reported by others, is unknown but may be related to depletion of high-energy phosphates. Additional prospective studies are desirable to confirm these intriguing findings.—R.C. Schlant, M.D.

Afterload Reduction: A Comparison of Captopril and Nifedipine in Dilated Cardiomyopathy

Pier G. Agostoni, Nicoletta DeCesare, Elisabetta Doria, Alvise Polese, Gloria Tamborini, and Maurizio D. Guazzi (Istituto di Cardiologia, Centro di Studio Ricerche Cardiovascolari del Consiglio Nazionale delle Ricerche, Univ. of Milan; and Fondazione "I. Monzino" and Istituto Ricerche Cardiovascolari "G. Sisini," Milan)

Br. Heart J. 55:391–399, April 1986   3–19

Nifedipine, 20 mg three times daily, and captopril, 50 mg three times daily, were added to an optimal regimen of digitalis and diuretics in a 16-

week, double-blind, randomized, crossover trial of 18 patients who had dilated cardiomyopathy. The peak response to both drugs occurred about 1.5 hours after administration. The mean exercise tolerance times and functional class during captopril treatment were significantly higher than baseline values or values with nifedipine therapy (Fig 3–5). In short-term usage, the systemic vascular resistance was consistently reduced during nifedipine treatment, cardiac output was raised, and the left ventricular (LV) filling pressure tended to fall. During prolonged treatment, however, cardiac output did not improve and the pulmonary capillary wedge pressure rose, even though the vasodilating action persisted. Changes in systemic vascular resistance after prolonged administration of capropril resembled those produced by nifedipine, but captopril improved LV performance, which may have been partially responsible for the increased functional capacity indicated by the reduced pulmonary capillary wedge pressure and increased cardiac output. The heart rate was increased during nifedipine therapy and reduced when captopril was given. Captopril treatment was associated with increased stroke index. The dimensions of the ventricular cavity were reduced by captopril therapy and increased by nifedipine; only captopril decreased the afterload (wall stress). The force-length relationship between LV end-systolic stress and end-systolic diameter was shifted to the left of baseline by captopril and to the right by nifedipine, suggesting a reduction in muscle contractility by nifedipine.

There were no dropouts as a result of side effects. Nifedipine caused headache in 5, palpitations in 11, increased body weight in 12, and enhancement of dependent edema in 11. Nifedipine also reduced the mean serum potassium concentration. Two patients taking captopril complained

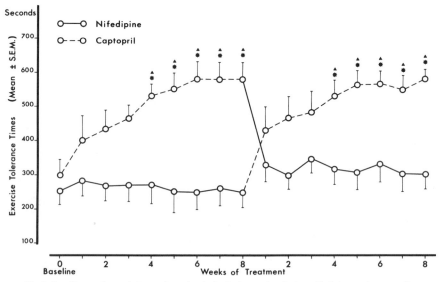

Fig 3–5.—Comparison of times of maximal physical capacity during nifedipine and captopril treatments. *Value significantly different from baseline value ($P < .01$); *Black triangle* is value significantly different from nifedipine treatment value ($P < .01$). (Courtesy of Agostoni, P.G., et al.: Br. Heart J. 55:391–399, April 1986.)

of slight and transient taste alteration; one had elevated serum creatinine and potassium levels. Therapeutic efficacy and a low frequency of adverse effects indicate captopril's usefulness in patients with decompensated dilated cardiomyopathies refractory to conventional treatment.

▶ This study clearly demonstrates the beneficial sustained effects of prolonged therapy with captopril when added to an optimal regimen of digitalis and diuretics in patients with dilated cardiomyopathy. These beneficial changes were in marked contrast to those seen with the use of nifedipine, which did not relieve symptoms and even made some patients worse. The mean heart rate was decreased by captopril but increased by nifedipine. This study supports the use of captopril, but not nifedipine, in patients with dilated cardiomyopathy who are refractory to conventional therapy.—R.C. Schlant, M.D.

Severe Functional Limitation in Patients With Hypertrophic Cardiomyopathy and Only Mild Localized Left Ventricular Hypertrophy
Paolo Spirito, Barry J. Maron, Robert O. Bonow, and Stephen E. Epstein (Natl. Heart, Lung, and Blood Inst., NIH Bethesda)
J. Am. Coll. Cardiol. 8:537–544, September 1986   3–20

Some patients with nonobstructive hypertrophic cardiomyopathy have severe symptoms but only mild, localized left ventricular (LV) hypertrophy. Ten such patients without significant LV outflow obstruction at rest but with moderate to severe functional limitation were studied. All were in New York Heart Association functional class III or class IV. All met echocardiographic criteria for hypertrophic cardiomyopathy. The mean age was 46 years, and the mean length of follow-up was 7 years. Seventeen patients with mild symptoms or none were also studied. Their morphological features were similar to those of the study group.

Serial studies showed an increase in LV end-diastolic cavity dimension and a decrease in ventricular septal thickness in severely symptomatic patients. Neither variable changed significantly in the asymptomatic or mildly symptomatic patients. Echocardiographic measurements were comparable in the two groups at the most recent evaluation. Both LV systolic function and LV diastolic function were impaired in most of the severely symptomatic patients. Five of the 10 patients and 11 of the 17 in the comparison group had a family history of hypertrophic cardiomyopathy.

In most severely symptomatic patients with nonobstructive hypertrophic cardiomyopathy who have only mild, localized LV hypertrophy, a progressive increase in LV cavity size, ventricular septal thinning, or both, occur in association with systolic and diastolic dysfunction. These changes could reflect progression of the primary cardiomyopathic process or myocardial ischemia.

▶ This study adds important data to the natural history of hypertrophic cardiomyopathy by identifying a subset of severely symptomatic patients with relatively mild, localized LV hypertrophy who often had abnormalities of both systolic and diastolic LV function. During the period of follow-up there was often a progressive increase in LV end-diastolic diameter or progressive ventricular septal thinning, or both. In the future it will be important to determine whether these changes result from myocardial ischemia or from progression of the basic cardiomyopathic process. Tanaka et al. (*Br. Heart J.* 55:575, 1986) recently emphasized the extent of fibrosis and myocardial fiber disarray in hearts with hypertrophic cardiomyopathy. They found that the percentage area of fibrosis increased from the outer to the inner third of the ventricular free wall. Such findings could also be related to an ischemic mechanism for the fibrosis. Interestingly, patients with dilated cardiomyopathy also have been reported to have more fibrosis in the endocardium (mean, 22%) than in the epicardium (mean, 14%) (Unverferth, D.V., et al.: *Am. J. Cardiol.* 57:816, 1986).—R.C. Schlant, M.D.

Pericardial Disease

Recurrent Acute Pericarditis: Follow-Up Study of 31 Patients
Noble O. Fowler and Daniel Harbin, III (Univ. of Cincinnati)
J. Am. Coll. Cardiol. 7:300–305, February 1986   3–21

It is difficult to determine the diagnosis, treatment, and prognosis of patients with recurrent idiopathic pericarditis. Although this disease is uncommon, it is not rare. A review was made of experience with recurrent acute pericarditis spanning 20 years and including 31 patients. Follow-up ranged from 2 to 19 years.

Twenty-four patients had idiopathic pericarditis, four had postoperative or posttraumatic pericarditis, two had postinfarction pericarditis, and one had recurrent pericarditis after anticoagulant-induced intrapericardial bleeding. In 24 patients (group I), recurrences were detected by ECG changes, echocardiographic evidence of pericardial fluid, or a pericardial rub as well as chest pain. In seven patients (group II), recurrences were demonstrated only by an increased white blood cell count, increased ESR, or fever in addition to pain. In 19 patients the duration of the active or recurrent process was at least 5 years, and in 7 the duration was at least 8 years. In the initial attack three patients experienced cardiac tamponade, but none had tamponade during recurrences. Immunoelectrophoresis demonstrated normal findings or minor deviations in 11 patients; B cell and T cell lymphocyte counts were normal in 10 patients and showed minor deviations in 3. Results of antinuclear antibody studies were normal in 19 of 22 patients and positive in low titer in 2.

Most patients required adrenal steroid therapy for pain relief, and steroid withdrawal was often difficult. Nine patients underwent pericardiectomy, but in only two did this procedure produce clear-cut relief. In this group of 31 patients, 22 of whom were observed for at least 5 years, recurrent attacks of chest pain were the only major disabling feature of the pericarditis.

▶ This is one of the larger and longer studies of patients with recurrent pericarditis, which was most often idiopathic. The study documents the chronicity of the syndrome in many patients despite adrenal steroid therapy or pericardiectomy. The latter procedure was often not successful in preventing recurrent attacks of chest pain (? mediastinitis), and its role is still uncertain.—R.C. Schlant, M.D.

Disturbances of Cardiac Rhythm and Conduction

Adverse Reactions to Antiarrhythmic Drugs During Therapy for Ventricular Arrhythmias

Thomas W. Nygaard, T. Duncan Sellers, Tracey S. Cook, and John P. DiMarco (Univ. of Virginia)
JAMA 256:55–57, July 4, 1986   3–22

Antiarrhythmic drugs may prevent potentially life-threatening arrhythmias in many patients, but they are not without risk because the drugs may themselves precipitate cardiac arrhythmias. To document the incidence of such adverse reactions to antiarrhythmic therapy, a review was made of experience with 123 consecutive patients with a history of sustained ventricular tachycardia (VT) or ventricular fibrillation (VF) who were evaluated prospectively. In addition to history, patients had also experienced VT or VF on programmed ventricular stimulation or spontaneously after withdrawal of antiarrhythmic therapy. During the trial drugs were introduced singly. Confirmation of the relationship of the adverse reaction to the drug was based on resolution of symptoms after reduction in dosage or discontinuation of the drug. Adverse reactions occurring at a serum level of more than 10% above the maximum derived therapeutic range were excluded, as were reactions that did not require specific therapy, dosage adjustment, or discontinuation of the drug.

Most patients were men and had atherosclerotic coronary artery disease. Half had an ejection fraction of less than 40%. The mean follow-up was 13.3 months. Only 1 of the 23 deaths was clearly related to a drug reaction, i.e., amiodarone pulmonary toxicity. A mean of two drugs per patient was tried, and 48% of patients had an adverse reaction. Side effects were slightly more frequent in patients aged 65 years or more, but they were not more common in patients with impaired ventricular function. Significant side effects occurred in 19% of quinidine trials, 24% of procainamide trials, 49% of mexiletine trials, and 44% of amiodarone trials. Nausea, vomiting, and diarrhea were more frequent with quinidine, whereas procainamide produced fever and a lupus-like syndrome along with nausea and vomiting. Mexiletine caused gastrointestinal upset and tremor, and amiodarone produced bradyarrhythmias resulting from sinus node suppression or atrioventricular block and hypothyroidism.

These data show a 20% to 50% incidence of toxic reactions to the various antiarrhythmic agents used, suggesting that the benefit-risk ratio should be considered carefully. Patients with life-threatening arrhythmias who require prophylaxis against recurrence may tolerate the side effects of these drugs more readily because the consequences of going without therapy are so grave. However, patients with less severe rhythm disturbances (e.g., ventricular premature beats) may gain little by antiarrhythmic treatment and yet be at high risk from the drugs themselves. Although a proarrhythmic effect was not considered an adverse reaction for this study, such effects have been reported with surprising frequency. Use of these potentially toxic agents in patients with only marginal indications for therapy may lead to significant morbidity.

▶ All physicians prescribing antiarrhythmic drugs should know that such therapy can potentially induce or worsen cardiac arrhythmias. Similar findings have been reported by several groups including Velebit et al. (*Circulation* 65:886, 1982) and Ruskin et al. (*N. Engl. J. Med.* 309:1302, 1983).—R.C. Schlant, M.D.

Findings on Ambulatory Electrocardiographic Monitoring in Subjects Older Than 80 Years
Jean-Pierre Kantelip, Evelyne Sage, and Pierre Duchene-Marullaz (Clermont-Ferrand and Aurillao, France)
Am. J. Cardiol. 57:398–401, Feb. 15, 1986   3–23

The diagnosis of cardiac arrhythmias in elderly patients is a common problem in medical practice, and use of the standard ECGs in older persons has been studied extensively. Although many studies have demonstrated physiologic and pathologic cardiac changes with age, only a few have described arrhythmias in normal elderly persons. This paucity of data results from difficulty in separating the effects of aging on the heart from those that result from unrecognized diseases. It was hypothesized that undetected significant coronary artery disease may be present in more than one fourth of persons older than 45 years. An attempt was made to determine the prevalence and frequency of cardiac arrhythmias in 44 women and 6 men older than age 80 without cardiovascular disease and with normal responses on ECGs who underwent 24-hour ambulatory monitoring.

During waking and sleeping periods, mean sinus rates were 78 beats per minute and 64 beats per minute, respectively, and heart rates ranged from 43 beats per minute to 180 beats per minute during the 24-hour period (Fig 3–6). Of the patients, 28% had supraventricular tachycardia and 12% had nocturnal sinus arrhythmia accompanied by sinus pauses of 1.8–2 seconds. One woman had a transient pattern compatible with atrioventricular dissociation. All of the patients had supraventricular ectopic contractions (SVECs). The frequency was less than 1 per hour in 25% of the patients and more than 20 per hour in 65%. Serious supraventricular tachyarrhythmias included, in one patient each, an episode of ectopic atrial tachycardia, a short run of atrial fibrillation, and flutter; several episodes of supraventricular tachycardia occurred in two patients. All of these were accompanied by more than 50 SVECs per hour. The number of ventricular premature contractions was more than ten per hour in 32% of the patients, and they were multifocal in 18%. There were

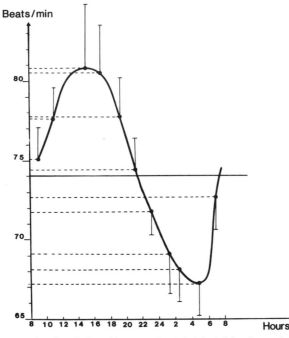

Fig 3–6.—Average circadian rhythm of heart rate in total male and female population. Vertical lines indicate mean ±SE of mean of hourly heart rate. (Courtesy of Kantelip, J. – P., et al.: Am. J. Cardiol. 57:398–401, Feb. 15, 1986.)

couplets in 8% (four patients) and a run of six ventricular premature contractions in 2% (one patient).

Sinus pause and atrioventricular block are unusual in persons older than age 80 years who have no apparent heart disease, but frequent SVECs and ventricular premature contractions are more common. This study emphasizes the difficulty in evaluating the normality of the ECG with portable monitoring in an older population.

▶ It is important for physicians to know the normal variations in ambulatory ECG recordings in many different subsets of patients, particularly when considering any of these individuals for pacemaker implantation. This is especially important in elderly patients in whom it may be difficult to obtain an accurate correlation between symptoms and ECG variations.—R.C. Schlant, M.D.

Characteristics and Prognosis of Lone Atrial Fibrillation: 30-Year Follow-Up in the Framingham Study

Frederick N. Brand, Robert D. Abbott, William B. Kannel, and Philip A. Wolf (Boston Univ. and Natl. Heart, Lung, and Blood Inst., NIH, Bethesda)
JAMA 254:3449–3453, Dec. 27, 1985   3–24

Lone atrial fibrillation (AF) occurs in the absence of coexistent heart disease, congestive heart failure, rheumatic heart disease, or hypertensive cardiovascular disease. Lone AF may be transient, or present as recurrent paroxysmal AF, or be chronic, which is less frequent. The incidence of lone AF was examined, as were the possible predisposing characteristics and prognosis in a cohort of 5,209 persons from the Framingham study.

Atrial fibrillation was diagnosed in 193 of 2,336 men and 183 of 2,873 women during the 30-year follow-up period. Generally, the incidence increased with age in both sexes. Lone AF occurred in 16.6% of the men and in 6% of the women with AF. Men with lone AF were older, a pattern not evident in women. Only serum cholesterol levels were associated with the appearance of lone AF; patients with lone AF had lower cholesterol levels than found in other patients with AF. However, the former were more likely to have had previous ECG abnormalities, e.g., nonspecific T-wave or ST-wave abnormalities and antecedent intraventricular block. On follow-up, the incidence of stroke was found to be significantly higher in the patients with lone AF, with an event rate more than four times that of the controls. As a consequence of the strokes, total cardiovascular disease occurred at a rate almost twice that of the controls. The association with stroke was similar for the two sexes.

These results confirm previous findings in showing that hypertension was not a risk factor for lone AF; only when associated with cardiac enlargement was there an increased propensity for AF. In contrast to the previous Framingham study, this analysis found no association of diabetes with AF or lone AF, perhaps because many such patients were removed from the study population because of preexisting cardiac conditions. There was no relationship to coffee intake or to alcohol consumption, particularly binge drinking, in the patients with lone AF, but the study patients were mostly elderly and did not consume much alcohol. The role of lone AF as a predictor of stroke was significant and calls into question the often presumed benign prognosis in this group. The decision to institute anticoagulant therapy in these patients must take into account the risk of stroke and the long-term hazards of anticoagulant therapy in otherwise healthy individuals. Routine ECG surveillance of elderly patients might improve detection of AF and lone AF. Although no overt underlying heart disease was present in these patients, their age alone might argue for clinically unobserved heart disease. Additional diagnostic tests may be needed to rule out heart disease.

▶ In this study approximately 40% of these older patients with lone AF had some type of overt cardiovascular disease after the diagnosis of AF during the follow-up period. A significant number sustained a stroke, which was presumably embolic. None of the patients in this study received anticoagulants. It is likely that a significant number of elderly patients with lone AF have primary conduction system disease as the cause of it, and many have associated dysfunction of the atrioventricular mode that restricts the ventricular response rate even without the use of digoxin, β-blockers, verapamil, or diltiazem. An increased risk of stroke in men with nonrheumatic AF has also been found in the Whitehall Study of London Civil Servants and the British Regional Heart Study (Flegel, K. M., et al.: *Lancet* 1:526–529, 1987). The decision of whether or not to give such elderly patients chronic anticoagulant therapy is difficult and obviously must be individualized. Echocardiography and 24-hour ambulatory ECG are occasionally of significant value in the management of these patients.—R.C. Schlant, M.D.

Characteristics and Prognosis of Incomplete Right Bundle Branch Block: An Epidemiologic Study
Youlian Liao, Linda Ann Emidy, Alan Dyer, John S. Hewitt, Richard B. Shekelle, Oglesby Paul, Ronald Prineas, and Jeremiah Stamler (Northwestern Univ., Univ. of Texas at Houston, Harvard Univ., and Univ. of Minnesota)
J. Am. Coll. Cardiol. 7:492–499, March 1986   3–25

Some believe that incomplete right bundle branch block (IRBBB) on the ECG has no prognostic significance when it is present without overt heart disease. In a prospective study of a cohort of 1,960 white men aged 40–56 years, the characteristics and prognostic significance of IRBBB without heart disease were examined.

Of the 1,960 men, 6.8% had evidence of incomplete block. Prevalence increased with age. During follow-up, IRBBB developed in 222 men, in about half within the first 4 years. The 11-year cumulative incidence was 13.6%, with similar incidence rates in all age groups. A greater proportion of men with IRBBB had left axis deviation of zero or less. Baseline left axis deviation was associated with an increased likelihood of IRBBB; for men with a baseline axis of -30 degrees or less, the incidence was 26.2%. Men with IRBBB at baseline or follow-up also had a greater chance of having left axis deviation. More men with IRBBB were smokers, compared with controls. During follow-up, complete RBBB developed in 17 men in an 11-year period. Patients with prevalent IRBBB had seven times the 11-year incidence of complete block than did those without. However, the age-adjusted death rates among men with IRBBB were similar to those in men without such block.

Judgments vary as to the nature and meaning of IRBBB, a common electrophysiologic finding. Some studies point to the condition as an abnormality of cardiac conduction, an intermediate phase between normality and complete block. Several findings of this study affirm this idea. The association of left axis deviation with IRBBB may support the concept. Patients with left axis deviation had a higher prevalence of myocardial fibrosis and myocardial infarction involving the anterior division of the left bundle branch. Some persons have mild slowing or delay of conduction, and fatal and nonfatal cardiac events may be increased in such persons. Although aging itself is associated with left axis deviation, the results in this study cannot be attributed to age alone. The previously reported association of greater body weight with left axis deviation was not found, but a relationship with smoking was evident. Coronary artery disease could easily result in conduction disturbances in the bundle branches and may play an etiologic role in the association between left axis deviation and IRBBB. Serial observations of ECG changes show increasing degrees of bundle-branch block in men who eventually experience complete block, suggesting incomplete block as a step toward complete block, an abnormality in the conduction system that can be manifest without overt heart disease.

▶ This is a valuable, large study of the natural history of IRBBB, which is usually considered a variant of only minor clinical significance. The present study emphasizes that the long-term mortality rates associated with coronary artery disease, cardiovascular diseases, and all causes for men with IRBBB were not statistically significantly greater than for those without IRBBB. It will be interesting to see the next 10-year follow-up of this carefully studied group of patients.—R.C. Schlant, M.D.

Incidence and Clinical Features of the Quinidine-Associated Long QT Syndrome: Implications for Patient Care
Dan M. Roden, Raymond L. Woosley, and R. Kirby Primm (Vanderbilt Univ.)
Am. Heart J. 111:1088–1093, June 1986   3–26

Quinidine therapy is one of the most common causes of the acquired long QT syndrome and torsade de pointes. Among 24 patients, 20 had torsade de pointes and 4 had marked QT prolongation but without torsade de pointes within 2 days of starting quinidine therapy. Eleven were being treated for atrial arrhythmias, and 13 were taking quinidine for isolated ventricular ectopic depolarization and short runs of monomorphic ventricular tachycardia. Of patients treated for atrial fibrillation, torsade de pointes developed in 75% after conversion to sinus rhythm. The most common cardiovascular disease identified was chronic hypertension, and 17 patients were taking potassium-wasting diuretics.

The average duration of quinidine therapy prior to syndrome recognition was 1–3 days. In four patients the syndrome developed after more than 1 year of quinidine therapy and in each case a clearcut complicating feature was identified, most commonly in association with hypokalemia. Plasma quinidine concentrations within 24 hours after syndrome recognition were in (or less than) the normal therapeutic range in more than 50% of the patients. In 20 patients (83%), at least one major associated risk factor was identified, including serum potassium values of less than 4.0 mEq/L (13 patients), high-grade atrioventricular block (4 patients), and marked QT prolongation (2 patients). The ECG features basically included absence of marked QRS widening, marked QT prolongation (by definition), and a stereo-typic series of cycle length changes just prior to onset of torsade de pointes. The latter commenced after the T wave of a markedly prolonged QT interval following a cycle that was markedly prolonged, usually by a postectopic pause. The risk of the syndrome developing was estimated as at least 1.5% per year.

Hypokalemia should be corrected prior to quinidine initiation, possibly obviating the need for this drug in certain patients. Initiation of quinidine therapy should be done under monitored circumstances in a hospital for 2–3 days. The QT intervals should be followed, particularly after a long cycle, and a Q peak T of more than 400 msec should indicate at least a reevaluation of patients and measurement of the serum potassium level.

▶ Of particular therapeutic importance is the relationship in patients between hypokalemia and the quinidine-associated long QT syndrome; most of these patients had torsade de pointes. It is significant that many of them had low plasma quinidine concentrations. In patients receiving quinidine (and probably other similar agents), one should either not use diuretics that may produce hypokalemia, or should frequently monitor the serum potassium level. Periodic monitoring of the QT interval should probably be performed in all patients in whom quinidine therapy is initiated.—R.C. Schlant, M.D.

Risk Factors for Sudden Unexpected Cardiac Death in Young Women in Rochester, Minnesota, 1960 Through 1974
C. Mary Beard, Marie R. Griffin, Kenneth P. Offord, and William D. Edwards (Mayo Clinic and Found.)
Mayo Clin. Proc. 61:186–191, March 1986   3–27

Coronary artery disease occurs less often in women than in men and consequently has been less well studied in women. However, accepted factors associated with an increased risk of coronary artery disease in men may also be found in women. Approximately 60% of deaths attributable to coronary artery disease occur suddenly, and the risk factors for sudden cardiac death are thought to be similar to those for other manifestations of coronary artery disease. An evaluation was made of alcohol use, the diagnosis of anxiety or tension states, and major psychiatric illness as possible risk factors for sudden unexpected death (SUD) in women younger than 60 years of age.

A case-controlled study of SUD as the initial manifestation of coronary artery disease was conducted in Rochester, Minnesota. Fifteen SUD cases were identified during the years 1960 through 1974. The risk factors among these cases were compared with those in two control groups—a population group of 60 (with four age-matched controls per case) and 59 women with myocardial infarction who were less than 60 years of age living in Rochester during the same period. The relative risks for the accepted coronary artery disease risk factors of ever smoking and hypertension were 8.6 and 5.7, respectively. When the SUD cases were compared with the myocardial infarction control group, the odds ratios were 1.2 for ever smoking and 0.8 for hypertension. Six of the 15 SUD cases had a diagnosis of alcoholism, as did only 2 of the 60 controls and 4 of the 59 myocardial infarction patients; thus, the relative risks were 12.0 and 4.8, respectively. In addition, ever married SUD cases were nulliparous or had fewer children more often than the controls of the myocardial infarction group. The combination of major psychiatric diagnosis and major tranquilizer use occurred with greater frequency among SUD cases than among controls, whereas comparison of SUD cases and myocardial infarction cases for this variable resulted in a relative risk of 0.7.

The elevated risks for the accepted coronary artery disease risk factors of smoking and hypertension for SUD found in this study agree with those reported in other studies of coronary artery disease in women. Nevertheless, the strikingly elevated relative risk of alcoholism for women with SUD in the present report deserves further study. It was hypothesized that the association between alcohol and SUD in young women could be a chance occurrence in this population, the results of systematic misclassification of alcohol-related deaths, or an actual and causal association.

▶ This study confirms the association between smoking or hypertension and the occurrence of SUD from coronary artery disease in women less than 60 years of age in Rochester, Minnesota. There was little evidence that any of the psychological variables evaluated were significantly more common among women with SUD than among controls. The possible relationship between SUD and a diagnosis of excess alcohol use is intriguing but needs to be confirmed in much larger studies. Although SUD was the initial manifestation of coronary artery disease in 15 women younger than 60 years of age, the initial manifestation was angina pectoria in 95 and myocardial infarction in 59 during the period of this study, 1960 through 1974. I wish the authors had been able to divide the smoking history into different categories, including former smokers who have quit for 5 or 10 years, because several studies have indicated that the risk of death from coronary disease decreases significantly in the years after cessation of smoking. In the present study, the only two groups were "never smoked" and "ever smoked."—R.C. Schlant, M.D.

Sudden Death and Its Relation to QT-Interval Prolongation After Acute Myocardial Infarction: Two-Year Follow-Up

Kevin Wheelan, Jhulan Mukharji, Robert E. Rude, W. Kenneth Poole, Nancy Gustafson, Lewis J. Thomas, Jr., H. William Strauss, Allan S. Jaffe, James E. Muller, Robert Roberts, Charles H. Croft, Eugene R. Passamani, James T. Willerson, and the MILIS Study Group (Univ. of Texas at Dallas, Parkland Mem. Hosp., Dallas, and cooperating institutions of the Multicenter Investigation of the Limitation of Infarct Size)
Am. J. Cardiol. 57:745–750, Apr. 1, 1986   3–28

Studies in survivors of acute myocardial infarction (AMI) recently report direct relationship between the risk of sudden death after hospital discharge, the frequency of ventricular ectopic activity, and the degree of left ventricular (LV) dysfunction as assessed by radionuclide ventriculography. It is thought that sudden death is caused usually by an arrhythmic event, most frequently ventricular tachycardia or ventricular fibrillation. An important factor in association with ventricular fibrillation and ventricular tachycardia is QT-interval prolongation. Knowledge of the electrophysiologic features associated with this event provided a rationale for investigation into the relationship between the QT interval and sudden death. An examination was made of the relationship between the variables of QT interval, LV ejection fraction, the presence or absence of frequent ventricular premature complexes, and sudden death in patients with AMI who were followed after hospital discharge.

The study group consisted of 533 patients who survived for at least 10 days after AMI and were followed for up to 24 months in the Multicenter Investigation of the Limitation of Infarct Size. Analysis of clinical and laboratory variables measured before hospital discharge indicated that the QT interval, either corrected or uncorrected for heart rate, did not contribute significantly to prediction of subsequent sudden death or total mortality. In this population, the occurrence of frequent ventricular premature complexes (more than ten per hour) on ambulatory ECG indicated patients at high risk of sudden death. In these patients, the mean QTc was 0.468 seconds among those who died suddenly and 0.446 seconds in survivors, but it was not statistically significant as an additional predictor of sudden death. These findings were not changed by consideration of the use of type I antiarrhythmic agents, digoxin, presence of U waves, and correction for intraventricular conduction delay. Although QT-interval prolongation occurs in some patients after AMI, a reduced LV ejection fraction (less than 0.40) and frequent ventricular premature complexes (more than ten per hour) are the most important factors for predicting subsequent sudden death in this patient population.

▶ This study from the MILIS group was unable to confirm previous reports from another large clinical trial, the Beta Heart Attack Trial (BHAT), which found (Peters et al.: *Circulation* 70 (Suppl. II):II–6, 1984) a significantly higher incidence of sudden death in patients with a corrected QT interval (QTc) of 0.45 or more, whether they were receiving propranolol or placebo. In the MILIS study, the authors found that the QTc most nearly achieved statistical significance as a predictor of subsequent sudden death only in those patients who were not taking type I antiarrhythmic agents. Some of the discrepancy may be because of the much smaller number of patients in the MILIS study, patient selection, the concomitant medications used, and difference in the technique of QT-interval measurement.—R.C. Schlant, M.D.

Electrophysiologic Characteristics of Ventricular Tachycardia or Fibrillation in Relation to Age of Myocardial Infarction

William G. Stevenson, Pedro Brugada, Ivo Kersschot, Bernd Waldecker, Manfred Zehender, Annette Giebel, and Hein J.J. Wellens (Univ. of Limburg, Maastrict, The Netherlands)
Am. J. Cardiol. 57:387–391, Feb. 15, 1986   3–29

Recent efforts to use programmed ventricular stimulation to predict arrthythmic events after acute myocardial infarction (AMI) have shown that initiation of sustained monomorphic ventricular tachycardia (VT) may not predict the occurrence of spontaneous VT or sudden death. Thus, it appears that although the electrophysiologic substrate of VT may be present, spontaneously occurring "triggering" mechanisms may not initiate VT; the substrate may change over time, or it may become incapable of producing a sustained arrhythmia. An attempt was made to determine if the ability of programmed stimulation to initiate VT was dependent on the age of the AMI at the time of electrophysiologic testing.

The incidence and characteristics of sustained VT initiated by programmed stimulation in relation to the time elapsed between AMI and electrophysiologic study was evaluated in 54 patients who experienced spontaneous episodes of sustained VT (42 patients) or ventricular fibrillation (VF) (12 patients) more than 3 days after a single AMI. In patients with VT, there were no significant differences in the incidence of initiation of sustained monomorphic VT among those evaluated 1–3 weeks (100%), 3–8 weeks (75%), 2–6 months (100%), 6–18 months (80%), or more than 18 months after AMI. The mean number of extrastimuli necessary to initiate VT did not differ among groups. Nevertheless, patients evaluated more than 4 weeks after the initial episode of VT had a lower incidence of inducible VT than those studied earlier [14 of 21 (71%) vs. 21 of 21 (100%)], although this was probably the result of earlier termination of the stimulation protocol because of initiation of polymorphic arrhythmias in those studied later. The 14 patients who were evaluated within 8 weeks of AMI had significantly faster VT rates (mean cycle length, 269 msec) than the 28 patients studied later (320 msec), possibly because there were more out-of-hospital presentations of VT in the later group. Although more patients studied within 3 weeks of AMI had anterior infarcts (100%), there were no other differences with regard to age, AMI location, or ejection fraction. Among patients with VF, five of seven (71%) who were studied for fewer than 8 weeks and three of five patients (60%) studied for longer than 8 weeks after AMI had inducible VT. The ability to induce sustained VT in patients with spontaneous episodes of sustained VT or VF after AMI appears unrelated to the interval between AMI and programmed stimulation.

▶ The results of this study are significant because they indicate that the presence of the electrophysiologic substrate for sustained VT in patients who have AMI and have an episode of sustained VT or fibrillation is independent of the interval between infarction and testing.—R.C. Schlant, M.D.

Survivors of Cardiac Arrest: Prevention of Recurrence by Drug Therapy as Predicted by Electrophysiologic Testing or Electrocardiographic Monitoring

Brian T. Skale, William M. Miles, James J. Heger, Douglas P. Zipes, and Eric N. Prystowsky (Indiana Univ., Indianapolis)
Am. J. Cardiol. 57:113–119, January 1986   3–30

Most sudden cardiac deaths in the United States are caused by ventricular fibrillation. In addition, approximately 25% of survivors of cardiac arrest unassociated with acute myocardial infarction (AMI) may have another episode of cardiac arrest within 1 year of the initial event. Programmed ventricular stimulation initiates ventricular tachycardias in many survivors of cardiac arrest, and drug suppression of ventricular tachycardia may be associated with a favorable long-term survival rate. However, ventricular tachycardia cannot be initiated in all patients, and some are not good candidates for serial electrophysiologic testing. Because of this, other potential markers of drug efficacy are necessary. This study sought to evaluate the clinical outcome in survivors of cardiac arrest in whom drug therapy was guided by electrophysiologic testing or continuous ECG monitoring.

The study group consisted of 44 men and 18 women who had been resuscitated from at least one cardiac arrest unrelated to AMI. At the time of the initial cardiac arrest, no patient was taking antiarrhythmic drugs, but 35 had coronary artery disease and 27 did not. Prior to drug treatment, control electrophysiologic studies induced ventricular tachycardia in 43 of 58 patients (74%) (30 of 35 with and 17 of 27 without coronary artery disease). When control continuous ECG monitoring was carried out for 48 hours, it was found that only 19 of 62 patients (31%) had spontaneous ventricular tachycardia, 5 of whom had no tachycardia induced at control electrophysiologic study. There was a mean follow-up of 22 months. Fourteen of 41 patients, 8 of 25 with and 6 of 16 without coronary artery disease, had ventricular tachycardia suppressed with drugs during serial electrophysiologic testing; moreover, none had a recurrent arrhythmic episode. Ventricular tachycardia was suppressed in 12 of 14 patients who were taking conventional drugs. Of 27 patients with ventricular tachycardia induced during all drug studies, 6 died of cardiac arrest and 4 had recurrent tachycardia. In 20 patients drug efficacy was guided by continuous ECG monitoring, and 4 of 9 in whom tachycardia and ventricular pairs were suppressed by drug therapy (as documented by continuous ECG monitoring for at least 48 hours) died of cardiac arrest. Overall, 26 patients were released with amiodarone therapy, 5 died of cardiac arrest, and 3 had recurrent sustained ventricular tachycardia.

In survivors of cardiac arrest, suppression of inducible ventricular tachycardia during electrophysiologic testing predicts a favorable outcome, whereas suppression of spontaneous ventricular tachycardia and repetitive beats during continuous ECG monitoring is often associated with recurrence of cardiac arrest. Furthermore, the risk of recurrent cardiac arrest or sustained ventricular tachycardia is significant if tachycardia is initiated during electrophysiologic study, even during amiodarone therapy.

▶ This study confirms the improved outcome of survivors of cardiac arrest who have inducible ventricular tachycardia on electrophysiologic study that can be suppressed by drug therapy, but patients in whom ventricular tachycardia could still be induced during all drug studies more often had recurrent cardiac arrest or symptomatic tachycardia. On the other hand, many patients who had suppression of spontaneous episodes of ventricular tachycardia during drug therapy also died suddenly. Ten patients had neither inducible nor spontaneous ventricular tachycardia. A previous report by Ruskin et al. (*Am. J. Cardiol.*

49:958, 1982) suggested a good prognosis in such patients, although Roy et al. (*Am. J. Cardiol.* 52:969, 1983) reported a continued risk of cardiac arrest. More and more such patients are being treated by external or internal automatic defibrillators, but to date there are no good large studies to support this growing practice. (See Abstract 3–36.) The clinical value of specialized electrophysiologic testing in patients who survive cardiac arrest is increasingly apparent, although the indications for such testing are still evolving. A recent symposium edited by Zipes and Rahimtoola (*Circulation,* 1987, in press) carefully reviewed current indications.—R.C. Schlant, M.D.

Plasma Norepinephrine in Exercise-Induced Ventricular Tachycardia
Neil M. Sokoloff, Scott R. Spielman, Allan M. Greenspan, Alan P. Rae, R. Stephen Porter, David T. Lowenthal, A.-Hamid Hakki, Abdulmassih S. Iskandrian, Harold R. Kay, and Leonard N. Horowitz (Likoff Cardiovascular Inst. and Hahnemann Univ., Philadelphia)
J. Am. Coll. Cardiol. 8:11–17, July 1986   3–31

A prospective evaluation was made of the relationship between plasma norepinephrine levels and exercise-related induction of ventricular tachycardia. Findings in 17 normotensive persons were analyzed, none of whom was taking antiarrhythmic, β-adrenergic blocking, or calcium channel blocking agents.

Seven patients had ventricular tachycardia only during ambulatory ECG monitoring (group 1); ten had ventricular tachycardia exclusively during exercise, recovery, or both. Demographic characteristics in each group were similar. There was no difference in exercise duration, left ventricular ejection fraction at rest, heart rate throughout the exercise protocol, rest QTc interval, change in QTc interval during exercise, presence of coronary artery disease, or exercise-related myocardial ischemia between the two groups. Thallium imaging detected myocardial ischemia in 20% of group 2 patients and in 14% of group 1 patients. Norepinephrine levels were above the limit of detection and closely paralleled the exercise level. Peak levels were observed either at peak exercise (10% in group 2 and 14% in group 1), or at 1 minute into recovery (90% in group 2 and 86% in group 1). Thus, no difference in plasma norepinephrine levels existed between the two groups.

Repeat testing for group 2 patients after maximal intravenous β-adrenergic blockade with propranolol showed a reduction in heart rate and plasma norepinephrine levels. No significant change in QTc interval at rest or in exercise duration was observed; ventricular tachycardia occurred in 10% of the patients.

This study demonstrated that plasma norepinephrine levels do not differentiate patients with exercise-induced ventricular tachycardia from patients in whom ventricular tachycardia occurs only during routine ambulatory monitoring. Propranolol was highly effective in abolishing exercise-induced ventricular tachycardia, although the exact mechanism cannot be determined on the basis of presented data. Patients with exercise-induced ventricular tachycardia may be more sensitive to plasma norepinephrine than are otherwise comparable patients.

▶ Although this study did not find that patients with exercise-induced ventricular tachycardia had higher than normal plasma levels of norepinephrine at rest or during exercise, it did show a decrease in plasma norepinephrine levels during propranolol treatment, and only one patient experienced ventricular tachycardia during exercise while taking propranolol. The results further document the beneficial antiarrhythmic effects of β-blocking drugs in selected patients.—R.C. Schlant, M.D.

The Role of Beta Blocking Agents as Adjunct Therapy to Membrane Stabilizing Drugs in Malignant Ventricular Arrhythmia
Geoffrey Hirsowitz, Philip J. Podrid, Steven Lampert, Joseph Stein, and Bernard Lown (Harvard Univ. and Brigham and Women's Hosp., Boston)
Am. Heart J. 111:852–860, May 1986   3–32

Certain complex forms of ventricular premature beats identify patients with coronary artery disease who are at increased risk of sudden cardiac death. Although antiarrhythmic drugs are frequently given to suppress these arrhythmias and to prevent sudden death, there are no data demonstrating that these drugs prolong life. Furthermore, classic antiarrhythmic drugs are often only partially or totally ineffective in suppression of ventricular arrhythmias in a given patient, and frequently the best therapeutic option is to use drug combinations. Although β antagonists have not been considered first-line therapy for malignant ventricular arrhythmia, these agents are beneficial in the management of certain ventricular arrhythmias. The role of β-blocking drugs as adjunct therapy with classic antiarrhythmic agents (membrane-stabilizing drugs) was evaluated in the short-term management of patients with ventricular arrhythmia.

The study group consisted of 54 patients who were evaluated by 24-hour ambulatory ECG monitoring and symptom-limited exercise testing. Patients underwent control studies without antiarrhythmic drugs; they were evaluated separately while taking membrane-stabilizing drugs and β-blocking agents and then during combination therapy. The combination of a β-blocking agent and a membrane-stabilizing drug abolished ventricular tachycardia and couplets in 83% and 86% of exercise tests in patients with this arrhythmia present during therapy with membrane-stabilizing drugs alone. When a β blocker was added to a membrane-stabilizing drug, it resulted in abolition of ventricular tachycardia and couplets in 43% and 20% of ambulatory monitoring studies. The frequency of ventricular premature beats was lowered by more than 50% in 65% of exercise tests and in 52% of monitoring studies. In this group of patients, β-blocking agents did not reduce ventricular arrhythmias when used alone.

The addition of a β blocker to a membrane-stabilizing drug substantially enhances suppression of ventricular arrhythmia, especially when assessed by exercise testing. This is thought to result from the synergistic drug effects of the combination rather than from the effect of the individual drugs. Patients who have a partial reduction in ventricular arrhythmia during treatment with any of the membrane-stabilizing drugs may benefit from the addition of a β blocker. Further prospective studies are needed for confirmation.

▶ It has been my experience and that of others that β-blocking agents do suppress ventricular arrhythmias (as well as some atrial arrhythmias) in many patients, including those with coronary artery disease. In the Beta Blocker Heart Attack Trial, which evaluated chronic propranolol therapy in patients after acute myocardial infarction, ventricular arrhythmias and sudden death were decreased by propranolol therapy (Lichstein et al.: *Circulation* 67 (Suppl. I):5, 1983). The study by Hirsowitz et al. indicates the value of adding a β-blocking agent to a membrane-stabilizing drug. The study used 24-hour ambulatory ECG monitoring and exercise testing to evaluate the patients. The conclusions seem clinically reasonable, although, of course, it would be helpful if they were confirmed by an appropriate clinical trial.—R.C. Schlant, M.D.

Flecainide: Steady State Electrophysiologic Effects in Patients With Remote Myocardial Infarction and Inducible Sustained Ventricular Arrhythmia

Charles R. Webb, Joel Morganroth, Sheila Senior, Scott R. Spielman, Allan M. Greenspan, and Leonard N. Horowitz (Likoff Cardiovascular Inst. and Hahnemann Univ., Philadelphia)
J. Am. Coll. Cardiol. 8:214–220, July 1986   3–33

Patients who survive a myocardial infarction are at risk of sudden cardiac death as a result of arrhythmia. Flecainide can suppress ventricular premature depolarizations and has been useful in patients with nonsustained ventricular tachycardia. The safety and efficacy of flecainide were examined in 24 patients with inducible sustained ventricular tachycardia. The drug dose was optimized by ambulatory ECG monitoring. The patients had sustained a myocardial infarction a mean of 8 years previously. All had reproducibly inducible sustained ventricular tachycardia by ventricular extrastimulus. Nine patients had experienced sudden cardiac death events and seven had sustained ventricular tachycardia. Most of the patients were male; the mean age was 65 years, and the mean left ventricular ejection fraction was 34%. Previous drug regimens had been unsuccessful or had not been tolerated. Flecainide was given in doses of 100–200 mg every 12 hours. Plasma concentrations were maintained at 1,000 ng/ml or lower.

Before flecainide administration, loss of consciousness or near-syncope occurred during the induced arrhythmia in 20 patients, angina in 2, and palpitation in 2. Cardioversion was required to terminate tachycardia in 13, pacing in 9, intravenous lidocaine injection in 1, and both lidocaine and pacing in 1. Holter monitoring showed means of 199 ventricular premature complexes (VPC) per hour, 406 VPC pairs per day, 19 nonsustained episodes of ventricular tachycardia per day, and 66 ventricular tachycardia complexes per day before drug treatment. Flecainide suppressed more than 80% of the VPC and all spontaneous ventricular tachycardia in 83% of the patients. No proarrhythmia effect was seen. The mean flecainide dosage was 144 mg every 12 hours; the mean plasma concentration was 583 ng/ml. Plasma concentrations and dosages in patients who did not respond to the drug were similar, but plasma concentrations in patients who experienced heart block were higher. Flecainide increased mean QRS, AH, and HV intervals; JT intervals were unchanged. Flecainide did not affect sinus cycle length, sinus node recovery time, atrial refractory period, atrioventricular node refractory period, or the mean right ventricular refractory period. In 22% of the 18 patients for whom complete data were available, flecainide prevented induction of sustained ventricular tachycardia; in all but 1 of the others, the cycle length was increased and correlated with the plasma drug concentration. Flecainide reduced the percentage of patients who lost consciousness during sustained ventricular tachycardia from 79% to 29%. There was no significant change in the mode of induction, however. Four patients who had no inducible ventricular tachycardia during flecainide treatment had no ventricular tachycardia or sudden cardiac death on follow-up. Of ten patients in whom ventricular tachycardia was still inducible, one died and four had nonfatal inducible tachycardia.

Flecainide is a potent suppressor of arrhythmia, although it does not necessarily suppress induction of ventricular tachycardia electrophysiologically. The data suggest that the drug may cause generalized slowing of myocardial conduction, indicating that cautious evaluation of patients with underlying His-Purkinje disease may be prudent before flecainide is administered. The authors' success rate with this drug compares favorably with that reported by others. In contrast with other reports, no proarrhythmia events were observed in this study, possibly because of avoidance of concomitant antiarrhythmia drug use and careful upward titration of flecainide. Holter monitor results were more abnormal than ventricular extrastimulation results, indicating that such stimulation may be a more sensitive indicator of the tendency for recurrent ventricular tachycardia. Patients without inducible arrhythmia during flecainide treatment have a better prognosis. Electrophysiologic study distinguishes patients for whom any recurrence is likely to be compatible with survival from those likely to have a fatal recurrence. Flecainide can be administered safely to patients with a history of remote myocardial infarction and inducible sustained ventricular tachycardia after a precise protocol for dose titration.

▶ As indicated by the results of this study, flecainide is a valuable addition to the medications available for the treatment of cardiac arrhythmias. Flecainide does have some negative inotropic actions, however (Roden and Woosley: *N. Engl. J. Med.* 315:36, 1986), and it would probably be prudent to avoid using it, if possible, in patients with compromised left ventricular function, i.e., an ejection fraction of less than 30%.—R.C. Schlant, M.D.

Long-Term Tolerance of Amiodarone Treatment for Cardiac Arrhythmias

Warren M. Smith, Wilhelm F. Lubbe, Ralph M. Whitlock, John Mercer, John D. Rutherford, and Anthony H. Roche (Green Lane Hosp., Auckland)
Am. J. Cardiol. 57:1288–1293, June 1, 1986   3–34

Amiodarone is an effective broad-spectrum antiarrhythmic agent. Its long half-life and minimal depressive effect on left ventricular (LV) function encourage administration to patients with LV impairment, or to those who are therapy resistant. However, despite its advantages, amiodarone is associated with many toxic side effects.

To assess the long-term tolerance of amiodarone, 155 men and 87 women (mean age, 58 years) were given a loading dose of 600–1,800 mg/day for 1–4 weeks. The maintenance dose was usually 400 mg/day for those with ventricular arrhythmias and 200 mg/day for those with supraventricular arrhythmias. During a mean follow-up period of 24 months, 56 patients died. The actuarial survival at 50 months for the entire group was 66% (Fig 3–7), and for the groups with supraventricular tachycardia and ventricular tachycardia/fibrillation, 74% and 52%, respectively.

With amiodarone therapy, arrhythmia was suppressed in 196 patients (81%). At assessment, only 81 patients were alive and still taking the drug. The actuarial probability of survival was 19% at 50 months in 143 patients (59%), forcing 64 (26%) to suspend therapy. Although amiodarone ef-

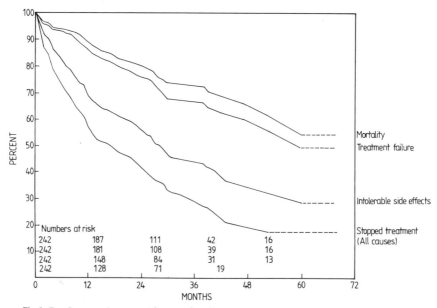

Fig 3–7.—Comparative actuarial curves for all patients treated with amiodarone. The highest curve is mortality irrespective of the status of amiodarone treatment. The second and third curves are surviving patients who discontinued amiodarone treatment because of arrhythmia recurrence and intolerable side effects, respectively. The lowest curve represents surviving patients in whom treatment is still being successfully continued. (Courtesy of Smith, W.M., et al.: Am. J. Cardiol. 57:1288–1293, 1986.)

fectively suppressed arrhythmia, mortality was high and long-term tolerance was poor. The outcome was somewhat better for patients with supraventricular tachycardia than for those with ventricular disturbances.

▶ This study, which is from a medium-sized hospital in New Zealand, reveals surprisingly high rates of mortality, treatment failure, or intolerable side effects in patients taking amiodarone therapy on a chronic basis. The toxic effects were similar to those previously reported, although pulmonary fibrosis was detected in only two patients, one of whom died. It is more apparent than previously that amiodarone should be used for the treatment of supraventricular or ventricular arrhythmias *only* after the failure of other antiarrhythmic agents.—R.C. Schlant, M.D.

Efficacy and Safety of Medium- and High-Dose Diltiazem Alone and in Combination With Digoxin for Control of Heart Rate at Rest and During Exercise in Patients With Chronic Atrial Fibrillation
Arie Roth, Earl Harrison, Gladys Mitani, Jordan Cohen, Shahbudin H. Rahimtoola, and Uri Elkayam (Univ. of Southern California)
Circulation 73:316–324, Feburary 1986   3–35

Traditionally, digitalis has been the drug of choice for control of ventricular rate in patients with atrial fibrillation. Although digitalis is useful at rest, it is less useful in the control of heart rate response to exercise or other stress-related situations. The direct effect of verapamil on slowing atrioventricular nodal conduction results in better control of the exercise heart rate in patients with atrial fibrillation. However, the use of verapamil is limited in patients with heart disease because of its negative inotropic effect and its interaction with digoxin. Diltiazem is another calcium-entry blocking agent that does not interact with digoxin. It has a favorable hemodynamic effect in patients with heart failure. An evaluation was made of the efficacy and safety of diltiazem alone and in combination with digoxin when used for control of heart rate in patients with chronic atrial fibrillation.

The study population consisted of 12 patients aged 34–57 years with chronic atrial fibrillation. Two doses of diltiazem were tested, medium (240 mg/day) and high (360 mg/day). The effect of the medium-dose diltiazem was comparable to the therapeutic dose of digoxin at rest but was superior during peak exercise. High-dose diltiazem provided better control of the heart rate than digoxin did, both at rest and exercise, but it was associated with side effects in 75% of the patients. Combined therapy with digoxin and diltiazem enhanced the effect of digoxin alone and led to substantially better control of the heart rate at rest and during peak exercise (Fig 3–8). The drop in heart rate, combined with the concomitant effect on blood pressure, resulted in a marked fall in the pressure-rate product at rest from $10,077 \pm 1,708$ mm Hg/minute with digoxin alone to $7,877 \pm 1,818$ mm Hg/minute after the addition of medium-dose diltiazem, and during exercise from $25,670 \pm 3,606$ to $18,349 \pm 4,115$ mm Hg/minute.

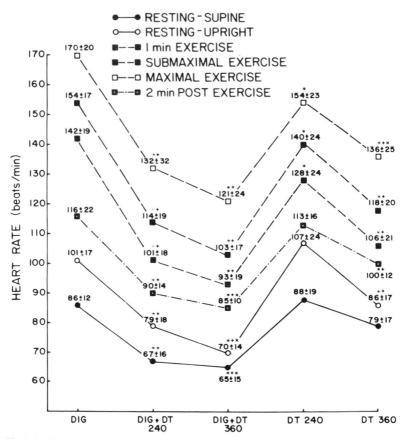

Fig 3–8.—Heart rate as measured at rest, during exercise, and at the recovery from exercise on the various therapeutic regimens studied. DIG = digoxin, DT 240 = diltiazem 240 mg per day, DT 360 = diltiazem 360 per day. *P < .05 vs. digoxin. †, P < .05 vs. DT 240. x, P < .05 vs. DIG + DT 360. (Courtesy of Roth, A., et al.: Circulation 73:316–324, February 1986. By permission of the American Heart Association, Inc.)

When therapy with digoxin combined with diltiazem was continued for 21 ± 8 days in nine patients, the drug combination maintained a persistent effect on heart rate and blood pressure without toxic manifestations or change in the serum digoxin or plasma diltiazem concentrations. Medium-dose diltiazem, when combined with digoxin, is an effective and safe regimen for the treatment of patients with chronic atrial fibrillation and enhances the digoxin-mediated control of heart rate both at rest and during exercise.

▶ An interesting study that, if confirmed in larger studies, demonstrates the usefulness of diltiazem to control the ventricular rate in patients with atrial fibrillation at rest and during exercise. In this study, the best control of the heart rate at rest and during exercise, and the least side effects, were achieved with combined therapy with digoxin and diltiazem.—R.C. Schlant, M.D.

The Automatic Implantable Cardioverter-Defibrillator: Efficacy, Complications, and Device Failures

Francis E. Marchlinski, Belinda T. Flores, Alfred E. Buxton, W. Clark Hargrove, III, V. Paul Addonizio, Larry W. Stephenson, Alden H. Harken, John U. Doherty, E. Wayne Grogan, Jr., and Mark E. Josephson (Univ. of Pennsylvania)
Ann. Intern. Med. 104:481–488, April 1986   3–36

It is thought that the automatic cardioverter-defibrillator is useful in the management of life-threatening ventricular arrhythmias. The 6-month and 12-month survival rates for sudden death in patients with the device appear to be approximately 95%. In addition, short-term morbidity and mortality reportedly are low. Experience with the cardioverter-defibrillator was reviewed, and its potential complications and modes of failure examined, in 26 male and 7 female patients aged 14–77 years who had refractory ventricular arrhythmias. Twenty-six received the automatic implantable cardioverter-defibrillator and seven received only a patch lead during surgery for arrhythmia. During a mean follow-up of 13 months the device discharged in ten patients for at least one episode because of a sustained ventricular arrhythmia, but no sudden deaths occurred. In 17 patients there were 31 complications, including postoperative refractory heart failure, erosion of the coronary artery, thrombosis of the subclavian vein, postoperative stroke after conversion of atrial fibrillation, atelectasis with pneumonia, symptomatic pleural effusions, and infection at the generator site. The cardioverter-defibrillator discharged in nine asymptomatic patients and failed to terminate ventricular fibrillation during postoperative testing in three; premature battery failure occurred in four. During chronic amiodarone therapy, slowing of tachycardia precluded or delayed arrhythmia sensing, as did unipolar ventricular pacing during ventricular fibrillation. The cardioverter-defibrillator can be lifesaving, but its potential complications and interactions with antiarrhythmic drugs and pacemakers must be considered when patients are selected.

▶ This is an interesting review of a relatively large series of patients treated by a new device that represents a major advance in the management of refractory ventricular arrhythmias. This instrument, first reported by Mirowski et al. (*N. Engl. J. Med.* 303:322, 1980) is undergoing continual improvement and refinement. Some of the problems associated with its use are reviewed in this paper. The following paper (Abstract 3–37) suggests additional areas for future improvement in such devices.—R.C. Schlant, M.D.

Dysrhythmias After Direct-Current Cardioversion

Bernd Waldecker, Pedro Brugada, Manfred Zehender, William Stevenson, and Hein J.J. Wellens (Univ. of Limburg, Maastrict, The Netherlands)
Am. J. Cardiol. 57:120–123, January 1986   3–37

Direct-current (DC) countershocks are often used to terminate life-threatening ventricular tachycardia (VT) and fibrillation (VF) as well as atrial fibrillation. Recently, an implantable defibrillator was developed that was shown to be useful for out-of-hospital management of malignant ventricular tachycardias. Nevertheless, a single DC shock may not interrupt VT/VF, and severe dysrhythmias may occur even after successful DC shocks. The effectiveness of immediate DC shocks for FT as compared with VF was evaluated and assessment made of which cardiac rhythm may occur after automatic DC discharges.

The results of DC shocks to interrupt VT (79 episodes) or VF (20 episodes) were analyzed in 62 patients studied with programmed stimulation of the heart. In addition, 13 episodes of atrial fibrillation were cardioverted in 13 patients. Clinical and arrhythmia characteristics were related to the success rate of DC shocks and were also related to postshock arrhythmias. Coronary artery disease was found in 56 patients and cardiomyopathy in 4; the other patients had no apparent structural heart disease. The success rate of transchest DC shocks for VT and VF appeared identical, and the first DC shock interrupted 80% of VT and VF episodes. All episodes were terminated by at least four DC shocks, and a single DC shock changed the morphological pattern or rate in four episodes of VT. Asystole after VT/VF (mean, 1,900 msec) was longer than after atrial fibrillation (1,150 msec); VT/VF recurred within 3 minutes after 26 of 99 initially successful DC shocks, requiring repeat shocks in two patients. Furthermore, ten patients required rate support pacing because of sinus bradycardia or high-degree atrioventricular block. Although antiarrhythmic drugs did not prevent postshock tachycardia, they did facilitate the development of bradycardia.

Reliable and continuous analysis of cardiac rhythm after discharge is mandatory to enable automatic devices to correct unsuccessful discharges or recurrent VT/VF. Demand pacing capability is desirable to prevent severe bradycardia after DC shocks in patients who receive antiarrhythmic drugs.

▶ The development of the implanted automatic defibrillator (Mirowski et al.: *N. Engl. J. Med.* 303:322, 1980) was a major advance in the therapy of highly selected patients with recurrent VR or VF. The results of this study of patients undergoing external defibrillation suggest that such automatic devices should be able to manage unsuccessful discharges or recurrent VT or VF, and, in patients receiving antiarrhythmic drugs, be able to correct severe bradycardia. The future undoubtedly will see rapid and marked advances in the capabilities of automatic implantable devices, including the ability to diagnose the dysrhythmia and automatically treat by defibrillation, overdrive pacing, or demand pacing.—R.C. Schlant, M.D.

Abnormal Signal-Averaged Electrocardiograms in Patients with Non-ischemic Congestive Cardiomyopathy: Relationship to Sustained Ventricular Tachyarrhythmias
David S. Poll, Francis E. Marchlinski, Rita A. Falcone, Mark E. Josephson, and Michael B. Simson (Univ. of Pennsylvania)
Circulation 72:1308–1313, December 1985

A high incidence of life-threatening ventricular arrhythmias and sudden cardiac death has been associated with congestive cardiomyopathy. However, no clinical predictors of sudden cardiac death have been identified. Signal-averaged ECG was developed as a technique for the noninvasive evaluation of intracardiac conduction. In patients with coronary artery disease the presence of abnormalities of the signal-averaged ECG (e.g., low voltage, high-frequency potentials late in the QRS complex, and prolonged duration of QRS has accurately identified patients with sustained ventricular tachycardia. Thus, this technique may be useful in identifying patients with nonischemic disease who are prone to ventricular arrhythmias. This hypothesis was tested by characterizing the signal-averaged ECG in 26 men and 15 women (mean age, 50 years) with nonischemic congestive cardiomyopathy with and without sustained ventricular arrhythmias.

Twelve of the 41 patients had sustained ventricular arrhythmia; 29 had no history of such arrhythmias. The mean ejection fractions were 30% and 24%, respectively. When these results were compared with those of signal-averaged ECGs in 55 normal individuals, it was found that the duration of filtered QRS was longest in patients with sustained ventricular arrhythmia (130.2 msec vs. 105.0 msec in the group without sustained ventricular arrhythmia and 95.9 msec in the normal group). The voltage in the last 40 msec of the filtered QRS was lower in the sustained ventricular arrhythmia group (11.3 μV) than in the group without sustained ventricular arrhythmia (53.5 μV) or the normal group (53.7 μV). In the sustained ventricular arrhythmia group, 83% of the patients had an abnormal signal-averaged ECG that was characterized by both a long duration of the filtered QRS and a late potential of low voltage level, whereas only 2% of normal persons and 14% of patients without sustained ventricular arrhythmias had an abnormal signal-averaged ECG. The signal-averaged ECG can identify patients with nonischemic congestive cardiomyopathy and sustained ventricular arrhythmias. However, the value of this test as a noninvasive predictor of risk in this patient population awaits prospective evaluation.

Improved Selection of Patients for Programmed Ventricular Stimulation by Frequency Analysis of Signal-Averaged Electrocardiograms
Bruce D. Lindsay, H. Dieter Ambos, Kenneth B. Schechtman, and Michael E. Cain (Washington Univ.)
Circulation 73:675–683, April 1986   3–39

Patients at risk of sustained ventricular tachycardia (VT) often are referred for electrophysiologic study. An attempt was made to determine whether frequency analysis aids identification of patients who will have sustained VT on programmed ventricular stimulation. Fast-Fourier transforms (FFTs) of signal-averaged ECGs were compared prospectively with the results of stimulation in 20 patients with sustained VT or cardiac arrest unrelated to new myocardial necrosis (group I) and 38 with nonsustained VT or episodes of syncope (group II). Sustained VT was not documented in group II. The FFT data were expressed as an area ratio quantifying the contributions of 20–50 Hz frequencies in the terminal QRS and S-T segment. Ratios higher than 20 were considered to be abnormal.

Sustained monomorphic VT was induced in 18 group I patients, all of whom had an area ratio higher than 20. Two patients in whom sustained VT was not induced had lower area ratios. Ventricular tachycardia was not inducible in any of 26 group II patients with normal FFT values. Sustained monomorphic VT was induced in 5 of the 12 patients with abnormal FFT values. The FFT values correctly predicted the outcome of programmed ventricular stimulation in 88% of all patients and in 82% of group II patients. The area ratio was independent of other determinants of inducibility, e.g., the left ventricular ejection fraction and past myocardial infarction.

Frequency analysis seems to be useful in identifying patients in whom sustained VT will be induced by programmed ventricular stimulation. This noninvasive procedure can be expected to improve the selection of patients at risk who require programmed stimulation.

▶ These two papers (Abstracts 3–38 and 3–39) further demonstrate the potential ability of signal-averaged ECGs in the detection of patients with nonischemic congestive cardiomyopathy and sustained VT, and of patients in whom sustained VT can be induced during programmed ventricular stimulation. Other reports have suggested that the test may be useful in the detection of patients at higher risk of death after acute myocardial infarction. The ultimate usefulness of this new experimental technique will have to await adequately controlled clinical trials. At present, it appears very promising.—R.C. Schlant, M.D.

Miscellaneous Topics

Comparison of Monounsaturated Fatty Acids and Carbohydrates for Lowering Plasma Cholesterol

Scott M. Grundy (VA Med. Ctr., Dallas, and Univ. of Texas at Dallas)
N. Engl. J. Med. 314:745–748, March 20, 1986   3–40

High levels of plasma cholesterol constitute a risk factor for coronary artery disease (CAD). The usual approach to preventing such disease involves a diet that is low in total fat, saturated fatty acids, and cholesterol. Such a diet is followed in many countries where the prevalence of CAD is relatively low, and this is taken as support for its usefulness. In contrast, there are certain countries (e.g., Italy and Greece) where the traditional diet is high in olive oil, and the total intake of fat can be substantial; however, both the levels of plasma cholesterol and the rates of CAD are relatively low.

Because olive oil is rich in oleic acid, a monounsaturated fatty acid, it was decided to compare the effects on plasma levels of lipids and lipoproteins of a liquid diet that was high in monounsaturates (High-Mono) and a diet that was low in fat (Low-Fat). Eleven patients in a metabolic ward were studied during three dietary periods, each of which lasted for

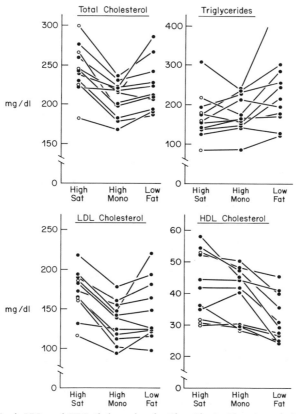

Fig 3–9.—Total, LDL, and HDL cholesterol and triglycerides in 11 patients during three dietary periods. Each point represents mean of six determinations. For High-Sat period *solid circles* represent mean values for study I and *open circles* those for study II. In High-Mono and Low-Fat periods diets for all patients were identical; thus *solid circles* represent values in both studies I and II. To convert values for cholesterol and triglycerides to millimoles per liter, multiply by 0.02586 and 0.01129, respectively. (Courtesy of Grundy, S.M.: N. Engl. J. Med. 314:745–748, March 20, 1986. Reprinted by permission of The New England Journal of Medicine.)

4 weeks. In the third dietary period patients received a diet that was high in saturated fatty acids (High-Sat).

The High-Sat and High-Mono diets contained 40% of their total calories as fat and 43% as carbohydrate; the Low-Fat diet contained 20% fat and 63% carbohydrate. To keep body weight constant, the total calorie intake was adjusted. When compared with the High-Sat diet, both the High-Mono and the Low-Fat diets lowered plasma levels of total cholesterol (by 13% and 8%, respectively) and the low-density lipoprotein (LDL) cholesterol level (by 21% and 15%, respectively). When compared with the High-Sat diet, the Low-Fat diet increased levels of triglycerides and substantially lowered plasma levels of high-density lipoprotein (HDL) cholesterol. Conversely, the High-Mono diet had no effect on levels of triglycerides or HDL cholesterol (Fig 3–9). The ratio of LDL to HDL cholesterol was also significantly lower when the High-Mono diet rather than the Low-Fat diet was followed. In short-term studies in which liquid diets are used and body weight is kept constant, a diet rich in monounsaturated fatty acids appears to be at least as effective in lowering plasma levels of cholesterol as a diet low in fat and high in carbohydrate.

▶ This study confirms prior studies (Mattson, F. M., Grundy, S. M.: *J. Lipid Res.* 26:194–202, 1985), which indicated that diets high in selected monosaturated fatty acids cause reductions in the plasma total cholesterol and LDL cholesterol levels, and that the reductions are essentially equivalent to those produced by diets high in polyunsaturated fatty acids. Both HDL and LDL cholesterol levels tended to decrease during the Low-Fat (20%) diet, whereas there was a greater fall in LDL cholesterol but little, if any, reduction in HDL cholesterol levels with the High-Mono diet, which contained 28% of calories as monounsaturated fatty acids (linoleic acid), 8% as polyunsaturated fatty acids (7.5% as oleic acid), and 4% as saturated fatty acid. In both instances, the reduction in LDL levels may be secondary to the increased activity of LDL receptors secondary to decreased intakes of saturated fatty acids. If confirmed, the studies suggest that diets high in monosaturated fatty acids, and especially oleic acid, the major fatty acid of olive oil, may be as effective as diets low in total fat, but relatively high in polyunsaturated fatty acids. In the meantime, one might use olive oil more freely in place of saturated fatty acids.—R.C. Schlant, M.D.

Effect of Activated Charcoal on Hypercholesterolaemia

Pasi Kuusisto, Vesa Manninen, Heikki Vapaatalo, Jussi K. Huttunen, and Pertti J. Neuvonen (Ilomantsi Health Ctr., Univ. of Tampere, Natl. Public Health Inst., and Univ. of Helsinki)
Lancet 2:366–367, Aug. 16, 1986   3–41

Seven patients with hypercholesterolemia were treated for 4 weeks with activated charcoal in a dosage of 8 gm three times daily. The plasma levels of total cholesterol and low-density lipoprotein (LDL) cholesterol decreased by 25% and 41%, respectively. The high-density lipoprotein cholesterol level increased by 8%. Body weight remained relatively constant. A small but significant fall in blood pressure was observed. Four weeks after completion of charcoal therapy, the total and LDL cholesterol values returned to pretreatment levels (Fig 3–10). No significant changes in serum triglycerides or hematologic variables were observed. With the exception of black-colored stools, no side effects were reported.

Activated charcoal adsorbs a wide range of substances, and it possibly adsorbed cholesterol in this study, interrupting the enterohepatic circulation. Additional studies should be undertaken to further assess the role of activated charcoal as a lipid-modulating agent.

▶ It is surprising that this simple and inexpensive therapy, which was first reported by Friedman et al. [*Kidney Int.* 13 (Suppl. 8):170, 1978], has not been more extensively evaluated. Although activated charcoal presumably binds or adsorbs dietary cholesterol and bile acids, as do cholestyramine or colestipol,

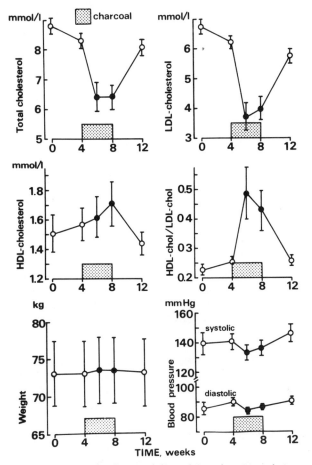

Fig 3–10.—Effect of 4 weeks' intake of activated charcoal (8 gm three times a day) on serum cholesterol level, body weight, and blood pressure in seven hypercholesterolemic patients. Results given as mean ± SEM. (Courtesy of Kuusisto, P., et al.: Lancet 2:366–367, Aug. 16, 1986.)

charcoal slightly raised the high-density lipoprotein-cholesterol level, an effect opposite to that usually produced by these other agents. Additional and larger studies would appear to be indicated, with particular attention to any harmful side effects of therapy with charcoal used for longer than 4 weeks.—R.C. Schlant, M.D.

Regression of Valvular Aortic Stenosis Due to Homozygous Familial Hypercholesterolemia Following Plasmapheresis

Ch. Keller, H. Schmitz, K. Theisen, and N. Zöllner (Universität München)
Klin. Wochenschr. 64:338–341, April 1986   3–43

Dermal lesions that are caused by hypercholesterolemia not associated with hypertriglyceridemia are reversible if treatment can markedly lower serum levels of cholesterol. Recent studies have also demonstrated the feasibility of diminishing tendon xanthomas with lipid-lowering therapy. However, there are few well-documented studies concerning reversion of cardiac or vascular pathology.

Man, 39, was seen initially at age 28 with hypercholesterolemia and xanthomatosis. Skin fibroblasts grown in culture indicated that the patient was homozygous (receptor defective) for familial hypercholesterolemia. He was treated with plasmapheresis every 2 weeks for 4 years. Plasmapheresis was carried out using a continuous flow cell separator; a 5% solution of human albumin substituted with potassium and calcium was used in exchange for 2.5 L of plasma from the patient. Immediately before treatment the patient was given heparin for anticoagulation, which was maintained during treatment. Platelet aggregation was suppressed with ACD-A solution at a 20:1 ratio. The left side of the heart and coronary arteries were visualized using the percutaneous femoral approach, and ECG and phonocardiographic studies were carried out with standard techniques.

Plasmapheresis led to a reduction in the serum level of cholesterol from 765 mg/dl to a mean of 320 mg/dl, and xanthomas of the Achilles tendons decreased from 17 mm to 12 mm on the right side and from 22 mm to 12 mm on the left. The tendon xanthomas on both hands became softer. There was also regression of the valvular stenosis as shown by echocardiography and cardiac catheterization.

The results obtained with plasmapheresis were in basic agreement with those reported by other investigators. However, there are individual differences in the receptor defect and in the clinical course of such patients that are not well understood.

▶ This is an intriguing case report of the use of plasmapheresis to treat a patient with homozygous familial hypercholesterolemia and the resultant decrease in tendon xanthomata and serum cholesterol level. The patient had a pressure difference of 20 mm Hg between the left ventricle and the ascending aorta in 1979 that was not present at catheterization in 1983. This is one of the few instances in which plasmapheresis has produced documented regression of this rare type of aortic stenosis.—R.C. Schlant, M.D.

Digoxin Therapy and Mortality After Myocardial Infarction: Experience in the MILIS Study
J.E. Muller, Z.G. Turi, P.H. Stone, R.E. Rude, D.S. Raabe, A.S. Jaffe, H.K. Gold, N. Gustafson, W.K. Poole, E. Passamani, T.W. Smith, E. Braunwald, and the MILIS Study Group (Brigham and Women's Hosp., Boston, and cooperating institutions of the Multicenter Investigation of the Limitation of Infarct Size)
N. Engl. J. Med. 314:265–271, Jan. 30, 1986   3–43

Certain studies have shown increased mortality in patients with myocardial infarction who are given long-term digoxin therapy. Others contend that the excess mortality seen in such patients can be accounted for by baseline differences in the two groups of patients. Thus, there still exists controversy about the putative hazards of digoxin in patients with myocardial infarction. Data obtained from the Multicenter Investigation of Limitation of Infarct Size (MILIS) were reviewed. All 903 patients enrolled had prior or confirmed myocardial infarction, and 281 were taking digoxin. An attempt was made to determine whether (1) patients taking digoxin had a higher mortality rate than those who were not using digoxin, (2) any mortality increase could be attributed to baseline differences, and (3) an ejection fraction of 40% or less and ventricular couplets or tachycardia constituted risk factors for a detrimental effect of digoxin therapy.

Of the 145 deaths, 78 occurred in patients taking digoxin (28% mortality) and 67 in the nondigoxin group (11% mortality). Most baseline differences between the digoxin and nondigoxin groups indicated a poorer overall prognosis for those taking digoxin. Also, 31% of patients taking digoxin had a prior infarction, and 50% had angina before the event. Complete data were available for 683 patients, in whom Coronary Artery Surgery Study analyses were carried out. Adjustment reduced the difference in survival between the digoxin and nondigoxin groups to a level that was not significant. In the suspected high-risk group (ejection fractions of 40% or less), mortality was analyzed for the 4-month period after infarction, the interval known to be detrimental for digoxin therapy. The unadjusted mortality rates in the digoxin and nondigoxin groups were 17% and 3%, respectively, a nonsignificant difference. After a year of follow-up, the difference in mortality remained nonsignificant.

Because of the difficulties with digoxin therapy, it would not be surprising if patients with myocardial infarction who also received digoxin were at greater risk. The therapeutic dose of digoxin is undesirably close to the toxic dose, and digitalis-induced arrhythmias in laboratory animals are more common after myocardial infarction. Also, there are long-standing uncertainties about the benefits of digoxin in certain subsets of patients with congestive heart failure (CHF). Those with more severe CHF and cardiomegaly showed more clinical benefit from digoxin than did those patients with mild disease and no cardiac enlargement. With regard to the appearance of increased mortality associated with digoxin therapy after myocardial infarction, these patients are given such treatment on the basis of clinical indications that may increase the risk of death regardless of the drug used.

Digoxin was not a significant predictor of mortality after myocardial infarction in this series. The data do not exclude any effect of digoxin, but they do suggest that there is no major hazard. A randomized trial of digoxin vs. placebo after myocardial infarction is the only way to prove the safety of digoxin definitively in such cases. Nonetheless, it would be wise to restrict digoxin use in postinfarction patients to those who are most likely to experience a benefit, i.e., patients with chronic CHF, a low ejection fraction, and left ventricular enlargement.

▶ This study confirms those of Ryan et al. (*Circulation* 67:735, 1983) and of Madsen et al. (*J. Am. Coll. Cardiol.* 3:681, 1984), both of which concluded that digoxin therapy after myocardial infarction does not, by itself, increase mortality, although patients who require digitalis have decreased myocardial function, which is known to be a major determinant of prognosis. This study should help to alleviate inappropriate fears about the use of digoxin in patients after myocardial infarction who have appropriate indications for such therapy.—R.C. Schlant, M.D.

Acute Cardiac Events Temporally Related to Cocaine Abuse
Jeffrey M. Isner, N. A. Mark Estes, III, Paul D. Thompson, Maria Rosa Cos-tanzo-Nordin, Ramiah Subramanian, Gary Miller, George Katsas, Kristin Sweeney, and William Q. Sturner (Tufts-New England Med. Ctr., the Miriam Hosp. and Brown Univ., Providence, Loyola Univ., Maywood, Ill., and the Medical Examiner's Offices of Suffolk County, Mass. and R. I.)
N. Engl. J. Med. 315:1438–1443, Dec. 4, 1986   3–44

Cocaine usage in the United States has reached epidemic proportions with more than five million persons reportedly using the drug regularly. There remains among many physicians the mistaken notion that the intra-nasal use of cocaine is safe. This view is challenged, however, by findings in 7 recent patients and in 19 others reported in the literature. The seven patients seen recently sustained a cardiac disorder that was related tem-porally to the nonintravenous use of cocaine. Six patients were using cocaine intranasally; the remaining patient was free basing the drug. Data concerning all seven are presented in the table.

Woman, 28, experienced cardiac symptoms (e.g., substernal chest pain, nausea, and diaphoresis) 6 hours after using cocaine when she took phenylpropranolamine and chlorpheniramine for insomnia. An ECG showed 8 mm of ST segment depres-sion and runs of ventricular tachycardia. A non-Q-wave infarction evolved. Cardiac catheterization several days later disclosed left ventricular anterolateral-wall hy-pokinesis, but coronary arteriograms were normal. In two of the other patients the outcome was fatal.

Most of the patients in this series were men. Several had factors that might have predisposed them to cardiac events, e.g., a high serum choles-terol level, myocarditis, and a myocardial bridge. A fresh occlusive throm-bus was found in one patient. The interval between cocaine use and the cardiac event ranged from "shortly after" to the same day. Because there are no specific clinical or pathologic markers for cocaine-induced cardio-toxicity, these data indicate only a temporal, not a causal, relationship.

Cocaine can increase the heart rate, blood pressure, and small vessel vasoconstriction, which are properties that could explain some of the cardiac events that occurred. Ischemia secondary to increased myocardial oxygen demand could precipitate arrhythmias, infarction, or aortic rup-ture, particularly in patients with preexisting cardiac abnormalities. Such effects might also occur, even in persons with normal hearts, by focal constriction of the medium-sized coronary arteries. Cardiac complications are not restricted to parenteral use of the drug; in fact, most of the effects occurred after intranasal use. Seizure activity is not a prerequisite for cocaine-related disorders, nor is underlying heart disease a precondition for a cardiac event after cocaine usage; at least 7 of the 26 patients had normal coronary arteriograms. Further, cardiac toxicity is not limited to

CLINICAL AND PATHOLOGIC FINDINGS ASSOCIATED WITH COCAINE ABUSE IN THE PRESENT SERIES

PATIENT No.	SEX/AGE	CARDIAC DISORDER	SEIZURE	FATAL	ROUTE	DOSE	TEMPORAL RELATION	ANGIOGRAPHIC FINDINGS	PATHOLOGICAL FINDINGS[†]
1	M/29	AMI	No	No	Intranasal	1 g	1 hr	—	—
2	F/28	AMI, VT	No	No	Intranasal	—	6 hr	Normal CA, ergonovine-neg	—
3	M/37	AMI, SD	No	Yes	Intranasal	—	—	—	Heart weight, 411 g; 100% LAD; 50% right CA; 25% LC
4	M/37	VT, VF	Yes	No	Intranasal	0.5 g	"Shortly after"	Normal CA; ergonovine-neg; EPS-neg	—
5	M/25	Myocarditis	No	No	Free base	—	"Day of admission"	—	—
6	M/20	SD	No	Yes	Intranasal	—	"Shortly before"	—	Heart weight, 287 g; normal CA; normal myocardium
7	M/23	AMI	No	No	Intranasal	—	11 hr	Normal CA; ergonovine-neg	—

*AMI = acute myocardial infarction, VT = ventricular tachycardia, CA = coronary artery, ergonovine-neg = negative response to administration of ergonovine, SD = sudden death, LAD = left anterior descending coronary artery, LC = left circumflex coronary artery, VF = ventricular fibrillation, and EPS = electrophysiologic study.

†The percentages refer to the extent of the narrowing in histologic cross-sectional area.

(Courtesy of Isner, J.M., et al.: N. Engl. J. Med. 315:1438–1443, Dec. 4, 1986. Reprinted by permission of The New England Journal of Medicine.)

those who consume massive doses of cocaine. The presence of a contaminant in the cocaine cannot be excluded as a cause of the cardiac effects, but the data nonetheless document that fatal and potentially fatal cardiac consequences are associated with cocaine usage.

▶ This report poignantly emphasizes the fact that even small amounts of intranasal cocaine may produce myocardial infarction, which can be fatal. Wiener et al. (*Am. J. Med.* 81:699, 1986) reported two patients with dilated cardiomyopathy attributed to cocaine abuse, and Mathias (*Am. J. Med.* 81:675, 1986) reviewed the literature reports of cocaine-associated myocardial ischemia, which may result from a potentiation of sympathetic activity. In the patients studied at our own institution (Smith, H. D., et al., in press), some patients had infarction with normal coronary arteries on coronary arteriography, whereas others appeared to have thrombus superimposed upon atheromata. The dangers of cocaine and all other abused drugs need even more emphasis by all of us.—R.C. Schlant, M.D.

Smoking as a Risk Factor for Recurrence of Sudden Cardiac Arrest
Alfred P. Hallstrom, Leonard A. Cobb, and Roberta Ray (Univ. of Washington and Harborview Med. Ctr., Seattle)
N. Engl. J. Med. 314:271–275, Jan. 30, 1986   3–45

Cigarette smoking is a major risk factor for coronary artery disease (CAD). The smoking behavior after cardiac arrest of 310 patients who had been habitual smokers at the time of arrest was evaluated to determine whether cigarette smoking is a risk factor for recurrent cardiac arrest. The mean age was 56 years. Patients with CAD were stratified into five prognostic groups according to mortality risk on the basis of recognized criteria.

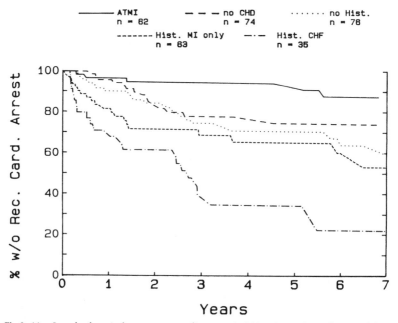

Fig 3–11.—Length of survival to recurrent cardiac arrest in 310 patients who at the time of the index event were habitual smokers. (Courtesy of Hallstrom, A.P., et al.: N. Engl. J. Med. 314:271–275, Jan. 30, 1986. Reprinted by permission of the New England Journal of Medicine.)

These included patients with CAD and acute transmural myocardial infarction at the index event, patients with no CAD, patients with CAD but no history of myocardial infarction or congestive heart failure before the index event, patients with CAD and a history of myocardial infarction, and patients with CAD and a history of congestive heart failure. The expected 1-year rates of recurrent cardiac arrest were 2%, 13%, 11%, 16%, and 40%, respectively, among the strata. Follow-up averaged 47.5 months.

Life-table analyses (Fig 3–11) showed that recurrent cardiac arrest occurred more frequently among patients who continued to smoke than among reformed smokers (27% vs. 19% at 3 years; $P = .038$ by one-sided test adjusted across strata). The survival patterns were similar in the four lower risk strata but were not affected in the highest risk stratum (patients with CAD and history of congestive heart failure). Mortality from other causes was similar in both groups. When patients were stratified into three cigarette consumption groups ($\frac{1}{2}$, $\frac{1}{2}$ to 1, more than 1 pack per day) and further subdivided into the five risk strata, survival analysis showed an enhanced significance ($P = .012$ by one-sided test adjusted across strata), suggesting a possible dose effect.

Long-term survival after resuscitation from out-of-hospital cardiac arrest is improved in reformed smokers. It is possible that continued smoking can accelerate the ongoing atherosclerotic process. However, the difference in early survival suggest that smoking may directly affect myocardial vulnerability to ventricular fibrillation in patients with established CAD.

▶ The message of this study reconfirms the benefit of discontinuing smoking in another subset of patients: those who have survived an episode of sudden cardiac arrest. The Framingham study (Kannel et al.: *Circulation* 51:606, 1975) also found a high incidence of smokers among victims of sudden cardiac arrest. The present authors suggest that one consequence of cigarette smoking and the cause of recurrent cardiac arrest may be enhanced myocardial vulnerability to ventricular arrhythmias, particularly ventricular fibrillation. In addition to this mechanism, I wonder whether or not effects of cigarette smoking on platelet activity may not be important in some of these patients. See the paper by Hammon and Oates (Abstract 3–46).—R.C. Schlant, M.D.

Interaction of Platelets With the Vessel Wall in the Pathophysiology of Sudden Cardiac Death
John W. Hammon and John A. Oates (Vanderbilt Univ.)
Circulation 73:224–226, February 1986   3–46

Sudden cardiac death is a major cause of death in industrialized nations. The essential pathophysiologic features relate to myocardial ischemia with ventricular fibrillation arising in a setting of severe coronary artery atherosclerosis. The most prominent cause of the malignant arrhythmias is acute mural thrombus. Most of the thromboses are associated with fissuring of an atherosclerotic plaque.

If plaque fissuring with attendant mural thrombosis is a trigger for many instances of sudden cardiac death, platelets must participate in the process. This hypothesis was tested by using a preparation in which the maximal activation of platelets could be achieved in a segment of the coronary circulation and one in which ventricular fibrillation frequently occurs, i.e., balloon occlusion of the circumflex coronary artery in the unanesthetized dog.

The incidence of ventricular fibrillation after circumflex occlusion was reduced from 53% to 6% by infusion of prostacyclin in doses that did not alter cardiac output or peripheral resistance. This finding led to evaluation of two structurally different inhibitors of thromboxane synthase in this preparation, RO 22-4679 and U-63557A. These drugs reduced ventricular fibrillation by 82% and 100%, respectively. Moreover, inhibition of ventricular fibrillation by U-63557A was attenuated by pretreatment with indomethacin, suggesting that a metabolite of the endoperoxide that accumulates during inhibition of thromboxane synthase is probably responsible for protection from ventricular fibrillation.

▶ This study lends further credence to the data implicating platelet-endothelial interactions in the pathogenesis of sudden cardiac death. It should serve as a stimulus for further basic and clinical research into the development and clinical use of medications that favorably influence platelets and the endothelium, particularly those that enhance the production of prostacyclin. There is good evidence that most patients who die suddenly of a malignant arrhythmia associated with coronary artery disease have an acute mural thrombosis. Davies and Thomas (*N. Engl. J. Med.* 310:1137, 1984) found thrombosis in 74% of such patients and further noted that the thrombosis was associated with fissuring of an atherosclerotic plaque in most instances. See the paper by Gewirtz et al. (Abstract 3–47) for more on platelets and myocardial ischemia.—R.C. Schlant, M.D.

Impaired Arteriolar Vasodilation Induced by Thrombosis of a Coronary Arterial Stenosis

Henry Gewirtz, Harvey Sasken, Manfred Steiner, and Albert S. Most (Rhode Island Hosp., Pawtucket Mem. Hosp., and Brown Univ., Providence)
Am. J. Physiol. 249:H1154–H1166, December 1985   3–47

Platelet aggregation at sites of atherosclerotic coronary artery lesions has been implicated in acute myocardial ischemia and infarction. The possible role of arteriolar vasospasm in the pathogenesis of regional myocardial ischemia in this setting is unknown. Studies were performed in closed-chest swine with an artificial left anterior descending (LAD) coronary artery stenosis of 82% that underwent spontaneous thrombosis to determine whether platelet aggregation and thrombus formation contribute to ischemia by impairing dilation of arterioles distal to the stenosis. The studies used U46619, a thromboxane A_2 mimetic, and UK 38485, a specific thromboxane synthetase inhibitor.

Endocardial blood flow in the distal LAD artery zone declined after occlusion, but distal endocardial resistance did not change at 5 minutes or 15 minutes. Distal epicardial resistance did decrease. Lactate extraction changed to production at 15 minutes. The arterial-anterior interventricular vein thromboxane B_2 difference changed from 13 to -16 pg/0.1 ml at 5 minutes.

The findings suggest that platelet aggregation and release at a spontaneously thrombosing coronary stenosis contribute to ischemia by reducing the coronary diameter and by impairing flow regulation in the distal portion of the endocardium. Distal embolization is not necessary for myocardial ischemia to occur in this setting. Interference with vasodilation in the distal coronary bed deprives the myocardium of an important defense mechanism.

▶ This study indicates that platelet aggregation at the site of a coronary arterial stenosis may contribute to myocardial stenosis by thrombus formation and by the release of thromboxane A_2 from aggregating platelets, which may facilitate both additional aggregation and distal arteriolar vasoconstriction. Distal embolization from the thrombus may also occur, although it was not demonstrated in this study. The phenomenon of intermittent platelet aggregation at the site of a partially obstructed vessel was described early by Folts et al. (*Circulation* 54:365, 1976).—R.C. Schlant, M.D.

Exercise: A Risk for Sudden Death in Patients With Coronary Heart Disease
Leonard A. Cobb and W. Douglas Weaver (Univ. of Washington and Harborview Med. Ctr., Seattle)
J. Am. Coll. Cardiol. 7:215–219, January 1986   3–48

Regular physical exercise has been widely advocated, at least in part because of its perceived health benefits. Regular exercise may help to prevent coronary artery disease (CAD) and its complications. However, the value of exercise in patients with known CAD has not been defined, and there are uncertainties about the effect of regular exercise in favorably altering the course of such patients. For example, exercise conditioning does not appear to have beneficial effects on extant coronary atherosclerosis, or on the incidence of reinfarction, complex ventricular arrhythmias, or mortality. An attempt was made to establish an estimate of the risk of sudden death associated with physical exertion, particularly in patients with CAD.

The normal heart is protected from lethal arrhythmias except in unusual conditions (e.g., profound electrolyte derangement or adverse drug reactions) and victims of sudden death almost always have underlying heart disease. However, one third of these individuals may be asymptomatic and unaware of underlying disorders. Ventricular fibrillation is the arrhythmia usually underlying the sudden cardiac death syndrome, particularly when exertion-related events occur. The specific factors that could cause the arrhythmia include coronary vascular spasm, local release of potent circulating substances (e.g., thromboxane), and arousal of the central and peripheral nervous system. Transient myocardial ischemia is a plausible cause for most episodes of exertion-related cardiac arrest in patients with CAD, and in one series premonitory warning symptoms were noted in only about a quarter of these patients; fewer than a third had new Q waves or enzymatic evidence of myocardial necrosis after resuscitation. Although there has been no large, prospective assessment of the role of exertion in precipitating cardiac arrest, reports indicate that exertion-related events may account for 10% to 30% of all sudden deaths. In retrospect, many reported individuals had symptoms that suggested the presence of heart disease; however, cardiac arrest was often the first recorded manifestation of it. Only limited data are available about the incidence of cardiac arrest in patients attending a cardiac rehabilitation program. However, the incidence of exertion-related cardiac arrest in cardiac rehabilitation programs is small and, because of the availability of rapid defibrillation, death rarely occurs.

The risk of exertion-induced cardiac arrest should be weighed against the perceived benefits and pleasures of physical exertion. Although it is not clearly defined, there is almost certainly a relationship between the intensity of exercise and the risk incurred for sudden death. The patient and the physician should both be informed and should make a determination concerning exercise based on individual considerations.

► These observations provide a basis for advising some patients with CAD to avoid vigorous and unsupervised exercise. For many patients, participation in low to moderate noncompetitive exercise is prudent. It is properly emphasized that physicians should consider if vigorous exercise is worth the risks in persons with CAD, whether or not the disease is evident. They also refute the common belief that exercise testing is useful in determining limits for exercise programs, and note that the available data do not support the contention that establishing such limits results in a safe conditioning program. All physicians interested in this problem should also read the latest book by Ernst Jokl, one of the world's authorities on exercise and cardiology: *Sudden Death of Athletes,* Charles C Thomas, 1985. It is a gem.—R.C. Schlant, M.D.

Radiation-Induced Coronary Artery Disease
Lillian D. Dunsmore, Marie A. LoPonte, and Richard A. Dunsmore (Ergon Cardiac Rehabilitation Ctr. and Paoli Mem. Hosp., Paoli, Pa.)
J. Am. Coll. Cardiol. 8:239–244, July 1986   3–49

The late development of coronary artery disease (CAD) occurred in three patients after middle to late 1960s conventional radiation therapy for Hodgkin's disease. Large areas of the heart were exposed to approximately 40 Gray (4,000 rad) to avoid geographic miss of disease.

CASE 1.—Female, 19, received radiation therapy in 1965 and again in 1970 when disease recurred. In 1974 the patient underwent cardiac catheterization after acute anterior myocardial infarction. This apparently represented accelerated atherosclerosis secondary to radiation castration, or possibly was radiation-induced CAD.

Case 2.—Male, 19, underwent total nodal irradiation in 1966. In 1968, chest radiography revealed pulmonary fibrosis along the medial aspects of the left and right upper lobes within the confines of the mediastinal irradiation portal, considered secondary to radiation therapy. Acute posterolateral and anterior myocardial infarction occurred in 1978 and, 2 months later, another insult to the infarcted areas caused the patient to stop his 15-year smoking habit. In 1983 the patient was hospitalized with a large pleural effusion, which showed severe left ventricular dysfunction and a large apical aneurysm. Cardiac catheterization revealed 80% stenosis of the left mainstem coronary artery, among other coronary artery compromisation. Bypass surgery was performed, but the patient died postoperatively. Autopsy and microscopic findings revealed intimal thickening with medial replacement, encroachment on the lumen, fibrotic hyalinization, and fibroblasts, believed to result from the effects of radiation on the coronary arteries.

Case 3.—Man, 32, underwent two courses of radiation therapy in 1970. The patient was hospitalized in 1973 for acute anterior myocardial infarction. Coronary artery disease was diagnosed, but bypass grafting was not considered.

The pathologic features of coronary arteries differ in patients exposed to radiation compared with nonirradiated patients who have typical atherosclerotic lesions. Coronary artery disease resulting from radiation therapy prior to 1979 may continue to appear during the next 20 years. The clinician should remain aware of this condition.

▶ Three patients had evidence of CAD 8, 12, and 4 years after receiving at least 40 Gray (4,000 rad) to large areas of the heart. The pathologic changes in the coronary arteries of the one patient who was examined were nonatherosclerotic. Ikaheimo et al. (*Am. J. Cardiol.* 56:943, 1985) reported acute, transient, and usually symptomless changes in cardiac function during the first 6 months after radiation therapy in 21 patients with breast cancer. The occurrence of such acute changes caused by radiation are easier to understand than are the late changes in the coronary vessels, myocardium, and pericardium, which may become apparent only many years after the radiation therapy.—R.C. Schlant, M.D.

The Effect of Weight Reduction on Left Ventricular Mass: A Randomized Controlled Trial in Young, Overweight Hypertensive Patients
(Univ. of New South Wales, Sydney)
N. Engl. J. Med. 314:334–339, Feb. 6, 1986   3–50

Left ventricular (LV) hypertrophy is a serious complication of sustained elevation of blood pressure that is associated with a higher risk of death from cardiovascular disease than the risk associated with hypertension alone. An increased total LV mass is also associated with an increased risk of cardiovascular events in patients with hypertension. Moreover, numerous reports have linked obesity to elevated blood pressure, and obesity is also associated with increased LV mass and wall thickness. Although weight reduction lowers blood pressure in overweight hypertensive patients, the effects of weight reduction on LV mass and wall thickness have not been defined. A comparison was made of the effects of weight reduction, metoprolol, and placebo on M-mode echocardiographic measurements of the thickness and mass of the LV wall in 41 young, overweight patients with hypertension.

By the end of the follow-up period, patients in the weight-reduction group had lost an average of 8.3 kg; their blood pressure had also decreased by an average of 14/13 mm Hg, as compared with 12/8 mm Hg in the metoprolol group and 9/4 mm Hg in the placebo group. Moreover, in the weight-reduction group interventricular septal and posterior wall thickness decreased by 14% and 11%, respectively, and the LV mass decreased by 20%. The decreases in interventricular septal and posterior wall thickness and in LV mass were markedly higher in the weight reduction group when compared with the metoprolol and placebo groups. Changes in weight, independent of changes in blood pressure, were directly associated with changes in LV mass. Weight reduction thus decreases LV mass in overweight hypertensive patients; control of obesity is thus important not only in the treatment of hypertension but also in prevention of LV hypertrophy.

▶ It has been known for a number of years that reduction of blood pressure in patients with hypertension produces decreases in the thickness of the ventricular septum and posterior LV wall and in the calculated LV mass. (Schlant, R. C., et al.: *Cardiovasc. Med.* 2:477, 1977). Subsequent studies indicated that repression was more likely to occur when the hypertension was controlled with β blockers, calcium channel blockers, converting enzyme inhibitors, or centrally acting agents than with arterial vasodilators or diuretics. This study documents the benefits of weight reduction in patients with systemic hypertension, both in helping to lower the blood pressure and in decreasing LV mass.— R.C. Schlant, M.D.

4 Coronary Artery and Other Heart Diseases, Heart Failure

Myocardial Infarction

Thrombolysis and PTCA

Effectiveness of Intravenous Thrombolytic Treatment in Acute Myocardial Infarction

Italian Group for the Study of Streptokinase in Myocardial Infarction (Istituto di Ricerche Farmacologiche "Mario Negri," Milan)

Lancet 1:397–401, Feb. 22, 1986   4–1

A trial was planned to test the effectiveness and safety of intravenously administered streptokinase early after myocardial infarction. The clinical benefit of intravenous infusion of the drug was assessed in terms of reduction of in-hospital and 1-year mortalities.

The study, a controlled, multicenter, unblinded trial with central randomization, included 11,712 patients in 176 coronary care units who were enrolled during a 17-month period. Patients hospitalized within 12 hours after onset of symptoms and with no contraindications to streptokinase therapy were randomized to receive the drug intravenously in addition to usual treatment. At 21 days, the overall hospital mortality was 10.7% in streptokinase recipients, and 13% in controls, and 18% reduction. The extent of beneficial effect appeared to be function of time from onset of pain to streptokinase infusion.

Intravenous infusion of 1.5 million units of streptokinase can be recommended as a safe treatment for all patients with no positive contraindications who can be treated within 6 hours after onset of pain. Retrospective pooled analyses suggest that the period of benefit may be longer, and this possibility is being tested in a major study. Although follow-up results are obviously of the greatest importance to provide the complete benefit profile of treatment, the striking decrease in in-hospital mortality must be regarded as a valuable result on its own. It means that substantially more patients can live to receive further pharmacologic and other treatments to improve outcome after myocardial infarction.

▶ This is a crucial study of thrombolytic therapy and needs careful review by all who treat patients with myocardial infarction. The Italian investigators deserve a great deal of credit for a beautiful study that has influenced the management of patients with acute myocardial infarction all over the world. Time is of the essence in instituting thrombolysis and, as noted in subsequent papers, the use of percutaneous transluminal coronary angioplasty in conjunction with thrombolytic therapy is gaining support. However, the fact seems clear that, given early, the intravenous administration of streptokinase may have a profound effect on mortality in patients with acute myocardial infarction, and this initial therapy can be given in hospitals without coronary arteriography facilities.—R.L. Frye, M.D.

Intravenous Recombinant Tissue-Type Plasminogen Activator in Patients With Acute Myocardial Infarction: A Report From the NHLBI Thrombolysis in Myocardial Infarction Trial
David O. Williams, Jeffrey Borer, Eugene Braunwald, James H. Chesebro, Lawrence S. Cohen, James Dalen, Harold T. Dodge, Charles K. Francis, Genelle Knatterud, Phillip Ludbrook, John E. Markis, Hiltrud Mueller, Patrice Desvigne-Nickens, Eugene R. Passamani, Eric R. Powers, A. Koneti Rao, Robert Roberts, Allan Ross, Thomas J. Ryan, Burton E. Sobel, Michael Winniford, Barry Zaret, and Co-Investigators (Natl. Heart, Lung, and Blood Inst., NIH, Bethesda)
Circulation 73:338–346, February 1986   4–2

Recombinant tissue-type plasminogen activator (rt-PA) is a means of fibrin-specific activation that holds promise of avoiding the systemic thrombolysis that complicates conventional intravenous treatment. The efficacy and safety of an infusion of rt-PA were studied in 47 patients seen within 7 hours of the onset of ischemic pain caused by acute myocardial infarction. In patients with significant luminal obstruction nitroglycerin was injected into the infarct vessel and, if obstruction persisted, a dose of 40 mg of rt-PA was infused intravenously in 1 hour, followed by 20 mg/hour for 2 hours. Infusion of heparin began 1 hour after the start of treatment with rt-PA and continued for 8–10 days.

Thirty-seven patients had total occlusion at the outset and 28 (78%) exhibited reperfusion during infusion of rt-PA. Reperfusion persisted at 90 minutes in 25 (68%) patients. Sustained perfusion of the infarct vessel was observed in 14 of 21 initially reperfused patients on follow-up angiography. Eight of nine patients with subtotal occlusion had sustained perfusion of the infarct vessel on late angiography. Significant bleeding occurred in 15 patients, usually in the form of a hematoma at the site of acute catheterization. Levels of fibrinogen and plasminogen fell significantly with rt-PA infusion, but the degradation of fibrin(ogen) products increased. However, no patient had a level of fibrinogen of less than 140 mg/ml.

The brief intravenous infusion of rt-PA can restore blood flow in many patients with acute infarction caused by total coronary occlusion. Some patients have reocclusion of the infarct vessel despite anticoagulation with heparin, and bleeding has occurred frequently.

▶ Subsequent studies have resulted in the use of a larger dose of rt-PA in the ongoing Thrombolysis in Myocardial Infarction (TIMI) trial, and the superiority of intravenous rt-PA in thrombolysis versus intravenous streptokinase has already been reported. The importance of the present study relates to documentation, in this early and small series of patients, of a high reocclusion rate (33%) after successful thrombolysis, and the hazards of bleeding when this agent is combined with heparin. All of this has contributed to recognition of the need for properly controlled studies of the effect of percutaneous transluminal coronary angioplasty in the infarct-related artery (and the timing of such a procedure) in patients receiving intravenous thrombolytic therapy. Phase II of the TIMI trial addresses these questions.—R.L. Frye, M.D.

Hemorrhage vs Rethrombosis After Thrombolysis for Acute Myocardial Infarction
Gerald C. Timmis, Eberhard F. Mammen, Renato G. Ramos, Seymour Gordon, V. Gangadharan, Andrew M. Hauser, Douglas C. Westveer, and James R. Stewart (William Beaumont Hosp., Royal Oak, Mich., and Wayne State Univ.)
Arch. Intern. Med. 146:667–672, April 1986   4–3

The systemic lytic state that regularly follows intracoronary or intravenous streptokinase administration is a major problem in thrombolysis for acute myocardial infarction. Bleeding after intracoronary thrombolysis may reflect the effects of circulating degradation products of fibrinogen and fibrin. The effect of the timing of heparin infusion on bleeding or reocclusion after intracoronary streptokinase administration was studied in 89 patients in whom heparin was infused immediately after streptokinase and 93 subsequent patients in whom heparin infusion was delayed for 12 hours. Thrombolysis was begun within 5 hours of the onset of acute infarction in both groups. Streptokinase was given in a dose of 200,000 international units in 1 hour. The heparin infusion was adjusted to maintain an activated clotting time of 150 seconds.

Twenty-two patients given heparin immediately after thrombolysis had bleeding. Bleeding was major in five patients, and caused one death. All 14 hemorrhages in those given heparin on a delayed basis were minor. Reocclusion occurred before discharge in 18% of those given heparin immediately and in 11% of those given heparin later. Reocclusion was somewhat less likely to occur in patients who bled than in those who did not. The bioassayable fibrinogen content was reduced for 20 hours after streptokinase infusion, independently of the occurrence of bleeding. Immunoassayable defibrinogenation, however, was much less striking.

Bleeding after thrombolysis with streptokinase appears to be related to the anticoagulant effects of fibrinogen degradation products interacting with heparin. It may be largely independent of hypofibrinogenemia. A 12-hour delay in administering heparin may reduce the risk of bleeding and have little effect on the risk of reocclusion.

► This paper is another example of the need for cardiologists to review their hematology in relation to coagulation and thrombolysis. The interaction of heparin with fibrinogen degradation products is proposed as the basis for excess bleeding after heparin therapy. It seems clear that bleeding is not related to absolute fibrinogen levels. As the authors note, the precision of knowing reocclusion rates with the delayed heparin approach is compromised by patient selection, but at least no gross problem with reocclusion could be identified.—R.L. Frye, M.D.

Analysis of Coagulation and Fibrinolysis During Intravenous Infusion of Recombinant Human Tissue-Type Plasminogen Activator in Patients With Acute Myocardial Infarction

Désiré Collen, Henri Bounameaux, Frans De Cock, Henri R. Lijnen, and Marc Verstraete (Univ. of Louvain, Belgium)
Circulation 73:511–517, March 1986   4–4

Human tissue-type plasminogen activator (t-PA) induces thrombolysis in the absence of systemic fibrinolytic activation in several animal models of coronary thrombosis. Coagulation and fibrinolysis were followed in 129 patients with evolving myocardial infarction, 64 of whom were randomly assigned to receive infused recombinant t-PA and 65, streptokinase. A dose of 0.75 mg of t-PA per kg was infused in 90 minutes. The dose of streptokinase was 1,500,000 international units (IU) in 60 minutes. All patients received 5,000 IU of heparin intravenously before the start of infusion.

The mean euglobulin fibrinolytic activity was 910 IU of t-PA per ml in the t-PA group and equivalent to 430 IU of t-PA per ml in the streptokinase group. The mean plasma fibrinogen concentration was 57% of baseline in the t-PA group at the end of infusion and 7% in the streptokinase group. The mean concentration of fibrinogen-fibrin degradation products increased to 0.75 mg/ml in the streptokinase group, but to only 0.1 mg/ml in the t-PA group. Plasma concentrations of α_2-antiplasmin, plasminogen, and factor V decreased significantly more in the streptokinase-treated patients.

Much less systemic fibrinolytic activation occurred with recombinant t-PA than with streptokinase in patients with acute myocardial infarction in this study. Increased fibrinogen breakdown was associated with successful recanalization. The extent of systemic activation of fibrinolysis occurring in t-PA-treated patients was probably overestimated.

▶ These studies of dose responses to thrombolytic drugs are crucial to clinical cardiologists as the use of these agents in patients with myocardial infarction increases. This t-PA in the doses studied clearly is associated with less activation of systemic fibrinolysis, but bleeding complications are not totally absent.—R.L. Frye, M.D.

A Prospective Randomized Clinical Trial of Intracoronary Streptokinase Versus Coronary Angioplasty for Acute Myocardial Infarction

William O'Neill, Gerald C. Timmis, Patrick D. Bourdillon, Peter Lai, V. Gan-

ghadarhan, Joseph Walton, Jr., Renato Ramos, Nathan Laufer, Seymor Gordon, M. Anthony Schork, and Bertram Pitt (Univ. of Michigan and William Beaumont Hosp., Royal Oak, Mich.)
N. Engl. J. Med. 314:812–818, March 27, 1986   4–5

Intracoronary streptokinase infusion is effective as coronary thrombolytic treatment, but its effect on subsequent left ventricular (LV) infarction remains to be established. A randomized, prospective, clinical trial was undertaken to determine if immediate amelioration of coronary stenoses by coronary angioplasty is more effective than thrombolytic recanalization with intracoronary streptokinase infusion in improving LV function after acute myocardial infarction (AMI). Of 56 patients seen within 12 hours of their first symptoms of AMI, 27 were randomly assigned to receive streptokinase in doses ranging from 250,000 to 350,000 units, and 29 underwent coronary angioplasty. Mean durations of symptoms and times to recanalization were similar in both groups. Treatment was defined as being successful if angiograms showed prompt opacification of the distal part of the vessel after therapy. Serial contrast ventriculograms were used to assess ventricular function before discharge.

Successful recanalization was achieved in 83% of angioplasty-treated patients and 85% of streptokinase-treated patients, not a significant difference. However, residual coronary stenosis was significantly reduced by a mean of 43% in the angioplasty group, compared with 83% in streptokinase group ($P < .001$). Residual stenosis of 70% or more was present in only 4% of the angioplasty patients, compared with 83% of the streptokinase patients ($P < .01$). Serial contrast ventriculograms showed that increases in global ejection fraction ($P < .001$) and regional wall motion ($P < .05$) were greater in the angioplasty group. Short-term follow-up after therapy showed no overall difference in the occurrence of postinfarction angina; however, patients with single-vessel disease were less likely to have postinfarction angina when treated by angioplasty, whereas those treated with streptokinase were more likely to have exercise-induced periinfarction ischemia on predischarge thallium scintigraphy (47% vs. 14%, $P < .05$), and were more likely to undergo subsequent elective angioplasty.

Coronary angioplasty is as effective as intracoronary streptokinase thrombolysis is in achieving early coronary recanalization. However, angioplasty is significantly more effective in alleviating the underlying stenosis of the infarct-related coronary artery, resulting in more effective preservation of ventricular function after therapy.

Prevention of Subsequent Exercise-Induced Periinfarct Ischemia by Emergency Coronary Angioplasty in Acute Myocardial Infarction: Comparison With Intracoronary Streptokinase
Anthony Y. Fung, Peter Lai, Jack E. Juni, Patrick D. V. Bourdillon, Joseph A. Walton, Jr., Nathan Laufer, Andrew J. Buda, Bertram Pitt, and William W. O'Neill (Univ. of Michigan)
J. Am. Coll. Cardiol. 8:496–503, September 1986   4–6

Predischarge submaximal exercise imaging with single-photon emission CT and ^{201}Tl-chloride was used to compare the efficacy of emergency angioplasty and the intracoronary administration of streptokinase in preserving left ventricular function in 28 patients seen within 12 hours of onset of symptoms of acute myocardial infarction. Fourteen patients underwent emergency coronary angioplasty with the use of Grüntzig catheters; 14 others received intracoronary infusion of streptokinase. Thallium studies were carried out within 7–20 days after admission. Peri-infarct ischemia was defined as the presence of a reversible thallium defect adjacent to a fixed defect on qualitative evaluation.

Reperfusion was achieved in 86% of patients who had angioplasty or were given intracoronary infusions of streptokinase. The mean residual stenosis of the infarct vessel at predischarge angiography was 44% in the angioplasty group and 75% in the streptokinase group. Nine percent of angioplasty patients had exercise-induced peri-infarct ischemia, compared with 60% of the streptokinase-treated patients. Only angioplasty patients had a significant increase in global left ventricular ejection fraction. Duration of exercise and the pressure-rate product achieved were similar in the two groups.

A significant number of patients with acute myocardial infarction have residual viable myocardium at risk after successful acute intervention, probably in relation to the degree of residual stenosis of the infarct vessel. Patients treated with intracoronary infusion of streptokinase may be at greater risk than those who have emergency coronary angioplasty. Further studies are needed to determine whether angioplasty, alone or combined with thrombolytic therapy, is superior in salvaging myocardium and promoting long-term survival.

▶ These two studies from Michigan (4–5 and 4–6) contain important data regarding thrombolysis and percutaneous transluminal coronary angioplasty (PTCA) in the setting of acute myocardial infarction. It seems clear in the first paper that PTCA was equally effective in recanalizing occluded coronary arteries, and that the underlying residual stenosis in the infarct-related artery was reduced as a result of PTCA. The sample size is too small to make any conclusions regarding mortality, and the authors' caution is well taken also regarding the functional correlates. Although there was a trend toward less angina and better left ventricular function in the angioplasty patients, the numbers are small. These encouraging data are consistent with several other studies noted in this section (Abstracts 4–6, 4–7 and 4–8).

The subsequent paper presents supporting evidence for the improved functional status of patients receiving PTCA during acute myocardial infarction. This is a crucial area for further investigation, because the implications for our health care system are profound. Fortunately, these questions are being addressed in several large trials.—R.L. Frye, M.D.

Percutaneous Transluminal Coronary Angioplasty After Thrombolytic Therapy: A Prospective Controlled Randomized Trial

Raimund Erbel, Tiberius Pop, Karl-Jürgen Henrichs, Klaus von Olshausen, Carl J. Schuster, Hans-Jürgen Rupprecht, Claus Steuernagel, and Jïgen Meyer (Mainz, Federal Republic of Germany)
J. Am. Coll. Cardiol. 8:485–495, September 1986   4–7

Percutaneous transluminal coronary angioplasty after successful thrombolysis is intended to reduce residual narrowing of the coronary lumina and thereby the risk of reocclusion. A prospective study was undertaken in 162 consecutive patients with acute transmural myocardial infarction who underwent combined intravenous and intracoronary thrombolytic therapy with streptokinase. Coronary angiography was repeated in multiple views, and vessels that remained occluded were recanalized; in 79 patients (group I) a 3F recanalization catheter was used, and in 83 (group II) a 4F Grüntzig balloon catheter. Intracoronary infusion of streptokinase was performed superselectively after reperfusion. Angioplasty was then done in group II patients only. The groups were clinically comparable at baseline.

Initial angiography showed an open vessel in 34% of group I and 25% of group II patients. Final reperfusion rates were 90% and 86%, respectively. Angioplasty was attempted in 69 of 71 group II patients, with a success rate of 65% and an occlusion rate of 3%. Reocclusion occurred in 20% of group I patients and in 14% of group II patients during the hospital stay. Angioplasty reduced coronary stenosis from 82% to 51% in group II patients. The rate of reocclusion in 45 patients who had successful angioplasty was 7%, compared with 32% in 22 patients in whom angioplasty failed. Regional left ventricular function improved only in group II patients who had anterior infarction. Hospital mortality in this study was 14% in group I and 8% in group II.

Combined thrombolysis and mechanical recanalization can provide a reperfusion rate of 90% in patients with acute myocardial infarction. Patients with anterior infarction have improved regional left ventricular function. Successful angioplasty lowers the rate of reocclusion.

▶ This is a well-designed trial that provides important new data on the importance of relief of high-grade residual stenoses in preventing reocclusion of arteries after successful thrombolysis. The improvement in regional left ventricular function seems clear in those with successful angioplasty. The practical challenge of providing early angiography for all appropriate patients soon after infarction is a serious one that demands additional data before implemented as health care policy.—R.L. Frye, M.D.

Preservation of Global and Regional Left Ventricular Function After Early Thrombolysis in Acute Myocardial Infarction

Patrick W. Serruys, Maarten L. Simoons, Haryanto Suryapranata, Frank Vermeer, William Wijns, Marcel van den Brand, Grits Bär, Chris Zwaan, X. Hanno Krauss, William J. Remme, Jan Res, Freek W.A. Verheugt, Ronald van Domburg, Jacobus Lubsen, and Paul G. Hugenholtz (Working Group on Thrombolytic Therapy in Acute Myocardial Infarction of the Netherlands Interuniversity Cardiology Inst., Rotterdam)
J. Am. Coll. Cardiol. 7:729–742, April 1986   4–8

Rapid restoration of coronary blood flow through thrombolysis can salvage myocardium and improve survival in animal models, but conflicting clinical results have been reported. The effects of myocardial reperfusion on left ventricular (LV) function were studied by analyzing systolic regional wall motion in 332 patients randomized to reperfusion or conventional coronary care. Studies were performed 2–8 weeks after onset of infarction, and angiographic findings were available after acute reperfusion in patients assigned to thrombolysis. Reperfusion was attempted by intracoronary streptokinase infusion. Conventional treatment was directed at rapidly achieving an "optimal" hemodynamic state, with no signs of LV failure or pulmonary wedge pressure of less than 12 mm Hg.

Significant preservation of LV function was observed after thrombolytic therapy, with an ejection fraction of 53%, compared with 47% in conventionally treated patients. Wall motion analysis indicated significant improvement of function in the infarct zone in patients with inferior and anterior infarction, and also significant changes in regional function in remote areas in the acute and chronic stages. Left ventricular function declined significantly over time in patients in whom thrombolysis failed.

Early reperfusion by thrombolysis can improve both regional and global LV function in patients with acute myocardial infarction. This probably explains the lower early and late mortalities associated with successful thrombolysis. Reperfusion may have to be supplemented by revascularization, as by angioplasty, to optimize the chance of full functional recovery.

▶ This multicenter trial on thrombolysis from The Netherlands has provided important data on the management of patients with acute myocardial infarction. The data reported in this paper are clearly presented, but changes in protocol during the course of the study cause some confusion and complicate the interpretation. However, as presented, the data support a conclusion of benefit in terms of LV function with successful thrombolytic therapy, and in a small number of patients, the advantages of percutaneous transluminal coronary angioplasty (PTCA) combined with thrombolytic therapy are suggested. Further study of PTCA in this setting is underway in several trials.—R.L. Frye, M.D.

General Topics

Intravenous Infusion of Magnesium Sulphate After Acute Myocardial Infarction: Effects on Arrhythmias and Mortality

L.F. Smith, A.M. Heagerty, R.F. Bing, and D.B. Barnett (Univ. of Leicester, England)
Int. J. Cardiol. 12:175–180, August 1986   4–9

Cardiac dysrhythmias cause much early mortality after acute myocardial infarction (AMI), and magnesium deficiency has been associated with serious dysrhythmias. A double-blind, placebo-controlled pilot study was undertaken to learn whether early magnesium sulfate therapy is of value in patients with AMI. The 200 patients received 65 mmole of magnesium sulfate in a 24-hour period, to double the serum magnesium concentration, or a placebo infusion of saline. Ninety-two patients given magnesium and 93 given placebo were evaluable. The groups were similar with regard to site of infarction, peak serum creatine phosphokinase activity, and early treatment.

Hypokalemia was found in six magnesium-treated patients and one given placebo. Magnesium treatment did not significantly alter the serum magnesium concentration in the first hour, but values about doubled within 6 hours. Seven placebo-treated patients and two given magnesium died in the first 24 hours; the difference was not significant. Ventricular dysrhythmias requiring treatment were less frequent in the magnesium-treated group. The total number of deaths and ventricular dysrhythmias was significantly less in magnesium-treated patients.

The therapeutic effect of magnesium sulfate might be enhanced by giving a bolus dose at the outset. Adverse reactions have not occurred, and magnesium may be given patients who have significant heart failure, in contrast with intravenous β blockade. Real benefit was apparent in this study, and a larger trial of magnesium sulfate in patients with AMI appears to be warranted.

▶ This is a provocative study. Similar results have been reported by Rasmussen (*Lancet* 1:234, 1986). Worthy of note is the potential of hypomagnesemia and torsade des pointe type of ventricular tachycardia in patients receiving cisplatin, an antitumor agent (Stewart, A. F.: *Am. J. Obstet. Gynecol.* 153:660, 1985).—R.L. Frye, M.D.

Effects of Full-Dose Heparin Anticoagulation on the Development of Left Ventricular Thrombosis in Acute Transmural Myocardial Infarction
Pascal Gueret, Olivier Dubourg, Alain Ferrier, Jean Christian Farcot, Michel Rigaud, and Jean-Pierre Bourdarias (Univ. of Paris-Quest, Boulogne Sur Seine, France)
J. Am. Coll. Cardiol. 8:419–426, August 1986   4–10

The role of full-dose heparin anticoagulation in preventing intraventricular thrombus formation was examined in a series of 90 patients with a first acute transmural myocardial infarction who were admitted within 12 hours (mean, 5 hours) of onset of symptoms. The 76 men and 14 women had a mean age of 53 years. Forty-six patients received heparin intravenously, and then subcutaneously, to maintain an activated partial thromboplastin time of 1.5–2.5 times normal.

Serial two-dimensional echocardiography showed no left ventricular thrombus in 44 patients with inferior infarction, 23 of whom received heparin. Twenty-one thrombi developed in patients with anterior myocardial infarction. The rates were 38% in patients given heparin and 52% in patients not given heparin, not a significant difference. No group differences were apparent in clinical variables, infarct size, hemodynamic impairment, or left ventricular function as judged from echocardiographic and cineangiographic findings.

Left ventricular thrombosis was not significantly reduced by full-dose heparin anticoagulation in patients with acute transmural myocardial infarction in this study. The value of giving heparin to all patients remains to be established, and it is still necessary to select patients at higher risk of subsequent thrombosis. Left ventricular thrombosis is relatively frequent in patients who have anterior infarction associated with early dyskinesia, but it is unclear whether the benefits of anticoagulation outweigh the risk of hemorrhage in these patients. Heparin prophylaxis does not appear to be worthwhile in patients with inferior infarction.

▶ This study is in conflict with that of Nordrehaug, J. C., et al. (*Am. J. Cardiol.* 55:1491, 1985) regarding the prevention of mural thrombus in patients with anterior infarction given heparin. However, the data seem clear from a number of studies that the risk of mural thrombus in inferior infarction is extremely small. Thus, the routine use of heparin in all patients with inferior infarction may not be worth the risk of bleeding.—R.L. Frye, M.D.

Haemostatic Function in Myocardial Infarction
A. Hamsten, M. Blombäck, B. Wiman, J. Svensson, A. Szamosi, U. de Faire, and L. Mettinger (Danderyd Hosp. and Karolinska Inst., Stockholm)
Br. Heart J. 55:58–66, January 1986   4–11

Young adults with ischemic heart disease comprise an ideal group in which to examine factors that are operative early in the course of atherogenesis and arterial thromboembolism. Blood coagulation and fibrinolysis were studied 3–6 months after myocardial infarction in 116 male and 32 female patients younger than age 45 years and in 136 age-matched and sex-matched controls. Most patients had no symptoms, or only mild angina in the early postinfarction period.

Plasma levels of fibrinogen and the fast inhibitor of tissue plasminogen activator were elevated in male patients, even after correction for levels of orosomucoid, blood group distribution, body size, and use of tobacco and alcohol. The capacity of plasminogen activator was reduced. Female patients had significantly increased levels of factor VIII, von Willebrand's factor, the fast inhibitor of tissue plasminogen activator, α_2-antiplasmin, and C1 inhibitor. Increased levels of factor VIII were related to a persistent inflammatory response. Multivariate analysis showed that male patients and controls were best distinguished by a combination of the levels of fibrinogen and tissue plasminogen activator inhibitor. For female patients the best distinction was with levels of von Willebrand's factor and the inhibitor. Male patients with multivessel coronary artery disease had higher levels of fibrinogen than those with single-vessel disease.

Disordered coagulation of blood and fibrinolysis may have considerable independent significance for the occurrence of myocardial infarction in young women because these conditions predispose to coronary thrombosis. The hemostatic changes seen in males may be primarily involved in the evolution of coronary atherosclerosis, but they also may have a role in precipitating infarction in patients with severe, widespread coronary atheromatosis.

▶ This is an excellent study of patients younger than 45 years of age after myocardial infarction with a very helpful review of literature relating to thrombosis research (12 of 42 references from the hematologic literature). It is essential that, as cardiologists, we develop more interaction with hematologists working in the field of thrombosis research. There is increasing interest in the inhibitor of tissue plasminogen activator and, as noted in this paper, young patients with myocardial infarction have elevated levels for this inhibitor. This invites a number of speculations regarding the significance of this finding not only in relation to a possible inability to lyse clots, but also in the pathogenesis of atherosclerosis.—R.L. Frye, M.D.

Pericardial Effusion in the Course of Myocardial Infarction: Incidence, Natural History, and Clinical Relevance
Enrique Galve, Herminio Garcia-Del-Castillo, Arturo Evangelista, Juan Battle, G. Permanyer-Miralda, and J. Soler-Soler (Ciudad Sanitaria "Vall d'Hebron," Barcelona)
Circulation 73:294–299, February 1986   4–12

Whether pericardial effusion after acute myocardial infarction (AMI) favors a diagnosis of subclinical pericarditis or is predictive of postinfarction syndrome is unclear. A study was carried out in 121 patients with AMI who underwent serial echocardiography prospectively 1, 3, and 10 days after admission and 3 and 6 months after discharge. Fifty-four patients with unstable angina, 57 without evident cardiovascular disease, and 35 who had cardiac operations were also evaluated.

Pericardial effusion was diagnosed echocardiographically in 28% of patients with AMI. On the third day after admission, 25% of survivors had pericardial effusion; it was found in 8% of patients with unstable angina and in 5% of those without heart disease. Effusion was considered to be mild in 88% of the patients and moderate in 12%. It did not correlate significantly with myocardial enzyme release or the need for resuscitation or electroconversion. Arrhythmias and conduction disorders were no more frequent in patients with effusion, and pericardial effusion was no more frequent in patients with pericarditis, regardless of the diagnostic criteria used. No patient had tamponade or required pericardiocentesis, and none had evidence of constrictive pericarditis. No patient surviving the acute phase of infarction experienced postinfarction syndrome. Pericardial effusion was not related to mortality in the hospital or at 6 months.

Pericardial effusion is frequent in patients with AMI, but it is generally mild and does not influence the outcome significantly. It need not lead to a change in heparin dosage.

▶ Many have opinions regarding the hazards of full-dose heparin in patients with pericardial effusion in the setting of AMI, but this important and carefully done study presents conclusions on this question based upon data. This study supports the conclusion that pericardial effusion is not a contraindication to the use of heparin in patients with myocardial infarction.—R.L. Frye, M.D.

Clinical and Prognostic Importance of Persistent Precordial (V₁–V₄) Electrocardiographic ST Segment Depression in Patients With Inferior Transmural Myocardial Infarction

Nicholas J. Lembo, Mark R. Starling, Louis J. Dell'Italia, Michael H. Crawford, Tuhin R. Chaudhuri, and Robert A. O'Rourke (Univ. of Texas at San Antonio and VA Hosp., San Antonio)

Circulation 74:56–63, July 1986   4–13

The clinical and prognostic significance of precordial ST segment depression during acute inferior transmural myocardial infarction is uncertain. The predictive value of precordial ST depression lasting for 24 hours or longer was examined in 43 men (mean age, 61 years) with a first acute inferior transmural infarction. Ten patients (group I) had persistent anterior precordial ST segment depression 24 hours after admission to coronary care, defined as 1 mm or more of depression in leads V_1–V_4. The other 33 patients (group II) did not have such ST depression.

Group I patients were older, and all were in Killip classes II–IV, compared with one third of group II patients. Average peak creatine kinase activity was more than twice as high in group I. Pulmonary wedge pressures were higher in group I, and cardiac indices were lower. The mean ejection fraction was 44%, compared with 53% in group II, and wall motion indices were higher in group I. Recurrent infarction was seen in 30% of group I patients and in no group II patient. One-year mortalities were 60% in group I and zero in group II. The most powerful predictor of 1-year mortality on univariate analysis was persistent precordial ST segment depression. Multivariate analysis yielded the same finding and also showed an elevated heart rate to be an important factor in 1-year mortality. Precordial ST segment depression that lasts for 24 hours identifies patients with acute inferior transmural myocardial infarction who are at increased risk of recurrent infarction and death within 1 year.

▶ This series clearly documents an adverse prognosis for patients with ST segment depression in the precordial leads persisting for 24 hours or longer after inferior wall myocardial infarction. Included in the paper is an excellent discussion of the basis for controversy regarding this question, as well as mechanisms for the depressed ST segments. Several other publications this year deal with this interesting problem (Quyyumi, A., et al.: *Lancet* 1:347, 1986; Stafford, A. N., et al.: *Aust NZ J. Med.* 16:378, 1986).—R.L. Frye, M.D.

Elevated CK-MB With Normal Total Creatine Kinase in Suspected Myocardial Infarction: Associated Clinical Findings and Early Prognosis
Robert A. Hong, Jonathan D. Licht, Jeanne Y. Wei, Gary V. Heller, Alvin S. Blaustein, and Richard C. Pasternak (Charles A. Dana Res. Inst., Beth Israel Hosp., and Harvard Univ., Boston)
Am. Heart J. 111:1041–1047, June 1986   4–14

Myocardial infarction has been confirmed in patients with normal serum levels of creatine kinase (CK) but with increased MB fractions. Data were reviewed on the hospital course of 347 consecutive patients hospitalized with suspected myocardial infarction to relate early morbidity and mortality to both the total peak level of CK and the MB fraction.

Sixty-four percent of the patients had both a normal total peak level of CK and a normal MB fraction. Nineteen percent had elevations of both values in a pattern that was diagnostic of typical infarction. The peak MB fraction alone was elevated in 12% of the patients; 5.5% had a flat or falling level of CK and CK-MB that was not diagnostic of an acute event. Patients with microinfarction in whom only the peak MB fraction was elevated were older than patients with normal values, and they had congestive heart failure more frequently. They required more intensive treatment over a longer period and had a higher in-hospital mortality of 7.5%. Hospital mortality in patients with macroinfarction was 29%.

Patients with microinfarction who present with a normal total level of CK but an elevated CK-MB fraction are at increased risk and require aggressive management and further evaluation. Treatment with β-blockers, nitrates, or antiarrhythmic agents may prove helpful in preventing reinfarction, or sudden death, or both, in patients with microinfarction.

▶ These observations are of great importance to the practicing physician to document the need for caution in ignoring these enzyme and isoenzyme patterns, particularly in patients with a high pretest likelihood of coronary artery disease. This is a frequent problem in patients after noncardiac surgery, a group not specifically addressed in this study; additional observations in this subgroup would be most welcome.—R.L. Frye, M.D.

Systemic and Transcardiac Platelet Activity in Acute Myocardial Infarction in Man: Resistance to Prostacyclin
Hiltrud S. Mueller, Parinam S. Rao, Mark A. Greenberg, Peter M. Buttrick, Ira I. Sussman, Howard A. Levite, Richard M. Grose, Vicente Perez-Davila, Janet E. Strain, and Theodore H. Spaet (Albert Einstein College of Medicine)
Circulation 72:1336–1345, December 1985   4–15

There is increasing evidence that platelets are important in the pathogenesis of acute ischemic heart disease. An attempt was made to characterize circulating platelets during acute myocardial infarction and the factors influencing platelet behavior. Fifty-nine patients with evolving infarction were studied. Twenty-two received an infusion of prostacyclin at a mean rate of 13 ng/kg/minute for 90 minutes. Both transcardiac platelet function and the response to prostacyclin were studied in 15 patients with anterior infarction.

Plasma concentrations of β-thromboglobulin and thromboxane B_2 were increased threefold and tenfold, respectively. A leftward shift of the thromboxane B_2-prostacyclin ratio was evident. Platelets circulating during evolving infarction were hyperaggregable with adenosine diphosphate and relatively resistant to prostacyclin. The content of platelet cyclic adenosine monophosphate (cAMP) and the cAMP response to prostacyclin were decreased. Platelet hyperreactivity was most marked early in the course of infarction and declined over time. "Ischemic" platelets produced twice the normal amount of thromboxane A_2 in response to arachidonic acid. The antiplatelet effect of prostacyclin was much reduced in patients with anterior infarction.

A proaggregatory environment is apparent in studies of platelet behavior during evolving myocardial infarction, with increased platelet reactivity in both the peripheral and the coronary circulations, and relative resistance to prostacyclin. Patients with acute infarction might benefit from suppression of platelet function. Conventional antiplatelet agents and prostacyclin, however, are probably inadequate by themselves. Alternatives include drugs that decrease catecholamine release; agents that block platelet α_2-adrenergic receptors; potentiators of prostacyclin effect (e.g., phosphodiesterase inhibitors) and drugs that reduce synthesis and/or the effects of thromboxane.

▶ This is a beautiful clinical investigation. The study is of interest both to those who manage patients with acute myocardial infarction and investigators interested in studying platelet function in the coronary circulation. This study critically analyzes the question of platelet activation as a result of blood withdrawal via catheters in the coronary sinus. The in vitro studies of platelet function documenting a "resistance" to PGI_2 are particularly interesting. The platelet is obviously a complex cell with multiple metabolic pathways and effects. As suggested by the investigators, a simplistic approach to only one aspect of platelet function is inappropriate.—R.L. Frye, M.D.

Diltiazem and Reinfarction in Patients With Non-Q-Wave Myocardial Infarction: Results of a Double-blind, Randomized, Multicenter Trial
Robert S. Gibson, William E. Boden, Pierre Theroux, Hans D. Strauss, Craig M. Pratt, Mihai Gheorghiade, Robert J. Capone, Michael H. Crawford, Robert C. Schlant, Robert E. Kleiger, Phillip M. Young, Kenneth Schechtman, M. Benjamin Perryman, Robert Roberts, and the Diltiazem Reinfarction Study Group
N. Engl. J. Med. 315:423–429, Aug. 14, 1986   4–16

The efficacy of the calcium channel blocker diltiazem, was examined in a randomized, double-blind trial conducted at nine centers in 1982. In all, 576 patients with acute non-Q wave infarction, documented symptomatically and enzymatically, were studied. Diltiazem was given to 287 patients in a dosage of 90 mg every 6 hours; the other 289 received placebo. Treatment began within 24–72 hours after onset of infarction and continued for up to 2 weeks unless the patient was discharged earlier. The treatment and control groups were well matched for clinical and laboratory variables.

Reinfarction occurred in 9% of the placebo group and 5% of those given diltiazem. Five of seven patients with second reinfarctions were in the placebo group. Postinfarction angina was comparably frequent in the two groups. Twenty placebo-treated patients and ten given diltiazem had refractory postinfarction angina. Cumulative 2-week mortalities from all causes were similar in the two groups. There were no differences in heart block. Five percent of diltiazem patients were withdrawn because of adverse reactions.

Treatment with diltiazem for up to 2 weeks after acute non-Q wave myocardial infarction protects against reinfarction and refractory angina. Diltiazem can be recommended as an effective prophylactic agent in these patients, but further studies of its long-term efficacy are warranted. Patients remain at risk of recurrent infarction, especially in the first year. There is evidence that non-Q wave infarction represents aborted Q wave infarction, and that a large mass of viable but jeopardized myocardium remains without the perfusion zone of the infarct vessel.

▶ This is a beautifully designed, conducted, and reported clinical trial. Such trials are most clear in settings where high event rates occur in the "control" group. Such is the case in non-Q wave infarction. Practitioners who apply these important data need to pay attention to dose levels of the drug used in the trial. It is my impression that, frequently, the drug is used in practice but not in the doses actually studied. Smaller doses may be effective, but it seems important to try to achieve the dose levels actually proven to be of benefit. It is also clear that diltiazem is not the entire answer to managing patients with non-Q wave infarction because reinfarction occurred in 5.2% of a highly selected group (64% of eligible patients were excluded because of a clinical judgment that treatment with a calcium channel blocker was indicated).—R.L. Frye, M.D.

Scintigraphically Detected Predominant Right Ventricular Dysfunction in Acute Myocardial Infarction: Clinical and Hemodynamic Correlates and Implications for Therapy and Prognosis
Prediman K. Shah, Jamshid Maddahi, Daniel S. Berman, Max Pichler, and H. J.C. Swan (Cedars-Sinai Med. Ctr., Los Angeles, and Univ. of California at Los Angeles)
J. Am. Coll. Cardiol. 6:1264–1272, December 1985   4–17

Although earlier studies indicated little hemodynamic disorder after right ventricular destruction in animals, clinical observations show low cardiac output and elevated right heart filling pressures after acute infarction with predominant right ventricular dysfunction. Forty-three patients who had scintigraphic evidence of predominant right ventricular dysfunction were studied. The right ventricle was dilated, with hypokinesia, akinesia, or dyskinesia of its free wall or apex, and the right ventricular ejection fraction was less than 0.39. The left ventricular ejection fraction was at least 0.45. All of the patients had acute inferior infarction.

Three fourths of the patients had a cardiac index of no more than 2.5 L/minute/sq m (average, 2 L/minute/sq m). The right ventricular ejection fraction had increased by at least 10% at follow-up in 79% of the 33 patients studied. The mean value rose from 0.30 to 0.40, with no significant change in mean left ventricular ejection fraction. More than half of the patients had bradycardia with hypotension, and 41% had low-output syndrome or shock. Six patients had complete atrioventricular block, and seven had early ventricular tachycardia or fibrillation. Two patients, both with ventricular septal rupture, died.

Predominant right ventricular dysfunction with nearly normal left ventricular function is often associated with low cardiac output. Volume loading alone is usually inadequate in these patients, necessitating added inotropic and vasoactive drug therapy. In-hospital complications are frequent, but short-term survival is excellent in the absence of such complications as septal, free wall, or papillary muscle rupture.

▶ This study clearly documents a higher rate of right ventricular dysfunction in the setting of myocardial infarction than might be expected clinically. Furthermore, the hemodynamic studies related to low cardiac output are of great practical value in emphasizing that one should not rely only on volume expansion in treating this not uncommon problem.—R.L. Frye, M.D.

Frequency and Significance of Induced Sustained Ventricular Tachycardia or Fibrillation Two Weeks After Acute Myocardial Infarction
Anil K. Bhandari, Jeffrey S. Rose, Adam Kotlewski, Shahbudin H. Rahimtoola, and Delon Wu (Univ. of Southern California, Puget Sound Cardiology Consultants, Everett, Wash., and Chang Gung Mem. Hosp., Taipei, Taiwan)
Am. J. Cardiol. 56:737–742, Nov. 1, 1985   4–18

There is some evidence that programmed ventricular stimulation may help to identify a subgroup of patients with acute myocardial infarction who are at high risk of sudden cardiac death. Responses to programmed stimulation were related to the ambulatory ECG, treadmill exercise, and angiographic findings in 45 patients evaluated a mean of 2 weeks after acute transmural infarction. The electrophysiologic protocol included burst ventricular pacing and one to three ventricular extrastimuli at two cycle lengths from the right ventricular apex, right ventricular outflow tract, and left ventricle.

Sustained monomorphic ventricular tachycardia was induced in 13 patients and ventricular fibrillation in 7 others (group I). Two extrastimuli sufficed to induce tachycardia-fibrillation in ten of these patients. A severe left ventricular wall motion abnormality was found in 70% of group I patients and 22% of patients without inducible tachycardia-fibrillation (group II). The groups did not differ significantly in sites of infarction, frequency or grade of ventricular ectopic rhythm on ambulatory monitoring, the double product on submaximal exercise, left ventricular ejection fraction, or number of obstructed coronary arteries. One sudden death occurred in each group during a mean follow-up of 10 months. One group I patient experienced spontaneous sustained ventricular tachycardia.

Electric induction of sustained ventricular tachycardia or fibrillation 2 weeks after acute myocardial infarction is associated with a higher risk of left ventricular wall motion abnormality, but its prognostic significance appears to be limited. Antiarrhythmia therapy does not appear to improve survival after myocardial infarction.

▶ Initial enthusiasm for the prognostic significance of programmed stimulation in patients early after myocardial infarction has waned. This study documents that patients with larger infarcts have a high rate of inducible ventricular tachycardia with an aggressive stimulation protocol, which did not correlate with the subsequent clinical course. The investigators clearly identify the problems of patient selection, sample size, and stimulation protocols in assessing the prognostic significance of electrophysiologic testing in patients early after infarction.—R.L. Frye, M.D.

The Prevalence and Clinical Significance of Residual Myocardial Ischemia 2 Weeks After Uncomplicated Non-Q Wave Infarction: A Prospective Natural History Study

Robert S. Gibson, George A. Beller, Mihai Gheorghiade, Thomas W. Nygaard, Denny D. Watson, Barry L. Huey, Sharon L. Sayre, and Donald L. Kaiser (Univ. of Virginia)

Circulation 73:1186–1198, June 1986   4–19

Non-Q wave infarction is generally thought to be associated with less necrosis and lower hospital mortality than Q wave infarction, but long-term survivals seem to be similar. Residual ischemic tissue may dispose to recurrent ischemia and infarction. This possibility was evaluated in a prospective study of 241 patients aged 65 and younger with acute uncomplicated myocardial infarction, none of whom had thrombolytic therapy or emergency angioplasty. Non-Q wave infarction was diagnosed in 87. The two groups were similar at baseline except for more frequent past angina and previous infarction in the group with non-W wave infarction. Norris coronary prognostic index scores were comparable in the Q wave and non-Q wave groups.

Lower peak creatine kinase activities and higher resting left ventricular ejection fractions indicated less necrosis in the non-Q wave group at baseline. Akinesia and dyskinesia were less evident in this group, and the patients had more patent infarct vessels. Thallium redistribution within the infarct zone on exercise was greater in the non-Q wave group. Cardiac mortalities were 8% in the Q wave group and 9% in the non-Q wave group during a median follow-up of 30 months. Reinfarction rates were 6.5% and 18%, respectively. Unstable angina requiring hospitalization was more frequent in the non-Q wave group. Bypass grafting or angioplasty was performed in 33% of non-Q wave patients, compared with 19% of the Q wave group. Nearly 90% of recurrent infarcts in the non-Q wave group involved the same area as the initial infarct, compared with 20% in the Q wave group.

Some patients with non-Q wave infarction, especially those with significant ischemia, should be considered for early cardiac catheterization and revascularization. Aspirin and calcium channel blockade should be evaluated in patients recovering from non-Q wave infarction.

▶ This study documents that patients with non-Q wave infarction represent an unstable group with a relatively high rate of reinfarction. Such a conclusion has been reported by other investigators. I agree with the conclusions of the authors that such patients are candidates for a more aggressive approach to revascularization early.—R.L. Frye, M.D.

Effect of Propranolol After Acute Myocardial Infarction in Patients With Congestive Heart Failure

Kul Chadda, Sidney Goldstein, Robert Byington, and J. David Curb (for the Beta Blocker Heart Attack Trial Res. Group), Heart Inst., New Hyde Park, N.Y.)

Circulation 73:503–510, March 1986   4–20

The Beta Blocker Heart Attack Trial is a multicenter, double-blind, randomized study of propranolol administration 5–21 days after myocardial infarction. Propranolol was assigned to 1,916 patients and placebo to 1,921, and the patients were followed for an average of 25 months. A history of congestive heart failure was present in 18% of the propranolol group and 19% of the placebo group. The daily dose of propranolol was 180 mg or 240 mg.

Definite congestive heart failure occurred in nearly 7% of both groups after randomization. Failure was considerably more frequent in patients with a history of heart failure before randomization. An increased cardiothoracic ratio at baseline predicted the occurrence of heart failure, as did an increased heart rate, diabetes, past myocardial infarction, older age, and more than ten premature ventricular beats per hour. Mortality was about 25% lower in propranolol-treated patients, whether or not congestive failure occurred. Propranolol reduced the occurrence of sudden death by 47% in patients with past heart failure and by 13% in the other patients.

Propranolol has beneficial effects on mortality and morbidity when given after acute myocardial infarction, without increasing the overall occurrence of congestive heart failure (Fig 4–1). In this series, patients with previous heart failure who were given propranolol had a greater reduction in total

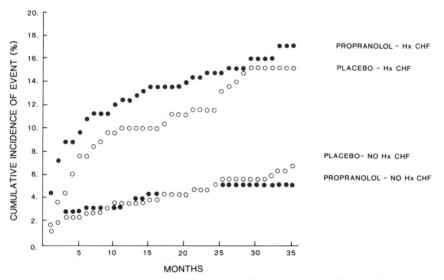

Fig 4–1.—Cumulative incidence of congestive heart failure (CHF) by prior history of CHF and by treatment group. (Courtesy of Chadda, K., et al.: Circulation 73:503–510, March 1986. By permission of the American Heart Association, Inc.)

mortality and coronary events without incurring an overall increased rate of heart failure. An increased incidence of congestive heart failure occurred in patients in the propranolol-treated group who had a history of prior heart failure. The drug may have antiarrhythmic or anti-ischemic effects in this setting.

Effect of Propranolol in Patients With Myocardial Infarction and Ventricular Arrhythmia
Lawrence M. Friedman, Robert P. Byington, Robert J. Capone, Curt D. Furberg, Sidney Goldstein, and Edgar Lichstein (for the Beta Blocker Heart Attack Trial Res. Group, Natl. Heart, Lung, and Blood Inst., NIH, Bethesda)
J. Am. Coll. Cardiol. 7:1–8, January 1986   4–21

The Beta Blocker Heart Attack Trial was a placebo-controlled, double-blind, randomized study of propranolol therapy in 3,837 patients, started 5–21 days after myocardial infarction. Propranolol was given in a daily dose of 180 mg or 240 mg to 1,916 patients; these patients and those given placebo were followed for 25 months on average. About 85% of patients had 24-hour ambulatory ECG monitoring at baseline. Arrhythmias were comparably distributed in the propranolol and placebo groups at the outset.

Both total mortality and sudden deaths increased with advancing grades of arrhythmia. Patients with arrhythmia who received propranolol did not have more frequent symptoms or adverse effects than those without arrhythmia. Antiarrhythmia drugs were prescribed more often for patients given placebo than for those given propranolol. There also were trends toward more frequent use of β blockers, diuretics, and digitalis in placebo-treated patients. Compliance with propranolol therapy declined as the severity of arrhythmia increased.

These findings fail to support the hypothesis that propranolol is of particular benefit to patients with past myocardial infarction who have ventricular arrhythmias. The presence of arrhythmia, however, can identify higher-risk patients in whom similar relative benefit will result in greater absolute benefit from propranolol therapy. Mechanisms other than the antiarrhythmia effect probably contribute to the reduction in mortality associated with propranolol administration.

▶ The Beta Blocker Heart Attack Trial has provided important data regarding the treatment of patients with myocardial infarction. These retrospective analyses of subgroups that might be considered at high risk are extremely important to the practicing physician. It is crucial for clinicians to understand that the greatest mortality reduction with β-blocker therapy after myocardial infarction occurs in those patients to whom one is uneasy about prescribing the drug (Furberg, C. D., et al.: *Circulation* 69:761, 1984). As noted in the paper on heart failure (Abstract 4–20), some patients with a history of heart failure may not tolerate the drug, but careful clinical observation while giving it usually allows its use with important benefit.

The paper dealing with ventricular arrhythmias is also of great interest. Although one might suppose that patients with ventricular arrhythmia on monitoring prior to randomization would derive the most benefit from propranolol, this was not the case. These observations thus stimulate further speculation and study of the mechanisms for mortality reduction with β-blocker therapy after myocardial infarction, observed now in multiple excellent trials [May, G. S.: *Circulation* 67(Suppl. I)]:46, 1983.—R.L. Frye, M.D.

Congestive Heart Failure

Effect of Vasodilator Therapy on Mortality in Chronic Congestive Heart Failure: Results of a Veterans Administration Cooperative Study

Jay N. Cohn, Donald G. Archibald, Susan Ziesche, Joseph A. Franciosa, W. Eugene Harston, Felix E. Tristani, W. Bruce Dunkman, William Jacobs, Gary S. Francis, Kathleen H. Flohr, Steven Goldman, Frederick R. Cobb, Pravin M. Shah, Robert Saunders, Ross D. Fletcher, Henry S. Loeb, Vincent C. Hughes, and Bonnie Baker (for the Veterans Administration Study Group, Univ. of Minnesota)

N. Engl. J. Med. 314:1547–1552, June 12, 1986   4–22

A Veterans Administration Cooperative Study was initiated to determine whether two widely used vasodilator regimens could alter mortality in patients with congestive heart failure. Men with stable chronic congestive heart failure undergoing treatment with digoxin and diuretics were assigned in a random, double-blind trial to treatment with prazosin, hydralazine plus isosorbide dinitrate, or placebo. The study included 642 patients: 284 had coronary disease and 358 did not. The mean follow-up was 2.3 years.

Life-table analysis revealed no differences in the three groups. A reduction in mortality was observed in those given hydralazine-nitrate compared with those given placebo during the entire follow-up period. This study provides data to support the hypothesis that treatment with hydrazaline-nitrate reduces mortality for 3 years. Mortality in the coronary heart disease group was higher than in the group without it, there was no evidence for a differential effect of therapy in the two groups.

Mortality among hydralazine-nitrate treated patients was reduced in comparison with that among patients in the placebo group during the entire follow-up period. These results suggest the use of hydralazine and isosorbide dinitrate to decrease mortality in patients with chronic congestive heart failure.

► This is truly a landmark study. Clinicians have debated the true survival benefits, if any, of vasodilator therapy. This beautifully designed, performed, and reported trial provides a clear answer. A specific combination of vasodilators improves survival, although mortality, as expected in this type of patient, remains high. The investigators have already answered the obvious question as to the effect of angiotensin converting enzyme inhibitors. A new trial is in progress and the results are eagerly awaited. The more profound effects of captopril on the neurohumoral consequences of heart failure stimulates optimistic expectations.—R.L. Frye, M.D.

Prognostic Importance of Serum Sodium Concentration and Its Modification by Converting Enzyme Inhibition in Patients With Severe Chronic Heart Failure
Wai Hung Lee and Milton Packer (Mount Sinai School of Medicine, New York)
Circulation 73:257–267, February 1986   4–23

Patients with severe chronic heart failure have a highly unfavorable long-term prognosis. Although a variety of clinical and hemodynamic variables have been identified that correlate with mortality, it is unclear that modification of these factors by inotropic, diuretic, or vasodilator drugs alters their prognostic import. Experimental observations suggest that high-risk variables reflect a more fundamental process that progresses inexorably despite therapeutic interventions. Treatment directed at amelioration of these variables may obscure their utility as prognostic markers without altering the natural history of the disease. The determinants of survival were analyzed in a large group of patients with severe chronic heart failure immediately before treatment with various vasodilators. The interaction of these prognostic variables with subsequent drug therapy was also evaluated.

The association of 30 clinical, hemodynamic, and biochemical variables with survival were analyzed in 203 consecutive patients with severe heart failure. All variables were assessed just before vasodilator drug treatment, and all patients were followed for 6–94 months.

By regression analysis, the pretreatment serum sodium concentration was the most powerful predictor of cardiovascular mortality. Hyponatremic patients had a substantially shorter median survival than did patients with a normal serum sodium concentration (164 days vs. 373 days). The unfavorable prognosis for hyponatremic patients appeared to be related to their marked elevation of plasma renin activity, because they fared significantly better when treated with angiotensin converting enzyme inhibitors than when treated with vasodilators that did not interfere with angiotensin II biosynthesis (median survival, 232 days vs. 108 days). In contrast, there was no selective benefit of converting enzyme inhibition on survival of patients with a normal serum sodium concentration, in whom plasma renin activity was low (mean, 1.9 ng/ml/hour).

The interaction among serum sodium concentration, drug treatment, and long-term outcome suggests that the renin-angiotensin system may exert a deleterious effect on survival of some patients with chronic heart failure that can be antagonized by converting enzyme inhibition, and provides a clinical counterpart for the similar prognostic role that has been postulated for angiotensin II in experimental heart failure.

▶ This is an important retrospective study of prognosis in patients with heart failure and continues the important contributions of Dr. Packer and his colleagues. The impact or prognosis of serum sodium renin levels and therapy with angiotensin converting enzyme inhibitors seems convincing. Whereas improved survival has been demonstrated in the VA trial with hydralazine and isordil as combined therapy (Abstract 4–22), the need for additional trials to test the observations reported in this paper is obvious. Such trials are in progress and their results are awaited with interest.—R.L. Frye, M.D.

Contribution of Vasopressin to Vasoconstriction in Patients With Congestive Heart Failure: Comparison With the Renin-Angiotensin System and the Sympathetic Nervous System

Mark A. Creager, David P. Faxon, Sally S. Cutler, Osvaldo Kohlmann, Thomas J. Ryan, and Haralambos Gavras (Boston Univ.)

J. Am. Coll. Cardiol. 7:758–765, April 1986   4–24

Increased vascular resistance may result from sympathetic stimulation and increased renin-angiotensin activity in patients with congestive heart failure, and it has been suggested that neurohypophyseal vasopressin secretion may be a contributing factor. The role of vasopressin in increased systemic vascular resistance was studied in ten men aged 50–78 years with chronic congestive heart failure. The average duration of symptoms was 23.5 months, and the average radionuclide left ventricular ejection fraction was 24%. The pressor effect of physiologic concentrations of vasopressin was examined by using a competitive antagonist of the vasoconstrictor action of vasopressin at the vascular V_1 receptors. The sympathetic nervous system was inhibited by phentolamine and the renin-angiotensin system by captopril.

The vasopressin antagonist decreased systemic vascular resistance in three patients who had plasma vasopressin concentrations of more than 4 pg/ml. The group average was 2.4 pg/ml. The plasma vasopressin concentration correlated with the decrease in resistance and serum sodium and creatinine concentrations. Captopril reduced systemic vascular resistance by 20%, especially in patients with high plasma renin activity. Phentolamine reduced vascular resistance by 34% on average, but the reduction did not correlate with the baseline norepinephrine concentration. All patients had elevated norepinephrine values, which correlated with both the baseline stroke volume index and the plasma renin activity.

Endogenous vasopressin apparently can contribute to elevated systemic vascular resistance in patients with chronic congestive heart failure. The sympathetic nervous system contributes to systemic vasoconstriction, and the renin-angiotensin system is often a determinant of systemic vascular resistance.

▶ An increasing interest is evolving in vasopressin activity in congestive heart failure. This paper by Creager et al. from Boston University is an important contribution and continues their important work in this area. It seems clear the high vasopressin levels in some patients with heart failure contribute importantly not only to renal abnormalities but to the high systemic vascular resistance in such patients. The potential of a vasopressin antagonist in therapy of heart failure awaits further study.—R.L. Frye, M.D.

Sodium and Water Excretion Abnormalities in Congestive Heart Failure: Determinant Factors and Clinical Implications
Bertrand Mettauer, Jean-Lucien Rouleau, Daniel Bichet, Carl Juneau, Claude Kortas, Jean-Noel Barjon, and Jacques de Champlain (Sacred Heart Hosp., Montreal)
Ann. Intern. Med. 105:161–167, August 1986   4–25

Renal hemodynamic and neurohumoral studies of patients with severe chronic congestive heart failure revealed a subgroup in whom neurohumoral activation is excessive and detrimental. The 66 patients (52 men), whose mean age was 61 years, were in New York Heart Association functional class III or class IV. Fifty-seven patients had ischemic heart failure, and nine had cardiomyopathy. Patients were taking a 2-gm sodium diet with fluid restriction at the time of study.

The patients generally had slight hyponatremia and renal impairment and moderate urinary sodium and water excretion abnormalities. The chief determinants of sodium excretion were activation of the renin-angiotensin system and ventricular function. Water excretion was most closely related to plasma and norepinephrine concentrations, renal function, and ventricular function. Of 31 patients with left ventricular stroke work indices of less than 20 gm-m/sq m, 20 also excreted less than 45% of a water load in 5 hours. These patients had especially marked neurohumoral activation and worse renal function than other patients. Patients with low stroke work indices had poorer survival than others on follow-up for 16–17 months, and those with low water excretion as well required more frequent hospitalization for worsening heart failure.

In patients with congestive heart failure, sodium excretion depends chiefly on the degree of ventricular functional impairment and activation of the renin-angiotensin system. Water excretion depends mainly on the plasma vasopressin and norepinephrine concentrations, renal function, and ventricular dysfunction. Patients with neurohumoral activation and marked abnormalities of sodium and water excretion have a less favorable clinical course.

▶ The neurohumoral response to heart failure is receiving increased attention. The study by Mettauer et al. provides new data on this problem, including studies of water metabolism and response of vasopressin. Not only are the data of interest in terms of the mechanism of the syndrome of heart failure, but as noted, prognosis is most adverse in those patients with the greatest activation of these compensatory mechanisms. Heart failure is obviously a complex physiologic state. However, the role of the kidney is frequently ignored by cardiologists. As noted in this study, the most dramatic renal abnormalities were found in patients with the most extensive left ventricular dysfunction. One wonders about the influence of cardiac receptors in this response, as the work of Thames (*Circ. Res.* 44:8, 1979) has provided intriguing insights to the interaction between cardiac receptors and reflex-induced modification of renal sympathetic nerve activity.—R.L. Frye, M.D.

Additive Effects of Dobutamine and Amrinone on Myocardial Contractility and Ventricular Performance in Patients With Severe Heart Failure

Joseph Gage, Howard Rutman, David Lucido, and Thierry H. LeJemtel (Albert Einstein College of Medicine)
Circulation 74:367–373, August 1986   4–26

Dobutamine therapy may adversely affect patients with limited coronary reserve, whereas amrinone, by decreasing loading as it increases contractility, tends to reduce myocardial oxygen utilization. The effects of dobutamine, alone and combined with amrinone, were studied in 11 patients with severe chronic congestive heart failure, six women and five men with a mean age of 54 years. All patients had functional class II to class IV symptoms despite digitalis and diuretic therapy. Dobutamine was infused at rates up to 15 μg/kg/minute to maximal cardiac output or until a 15% rise in heart rate or a 15% decrease in mean arterial pressure occurred, or complex ventricular arrhythmia developed. Amrinone was then given in a bolus of 1.5 mg/kg, if the cardiac index did not increase by 20% and the left ventricular end-diastolic pressure did not fall to less than 12 mm Hg, a bolus of 0.75 mg/kg was given.

Both dobutamine and amrinone, given alone, significantly increased the differential left ventricular pressure (dP/dt) and performance. The addition of amrinone to dobutamine led to a further increase in dP/dt and cardiac index, the latter increasing from a mean of 3.0 to a mean of 3.6 L/minute/ sq m. The mean left ventricular end-diastolic pressure fell further from 18 mm Hg to 15 mm Hg with combined treatment. The heart rate increased slightly, compared with either drug given alone; systemic arterial pressure did not decline further. The addition of amrinone to any dose of dobutamine produced lower systemic vascular resistance than did either drug used alone.

Combined treatment with dobutamine and amrinone leads to additive improvement in ventricular performance in patients with severe congestive heart failure. A marked reduction in ventricular loading occurs with only a modest rise in heart rate. This should preclude a significant increase in myocardial oxygen demand. Combined treatment may be especially useful in patients with critical coronary obstruction and left ventricular dysfunction.

▶ This study clearly documents the beneficial additive effects of dobutamine combined with amrinone in the treatment of severe heart failure. The rationale for this potentiation of effects is well presented. In many patients with profound heart failure, there is a sense of frustration regarding further pharmacologic support, particularly if the heart failure is in a setting of potential reversibility or definitive therapy. These data provide a rational and well-documented basis for combining dobutamine and amrinone in such settings.—R.L. Frye, M.D.

Differential Long-Term Intrarenal and Neurohumoral Effects of Captopril and Prazosin in Patients With Chronic Congestive Heart Failure: Importance of Initial Plasma Renin Activity

Bertrand Mettauer, Jean-Lucien Rouleau, Daniel Bichet, Claude Kortas, Christiane Manzini, Gérard Tremblay, and Kanu Chatterjee Hôpital du Sacré-Coeur, Montréal, and Univ. of California at San Francisco)
Circulation 73:492–502, March 1986   4–27

Tolerance to vasodilators develops in some patients for reasons that are unclear, and the long-term effects of these drugs on compensatory neurohumoral mechanisms remain to be elucidated. The effects of captopril, which has extensive renal and neurohumoral effects, and prazosin, which does not, were compared in 50 patients with congestive heart failure. Studies were done with infusion of a 15-ml/kg water load before and 2 days and 30 days after assignment to treatment. Prazosin was given in daily doses of 4–20 mg, and captopril in daily doses of 25 mg or 50 mg. Patients continued a 2-gm sodium diet during treatment.

Most patients had severe heart failure and evidence of compensatory neurohumoral stimulation. Prazosin and captopril led to similar hemodynamic changes. Captopril increased creatinine clearance and excretion of a water load after a month of treatment. Sodium excretion also increased, and the plasma catecholamine concentrations declined. Plasma aldosterone concentrations decreased, but vasopressin values were unchanged. Benefits were more apparent after a month of treatment than after 2 days. Prazosin increased water excretion, but the other effects were not observed. Prazosin decreased pulmonary capillary wedge pressure in patients with lower renin concentrations and decreased the plasma epinephrine level in this group.

Captopril normalizes overstimulated compensatory mechanisms more than does prazosin in patients with chronic heart failure. Similar hemodynamic changes nevertheless are seen with these vasodilators. The neurohumoral effects of captopril may help to explain why less tachyphylaxis is observed with this drug than with other vasodilators.

▶ This is a beautiful study of heart failure that clearly demonstrates the long-term advantages of captopril versus prazosin, though hemodynamic improvement is similar. High renin levels were associated with loss of effectiveness of prazosin but not captopril. Captopril was clearly superior in terms of improving renal function, presumably as a result of intrarenal blockade of effects of angiotensin II and improvement in renal blood flow. Enhancement of sodium exertion with captopril relates to both of the above as well as to a reduction in sympathetic outflow.

The study emphasizes the differences between vasodilators: prazosin, which has no direct renal and/or neurohumoral effects, versus captopril, which does influence these other systems over and above its general vasodilating effects.—R.L. Frye, M.D.

Atrial Natriuretic Peptide and Atrial Pressure in Patients With Congestive Heart Failure
Anthony E.G. Raine, Paul Erne, Ernst Bürgisser, Franco B. Müller, Peter Bolli, Felix Burkart, and Fritz R. Bühler (Univ. Hosp., Basel, Switzerland)
N. Engl. J. Med. 315:533–537, Aug. 28, 1986   4–28

There is some evidence that atrial natriuretic peptide concentrations in venous plasma may be elevated in patients with congestive heart failure and supraventricular tachycardia. The primary stimulus for the secretion of atrial natriuretic peptide may be atrial distention which is seen in both of these conditions. Whether there is any relationship between atrial pressure and the release of atrial natriuretic peptide was investigated by examining cardiac patients with normal and elevated left and right atrial pressures.

In 26 patients with heart disease, venous plasma concentrations of atrial natriuretic peptide were measured during diagnostic cardiac catheterization. Eleven patients had normal atrial pressures (group 1) and 15 had elevated pressures (group 2), including 11 who had elevated pressures in both atria.

A mean atrial natriuretic peptide concentration of 48 pmole/L was found in patients with cardiac disease but normal atrial pressures. Concentrations were increased twofold (mean, 87 pmole/L) in patients with heart disease and elevated atrial pressures. A mean concentration of 17 pmole/L was found in healthy volunteers. When all patients were considered together, peptide concentrations in right atrial plasma were significantly higher than in the venous plasma, consistent with secretion of peptide into the right atrium. Plasma concentrations of atrial peptide in the right atrium at rest were related to the mean right atrial pressure at rest. During exercise, patients with normal resting atrial pressures had a higher absolute increase in right atrial peptide concentration than did patients with congestive failure. Release of atrial natriuretic peptide is at least partly regulated by right and left atrial pressures.

▶ This interesting paper documents the elevation of atrial natriuretic peptide in the plasma of patients with heart failure, and it seems both atria participate in the release of these peptides. The pressure measurement correlations with peptide levels are interesting. Work in Burnett's laboratory suggests that it is not just intracavitary pressure but a transmural pressure gradient, or "stretch," that is the primary stimulus for release of these peptides. There is an enormous amount of work ongoing with regard to the pathophysiology of atrial naturetic peptides. These efforts should provide us with new insights into not only the mechanisms of heart failure, but control of the circulation in general.—R.L. Frye, M.D.

PTCA

Results of Percutaneous Transluminal Coronary Angioplasty by Multiple Relatively Low Frequency Operators
Andrew S. Jacob, Augusto D. Pichard, Susan D. Ohnmacht, and Joseph Lindsay, Jr. (Washington Hosp. Ctr. and George Washington Univ.)
Am. J. Cardiol. 57:713–716, Apr. 1, 1986   4–29

Success rates in percutaneous transluminal coronary angioplasty (PTCA) have improved from about 60% to nearly 85%, and part of this success appears to result from physician experience. The results of PTCA obtained by a number of physicians, often with relatively little experience in this procedure, were reviewed. Procedures were done in a catheterization laboratory where an experienced team assists in one to four angioplasties a day. A movable guidewire system was used in nearly all instances. Each operator was assisted by members of a team that consisted of technicians, a nurse, a PTCA fellow, and the laboratory director.

Sixteen physicians performed 131 PTCAs in a 1-year period in 1983–1984; 279 procedures were performed in the subsequent 10 months. Mean number of procedures per physician per month increased from 0.7 to 1.7. Success, defined as improvement of at least 20% in visually estimated diameter of stenosis, was obtained in 76% of patients in 1983–1984 and in 84% in 1984–1985, not a significant change. (Emergency coronary artery bypass surgery declined from 11% to 5.4%.) In the later period success rates were nearly identical whether two or fewer angioplasties or more than two procedures were done each month.

These results may reflect the performance of the laboratory PTCA team and the assistance of more experienced physicians, as well as the performance of the individual operator. Although better results may be obtained by frequent operators in a larger sample, excellent results were achieved without limiting privileges to those who have the greatest experience with angioplasty. Similar results cannot be expected from a laboratory with less experienced support personnel or without the assistance of experienced PTCA operators.

Percutaneous Transluminal Coronary Angioplasty: View of a Single Relatively High Frequency Operator
Geoffrey O. Hartzler (St. Luke's Hosp., Kansas City, Mo.)
Am. J. Cardiol. 57:869–872, Apr. 1, 1986   4–30

Percutaneous transluminal coronary angioplasty (PTCA) is much more complex than coronary angiography and requires greater manipulative skills. The risks of morbidity and mortality are also greater with angioplasty. The experience of the operator remains the single most important assurance of successful and uncomplicated angioplasty. A definite "learning curve" exists for the primary operator and the laboratory staff. Operators with case volumes that exceed 150 procedures have exhibited continued improvement and a relatively high primary success rate. The technology of angioplasty is not static and continued exposure to improved techniques and equipment is necessary. Prolonged training, ongoing experience, and sophisticated support personnel all are necessary for optimal performance.

Too many institutions have permitted operators without a high level of basic skill and experience in routine cardiac catheterization to perform angioplasty. An initial procedural base of at least 750–1,000 unsupervised coronary angiograms after completion of formal training will help to select candidates for training in performing angioplasty. More than ten "assisted" angioplasty procedures are needed before an operator begins an unsupervised program. The increasing number of patients who have repeat angioplasties has contributed to the trend in improving the primary success rate. The prevalence of acute coronary occlusion and emergency bypass surgery continue to be excessive.

Limitation and restriction of PTCA "privileges" would seem to be appropriate. Two to three skilled invasive cardiologists at a given institution should be able to perform PTCA. They in turn will share their experience in teaching local and regional colleagues.

Percutaneous Coronary Angioplasty: Influence of Operator Experience on Results
Gary S. Roubin, John S. Douglas, Jr., and Spencer B. King, III (Emory Univ.)
Am. J. Cardiol. 57:873–874, Apr. 1, 1986   4–31

Grüntzig was concerned that his method of percutaneous transluminal coronary angioplasty (PTCA) would be misused by overenthusiastic and inadequately trained operators. None of his first 2,000 electively treated patients died of a cause attributable to the intervention. The proper selection of patients probably is the chief determinant of success, regardless of the extent of the experience of the operator. If, as is uncertain, most patients in the study of Jacob et al. (Abstract 4–29) had discrete proximal lesions with favorable anatomical features, the results indicate that operator inexperience probably led to unsatisfactory results in 10% of the patients. With current technology even relatively inexperienced operators with a high volume can expect success rates of 90% to 95% in carefully selected patients.

Successful PTCA requires that the operator have both the clinical judgment and technical skills required to deal rapidly with any potential problem. Teaching should consist of a structured 1-year PTCA program, which should be given after 2–3 years of formal training in cardiology that includes extensive experience in angiography. Selection of patients is emphasized in the PTCA course. "Demonstration" courses are potentially useful. More formal training in angioplasty is necessary as the practice increases in complexity and the procedure is applied to a larger proportion of patients who have obstructive coronary artery disease.

▶ The paper reviewed in Abstract 4–29 was selected to emphasize the problem of training and maintaining skills in PTCA. The authors are appropriately cautious about the interpretation of their observations. The study really does not address individual results dealing with comparable lesions. I can frankly see no reason for someone to do one angioplasty per week and try to justify such an experience with that of experts. Every other technical or mechanical skill depends on maintenance of a level of activity and practice that allows one to be confident of providing the best for the patient. The experts in angioplasty must help to define these levels, and arbitrary revisions will need to be made. Data such as are presented in this study do not constitute an excuse for the casual performance of angioplasty. I thus strongly support the views expressed in the subsequent editorials on this paper (Abstracts 4–30 and 4–31).—R.L. Frye, M.D.

Restenosis After Successful Coronary Angioplasty in Patients With Single-Vessel Disease
Pierre P. Leimgruber, Gary S. Roubin, Jay Hollman, George A. Cotsonis, Bernhard Meier, John S. Douglas, Spencer B. King, III, and Andreas R. Gruentzig (Emory Univ.)
Circulation 73:710–717, April 1986   4–32

Restenosis has been reported in 17% to 47% of patients undergoing percutaneous transluminal coronary angioplasty (PTCA); little is known about the factors disposing to recurrences. Risk factors for restenosis were studied in 998 patients undergoing elective first PTCA for single-vessel coronary artery disease between 1980 and 1984. The procedure was angiographically and clinically successful in all, and angiographic follow-up was available. Restenosis was defined as stenosis of more than 50% diameter observed at follow-up angiography.

Restenosis occurred in 30% of the study group. When defined as a loss of half or more of the gain achieved at PTCA, the rate was 32%, and the rate of an increase in stenosis of 30% or more was 27%. Patients with unstable angina had a higher rate of restenosis. Men had restenosis more often than women, but the difference was not significant. Restenosis was most frequent after PTCA in the left anterior descending coronary territory. The lowest rates of restenosis were associated with post-PTCA stenosis of 30% or less and with a transstenotic pressure gradient of 15 mm Hg or less. Multivariate analysis showed the vessel dilated at PTCA to be the most significant factor, followed by the degree of stenosis at baseline. Restenosis was infrequent when follow-up angiography was performed after more than a year.

The risk of restenosis after PTCA of single-vessel coronary disease is reduced if the initial angiographic and hemodynamic results are optimal. Because the extent of arterial dissection is not controllable, the goal should not be to produce evident intimal disruption. Pharmacologic means of reducing recurrences of obstructive plaque are probably the most likely to lower the occurrence of restenosis after PTCA. Patients with residual stenosis of more than 30% and a final transstenotic gradient of more than 15 mm Hg should be followed closely.

▶ This sobering report reflects the critical and scientific approach to PTCA that Gruentzig promoted. These results concerning restenosis should stimulate a critical analysis of each individual patient in terms of indications for angioplasty, because there is little reason to do a procedure that results in a 30% failure rate in a period of 6 months if, in fact, the outlook for that patient is otherwise excellent. The biology of restenosis remains intriguing, and a number of trials are ongoing in an attempt to define the best pharmacologic approach to helping alleviate this problem. The remolding of the internal structure of the artery after angioplasty that allows those in whom restenosis does not develop to enjoy a prolonged period without progression of disease in the dilated area is an intriguing process.—R.L. Frye, M.D.

Measurement of Transstenotic Pressure Gradient During Percutaneous Transluminal Coronary Angioplasty

H. Vernon Anderson, Gary S. Roubin, Pierre P. Leimgruber, William R. Cox, John S. Douglas, Jr., Spencer B. King, III, and Andreas R. Gruentzig (Emory Univ.)
Circulation 73:1223–1230, June 1986 4–33

A decrease in the measured pressure gradient after percutaneous transluminal coronary angioplasty (PTCA) should reflect a lessening of the obstruction if the heart rate and blood pressure are relatively constant, and the gradient at the end of the procedure should help predict later angiographic measurements. To determine the relationship between the transstenotic pressure gradient, diameter of the stenosis, and length of the lesion, as well as the reliability of changes in pressure gradient in predicting changes in diameter of the stenosis induced by dilatation, data were reviewed in 4,263 angioplasties of single discrete coronary lesions performed from 1980 to 1985.

The initial diameter of the stenosis exceeded 70% in 63% of the lesions. The post-PTCA diameter was less than 30% in 63% of lesions and less than 50% in 93% of lesions. The mean transstenotic pressure gradient was 51 mm Hg before PTCA and 12 mm Hg afterward. The gradient was reduced by more than 30 mm Hg in 74% of the lesions. Reductions in stenosis and the pressure gradient were nonlinearly related; the change in diameter of the stenosis was proportional to the square root of the change in pressure gradient. A final gradient of 15 mm Hg or less predicted a final post-PTCA diameter of 30% or less, with a sensitivity of 75% and a specificity of 29%.

These findings suggest that a reduction in the pressure gradient across a coronary artery narrowing is directly proportional to an increase in the cross-sectional area of the stenosis. The length of the lesion was unrelated to the pressure gradient in the present study. Both the reduction in pressure gradient and the final postangioplasty gradient are useful indicators of the initial angiographic outcome.

▶ This study from Emory of their large experience with PTCA is a valuable contribution to our knowledge regarding hemodynamics of focal coronary arterial lesions and the theoretical and practical problems of interpretation of such data. Despite the relationships described, routine measurement of the gradient across the dilated lesion post PTCA seems infrequently performed now.—R.L. Frye, M.D.

Primary Angiographic Success Rates of Percutaneous Transluminal Coronary Angioplasty
H. Vernon Anderson, Gary S. Roubin, Pierre P. Leimgruber, John S. Douglas, Jr., Spencer B. King, III, and Andreas R. Gruentzig (Emory Univ.)
Am. J. Cardiol. 56:712–717, Nov. 1, 1985   4–34

Since the introduction of percutaneous transluminal coronary angioplasty (PTCA) in 1977, three distinct periods in the design of catheter systems are recognizable. In the earliest period, PTCA was performed with a double-lumen, balloon-tipped catheter with a fixed, flexible guidewire at the tip, just in front of the balloon. The second period was characterized by the introduction of the independent, steerable guidewire and a steerable catheter system. Most recently, the low-profile catheter was introduced. To determine whether changes in the primary angiographic success rate of PTCA were related to changes in catheter design, results were reviewed in 2,969 patients who underwent single-vessel PTCA of a native coronary artery from June 1981 to August 1984. The patients were categorized according to the period during which PTCA was performed.

A learning curve effect was discernible in the early performance of PTCA. The early PTCA attempts, which represented the steeply rising segment of the learning curve, were excluded from later analysis. Abrupt changes characteristic of the learning curve were not reflected in later monthly primary success rates, even at the points at which the steerable and low-profile catheters were introduced. The proportion of single-vessel PTCA attempts in the three major coronary arteries varied during each of the three periods. In each the left anterior descending (LAD) coronary artery accounted for most attempts, although its percentage of the total decreased significantly. The percentage of all PTCA attempts in the right coronary artery (RCA) did not change significantly. The percentage of attempts in the left circumflex artery increased significantly. The primary success rates for the three coronary arteries considered together were 88% in period I, 90% in period II, and 92% in period III. The percentage of lesions that could not be reached fell from 3% to 2% with the advent of the steerable catheter. Introduction of the steerable catheter system did not significantly increase the primary success rate of PTCA attempts on the LAD artery, but it was accompanied by significant improvement in the success rate in PTCA attempts on the RCA from 78% to 88% ($P < .005$). Neither introduction of the steerable catheter nor addition of the low-profile catheter significantly improved primary success rates in PTCA attempts on the LAD artery from 90% to 94% ($P < .005$), but it did not influence success rates in the RCA. The percentage of failures caused by the inability to reduce the stenosis in any of the three vessels was not affected by the introduction of the steerable catheter or by the addition of the low-profile catheter. Although there were significant differences in the ability to reach and cross stenoses among the three major coronary arteries before the steerable and low-profile catheters became available, these differences no longer exist. Technical improvements and operator experience have made stenoses in all three major coronary arteries equally accessible, and primary success rates and reasons for failure of PTCA in these arteries are now similar.

▶ This article will be of interest to those performing angioplasty as well as those referring patients for this procedure. The technical achievements in catheter design are quite remarkable and obviously of great importance. The judgment and skill of the operator, however, remain critical to overall success.— R.L. Frye, M.D.

Clinical and Angiographic Assessment 6 Months After Double Vessel Percutaneous Coronary Angioplasty
Luis Adolfo Mata, Xavier Bosch, Paul R. David, Hans J. Rapold, Thierry Corcos, and Martial G. Bourassa (Montreal Heart Inst.)
J. Am. Coll. Cardiol. 6:1239–1244, December 1985   4–35

Percutaneous transluminal coronary angioplasty is an accepted means of treating selected patients with single-vessel disease. Its efficacy in double-vessel coronary disease (at least 50% diameter stenosis) was assessed in 74 patients. They were among 769 patients undergoing coronary angioplasty between 1980 and 1984. The 58 men and 16 women had a mean age of 52 years. Sixteen patients had previous myocardial infarction. None had totally occluded arteries. Nearly half of the 148 attempts were in the left anterior descending artery.

Both lesions were treated successfully in 85% of the patients. The only serious complication was a myocardial infarction in one patient. Twenty-seven patients were asymptomatic 6 months after angioplasty. Five patients had class III effort angina, and two had an episode of unstable angina. Two patients had infarction during follow-up. One patient had coronary bypass grafting. Follow-up coronary angiography, performed a mean of 5.5 months after angioplasty, showed restenosis in 23% of evaluable segments. Half of the patients with angina had restenosis. Restenosis was associated with right coronary disease, the degree of residual stenosis, and calcific stenosis.

Double-vessel coronary stenosis may be managed by percutaneous angioplasty in selected patients with a high primary success rate and a low rate of complications. The rate of restenosis per patient, however, is greater than in single-vessel angioplasty. The use of medication to limit restenosis remains an area of interest.

▶ Multivessel percutaneous transluminal coronary angioplasty is being applied widely, and these carefully studied patients provide support for the use of this procedure to relieve symptoms and myocardial ischemia. Such an approach is particularly valuable in patients with double-vessel disease in whom one would like to delay surgery until all three arteries need a bypass procedure. Restenosis continues to be a major problem.—R.L. Frye, M.D.

Unstable Angina

▶ The series of studies in this section are of particular interest because they deal with the problem of mechanisms that may account for the sudden change in the clinical stability of the patient with coronary artery disease.

The postmortem studies of Davies et al. (Abstract 4–36) show the importance of platelet emboli apparently from proximal lesions with plaque fracture and thrombosis in patients dying suddenly of coronary artery disease. Similar findings have been reported by Falk (*Circulation* 71:699, 1985). Both studies found these lesions most commonly in patients with unstable angina prior to death.

Ambrose et al.'s coronary arteriographic analysis of lesions in patients with unstable angina independently identifies lesion characteristics that are more common in patients with unstable angina (Abstract 4–37). Thus, the focus now is on plaque instability with thrombus formation and platelet embolization as a major mechanism for changing the course of patients with coronary artery disease. The biology of the interaction of lesion and blood is obviously complex and will be the focus of increased investigations.

The third paper in this section by Fitzgerald et al. (Abstract 4–38) is another important contribution to these issues. Fitzgerald and colleagues have emphasized proper analytical methods and study design in attempting to assess the role of platelet activation in patients. This paper is fundamental to our understanding of the pathophysiology of unstable angina. The observations with angioscopy by Sherman et al. (Abstract 4–39) further support the overall concept of acute thrombosis at sites of atherosclerotic plaques in unstable patients with coronary artery disease.

Another paper of interest to those concerned in this area is that by Hammon and Oates (*Circulation* 73:224, 1986). Note also the paper in the section on myocardial infarction relating to activation of platelets in patients with myocardial infarction (Mueller, H.S., et al.: *Circulation* 72:1336, 1985).

Intramyocardial Platelet Aggregation in Patients With Unstable Angina Suffering Sudden Ischemic Cardiac Death
Michael J. Davies, Anthony C. Thomas, Paul A. Knapman, and J. Robert Hangartner (St. George's Hosp. Med. School, London)
Circulation 73:418–427, March 1986   4–36

Autopsy studies have demonstrated myocardial platelet aggregates in up to half of sudden ischemic deaths, but these have been ascribed to spontaneous intravascular agglutination of hyperactive platelets. Platelet masses were sought in the small myocardial vessels in patients dying within 6 hours of onset of pain or other symptoms of a fatal attack, in whom no cause of death other than atheromatous coronary stenosis was apparent. Ninety patients with coronary stenosis of more than 75% were included. All had been leading normal lives and had not seen a physician in the 2 weeks before death.

Plaque fissures were present in all but four patients, and intravascular masses of platelets were present in 30% in myocardial segments downstream from fissured plaques. Exposed mural thrombi were present in all but one of these patients. Other myocardial segments were free from emboli, with one exception. Most platelet aggregates had a minimal or absent fibrin component. The masses were found in precapillary arterioles and arteries up to 1 mm in diameter; they usually occluded the vessel. Platelet emboli were more frequent in patients who had episodic chest or arm pain in the 2 weeks before death. Multifocal microscopic myocardial necrosis was associated with the presence of platelet fibrin aggregates.

Myocardial platelet aggregates appear to reflect an embolic phenomenon and may be a cause of unstable angina. Myocardial necrosis from emboli could precipitate sudden death from ventricular fibrillation.

Angiographic Evolution of Coronary Artery Morphology in Unstable Angina
John A. Ambrose, Stephen L. Winters, Rohit R. Arora, Angie Eng, Albert Riccio, Richard Gorlin, and Valentin Fuster (Mount Sinai Med. Ctr., New York)
J. Am. Coll. Cardiol. 7:472–478, March 1986   4–37

An eccentric convex coronary stenosis with a narrow neck resulting from overhanging edges or irregular, scalloped borders, or both, has been found at coronary angiography in most patients with unstable angina. The evolution of lesions producing unstable angina was studied in 25 patients with previously stable angina who had an acute episode of unstable angina (group I) and in 21 patients with fairly stable symptoms between catheterizations (group II). The groups were similar in age and sex distribution. The mean intervals between angiographic studies were 30 months in group I and 25 months in group II.

Coronary disease progressed in 76% of group I and 33% of group II patients. Eight lesions in group I progressed to complete occlusion. Most group I lesions were insignificant initially, involving less than 50% stenosis, whereas most group II lesions that progressed were significant on initial angiography. Eccentric lesions were found in most group I patients with progression to less than complete occlusion, but in no group II patient with progression.

Progression of coronary artery disease is a frequent finding in patients with a history of stable angina who are reevaluated after an acute episode of unstable angina. Progression usually evolves from previously insignificant stenosis in these patients. The eccentric coronary lesion is the most common finding in progressive disease. It may represent a disrupted atherosclerotic plaque, a partially lysed thrombus, or both. The lesion appears to be a major cause of unstable angina.

Platelet Activation in Unstable Coronary Disease
Desmond J. Fitzgerald, Louis Roy, Francesca Catella, and Garrett A. Fitz-Gerald (Vanderbilt Univ. and Inst. of Cardiology, Quebec City)
N. Engl. J. Med. 315:983–989, Oct. 16, 1986   4–38

There is evidence that periodic platelet activation occurs in patients with unstable angina and may eventually lead to coronary occlusion by thrombus formation or by platelet release of vasoactive substances. Thromboxane A_2 formation and prostacyclin biosynthesis were studied by using urinary estimates of the metabolite 2,3-dinor-6-keto-prostaglanding $F_{1\alpha}$ in 36 patients hospitalized with chest pain. Sixteen patients had unstable angina, 14 had a diagnosis of myocardial infarction, and 6 had noncardiac chest pain. All 11 patients with unstable angina who underwent coronary angiography had coronary artery disease.

Peak urinary concentrations of prostacyclin metabolite and thromboxane B_2 were higher in patients with noncardiac chest pain than in nonhospitalized controls. Prostacyclin metabolite values were highest in the patients with myocardial infarction (Fig 4–2). Urinary metabolite values correlated with plasma creatine kinase activities. The increase in thromboxane B_2 was most marked in the patients with unstable angina. Urinary metabolite values were normal at rest in patients with stable coronary artery disease and were not altered by exercise-induced myocardial ischemia.

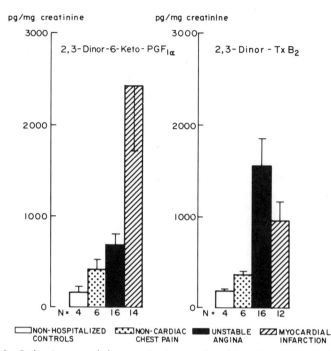

Fig 4–2.—Peak urinary metabolite excretion in controls and in patients with unstable angina or myocardial infarction. Peak 2,3-dinor-6-keto-prostaglandin $F_1\alpha$ excretion was highest in patients with myocardial infarction ($P < .025$ vs. patients with unstable angina and $P < .01$ vs. controls), whereas 2,3-dinor-thromboxane B_2 excretion was highest in patients with unstable angina ($P < .05$ vs. patients with myocardial infarction and $P < .01$ vs. controls). PG, prostaglandin; and Tx, thromboxane. Means ± SEM are shown. (Courtesy of Fitzgerald, D.J., et al.: N. Engl. J. Med. 316:983–989, Oct. 16, 1986. Reprinted by permission of The New England Journal of Medicine.)

Increased thromboxane biosynthesis is probably an event of primary importance in unstable angina, not merely a result of myocardial ischemia. Observed increases in thromboxane and prostacyclin synthesis have usually coincided with episodes of ischemia. Prostacyclin generation may modify platelet activation within coronary vessels. If so, clinical benefit from high-dosage aspirin treatment would be augmented by the use of selective inhibitors or pharmacologic antagonists of thromboxane A_2 or both.

▶ This is an extremely important study from an outstanding group of clinical investigators. Fitzgerald and his colleagues emphasize the crucial role of proper analytic methods and sampling artifacts in the attempt to study prostaglandin metabolism in clinical investigations. This paper is fundamental to our understanding of platelet activation in the pathogenesis of the clinical instability of the patient with coronary artery disease.—R.L. Frye, M.D.

Coronary Angioscopy in Patients With Unstable Angina Pectoris

C. Todd Sherman, Frank Litvack, Warren Grundfest, Myles Lee, Ann Hickey,

Aurelio Chaux, Robert Kass, Carlos Blanche, Jack Matloff, Leon Morgen-stern, William Ganz, H.J.C. Swan, and James Forrester (Cedars-Sinai Med. Ctr., Los Angeles, and Univ. of California at Los Angeles)
N. Engl. J. Med. 315:913–919, Oct. 9, 1986   4–39

Why marked changes occur in the pattern of anginal pain is unknown, but acute intimal pathologic change may be more frequent in unstable angina than is apparent from coronary angiography. High-resolution flexible fiberoptic angioscopy was used to determine the frequency of complex atheroma and thrombus in patients scheduled for coronary bypass grafting. In all, 32 coronary vessels were examined in ten patients with stable coronary disease and ten with unstable angina.

All seven patients with rest angina had thrombus in the offending vessel. No thrombus was found in the arteries of patients with stable angina or in nonoffending arteries in those with unstable angina. Thrombi ranged from partially to completely occlusive and often were found on the distal side of an obstruction at angiography. All three patients with accelerated angina had a complex plaque in the offending artery; none had thrombus. One patient with rest angina had a complex plaque as well as thrombus, at separate sites in the offending artery. Angiography detected only one of four complex plaques and one of seven thrombi, but it correctly demonstrated the absence of such pathologic processes.

Both acute thrombi and ulcerated, hemorrhagic endothelium characterize acute ischemic syndrome, whereas the absence of such lesions is typical of stable coronary artery disease. The angioscopic findings in this investigation suggest the need for systematic studies of the risks and benefits of anticoagulant, antiplatelet, and thrombolytic treatments in patients with unstable coronary syndromes.

▶ These are really exciting observations. The technologic advances that allow such visualization of intraluminal pathology represent a major step forward, and the observations on pathogenesis of unstable angina are consistent with the prior papers in this section. The field of intraluminal therapy is quite active, and the best technique for dealing with atheromatous plaques remains unsettled. The work with lasers, roto-rooters, and other approaches will be facilitated by the ability to visualize the internal structure of the artery with angioscopy.—R.L. Frye, M.D.

Silent Ischemia as a Marker for Early Unfavorable Outcomes in Patients With Unstable Angina
Sidney O. Gottlieb, Myron L. Weisfeldt, Pamela Ouyang, E. David Mellits, and Gary Gerstenblith (Francis Scott Key Med. Ctr., Baltimore, and Johns Hopkins Univ.)
N. Engl. J. Med. 314:1214–1219, May 8, 1986   4–40

Unstable angina is characterized by symptoms of recent onset, a crescendo pattern, or the occurrence of symptoms at rest. High incidences of

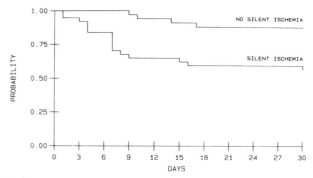

Fig 4–3.—Kaplan-Meier curves comparing cumulative probabilities of not experiencing myocardial infarction or revascularization for recurrent angina during 30 days for 37 patients with silent ischemia (group I) and 33 patients without it (group II), as detected by continuous ECG monitoring (P < .002). (Courtesy of Gottlieb, S.O., et al.: N. Engl. J. Med. 314:1214–1219, May 8, 1986. Reprinted by permission of The New England Journal of Medicine.)

sudden death, myocardial infarction, and persistent angina requiring revascularization are associated with medically treated patients with angina at rest. These patients also have the poorest short-term and long-term prognoses. Patients with stable and unstable angina have a high incidence of silent myocardial ischemia, defined by the occurrence of ischemic ECG changes without accompanying symptoms. A study was conducted to determine the presence and extent of silent ischemia in 70 patients with unstable angina treated in the coronary care unit with an intensive medical regimen.

Two double-blind, randomized, placebo-controlled trials were carried out to assess β blocker and calcium channel blocker efficacy in the treatment of unstable angina. Two-channel continuous ECGs were obtained during the first 2 days after a patient had started drug therapy to quantify the frequency and duration of asymptomatic ischemic episodes, defined as a transient ST segment shift of at least 1 mm. The patients were followed for 1 month to determine the occurrence of death, infarction, or revascularization to relieve symptoms.

Thirty-seven patients experienced 205 silent ischemic episodes detected by continuous ECGs. The mean duration of each episode was 20 minutes (Fig 4–3). More than 90% of episodes were asymptomatic. Of the 37 patients, 29 had only silent ischemia; the other 8 had symptoms associated with at least one episode. No evidence of ischemia during the 2-day monitoring was found in the other 33 patients enrolled in the study. During the 1-month follow-up, 7 patients had myocardial infarction and 13 required revascularization for recurrent symptoms. No cardiac deaths occurred. Six of the 7 patients with infarction were in the silent ischemia group, as were ten revascularized patients.

▶ This is an important study related to the management of patients with unstable angina as well as to the overall problem of silent ischemia. Clinicians need to be aware that, despite good control of symptoms, recurrent ischemia may be observed with this type of monitoring, as clearly demonstrated by Gottlieb and associates. In this subgroup of patients, adequate control of symptoms with drugs was not sufficient to prevent a high rate of cardiac events as defined for the purpose of this study. The impact of revascularization procedures on silent ischemia needs documentation, and I have no doubt that such trials will be forthcoming in the future.—R.L. Frye, M.D.

Effect of the Addition of Propranolol to Therapy With Nifedipine for Unstable Angina Pectoris: A Randomized, Double-blind, Placebo-Controlled Trial
Sidney O. Gottlieb, Myron L. Weisfeldt, Pamela Ouyang, Stephen C. Achuff, Kenneth L. Baughman, Thomas A. Traill, Jeffrey A. Brinker, Edward P. Shapiro, Nisha Chibber Chandra, E. David Mellits, Susan N. Townsend, and Gary Gerstenblith (Francis Scott Key Med. Ctr., Baltimore, and Johns Hopkins Univ.)
Circulation 73:331–337, February 1986   4–41

β Blockers are useful in patients with stable demand angina, but their use in those with resting angina is controversial. A double-blind trial was conducted to determine whether the addition of propranolol to nitrate and nifedipine therapy is beneficial to patients with unstable resting angina. Forty-two of 81 such patients were assigned to receive propranolol, and the other 39 received placebo. Most patients were in a coronary care unit at randomization. Nearly 80% had double-vessel or triple-vessel coronary disease. All patients received intravenous or long-acting nitrate therapy orally or topically, as well as nifedipine. Study patients received 40 mg of propranolol every 6 hours.

Four patients, two taking propranolol, were withdrawn because of side effects. Propranolol did not significantly influence the incidence or cumulative probability of cardiac death, myocardial infarction, or persistent ischemia necessitating angioplasty or bypass. Fifteen propranolol-treated patients and 19 given placebo required increased study medication because of recurrent angina. Propranolol-treated patients had a lower risk of recurrent resting angina, and ECG monitoring showed fewer daily ischemic episodes and shorter episodes in the propranolol treated group.

The addition of propranolol to nitrate and nifedipine therapy reduces the occurrence of resting angina and silent myocardial ischemia in patients with unstable angina. No significant change in the risk of infarction or cardiac death is evident. Propranolol may help by lowering heart rate and myocardial oxygen demand in this setting.

▶ Clinicians have worried about the use of propranolol in the setting of unstable angina because of its potential to trigger coronary arterial spasm. This trial clearly demonstrates the beneficial effects of β blockade when added to nitrates or nifedipine by providing better control of heart rate.— R.L. Frye, M.D.

CV Mortality and Epidemiology

Coronary Heart Disease Death, Nonfatal Acute Myocardial Infarction and Other Clinical Outcomes in the Multiple Risk Factor Intervention Trial
S.B. Hulley for the Multiple Risk Factor Intervention Trial Research Group (San Francisco Gen. Hosp.)
Am. J. Cardiol. 58:1–13, July 1, 1986   4–42

The Multiple Risk Factor Intervention Trial (MRFIT) was a randomized clinical study of 12,866 middle-aged men with high levels of risk factors for coronary heart disease (CHD) in which a special intervention program and usual care were compared. The program was intended to control serum levels of cholesterol, blood pressure, and cigarette smoking. The last major prespecified end point was the occurrence of a first major event that was caused by CHD, either nonfatal acute myocardial infarction or death.

Follow-up for 7 years showed that first major events were slightly less frequent in men who were assigned to the special intervention program than in those who were assigned to usual care. The relative differences, however, were not statistically significant. Regression analyses within the two groups indicated that the cholesterol and smoking interventions both reduced the number of first major events and were significantly associated with decreases in the CHD. Lowering blood pressure was not associated with a decrease in the rate of CHD. Nominally significant decreases in angina, congestive heart failure, and peripheral arterial disease were observed in the special intervention group.

The lack of a significant overall difference in rates of CHD between the special intervention and usual care groups in the MRFIT may reflect a combintion of expected beneficial effects from the cholesterol and smoking interventions and unexpected heterogeneous effects of antihypertensive intervention. There is evidence that this intervention may have benefited some patients but had adverse effects on others.

▶ This is an important analysis of the MRFIT. The initial results were reported by these researchers in 1982 (*JAMA* 248:1465, 1982). In the first reports, substantial risk factor reductions in the three main risk factors were noted in both the usual care and special intervention groups; the 7% relative difference in mortality between the two groups was not statistically significant, however. Total deaths and deaths from all cardiovascular causes were also essentially the same. The current report deals with the occurrence of nonfatal acute myocardial infarction or CHD death, as well as other prespecified cardiovascular end points. It is interesting that, once again, there is a nonsignificant difference between the special intervention and the usual care groups in terms of the rate of occurrence of a first major CHD event. One of the most interesting aspects of the MRFIT has been the finding of an adverse effect of blood pressure lowering in the special intervention group among those who had an abnormal baseline ECG and were given hydrochlorothiazide.

The breakdown of the analysis to include specific subgroups is helpful and does document, as do other reports, that the major benefits of these prevention programs occur in patients identified as being at high risk, i.e., those with high cholesterol levels or active cigarette smokers; it is in these two subgroups in particular that this trial does show a benefit in terms of reducing CHD rates. I think these findings are of real importance for the practicing physician, and they need to be considered carefully.—R.L. Frye, M.D.

European Collaborative Trial of Multifactorial Prevention of Coronary Heart Disease: Final Report on the 6-Year Results
G. Rose for the WHO European Collaborative Group (London School of Hygiene and Tropical Medicine)
Lancet 1:869–872, Apr. 19, 1986   4–43

Preliminary results from the World Health Organization (WHO) European Collaborative Trial of Multifactorial Prevention of Coronary Heart Disease gave some indications of reduced rates of coronary heart disease (CHD). The first complete results from all centers are now available. About 60,000 working men aged 40–59 years living in Belgium, Italy, Poland, and the United Kingdom entered the trial. Half received advice on a cholesterol-lowering diet, the control of smoking, overweight, blood pressure, and regular exercise.

Risk factor interventions were associated with a 10% reduction in total CHD and a 7% decline in fatal CHD. Nonfatal myocardial infarctions decreased by 15%, and total deaths decreased by 5%. Benefit correlated significantly with the extent of change in risk factors. Results were comparable in all countries. Multiple logistic analysis showed that the observed reduction in total CHD was 62% of that predicted.

The WHO Collaborative Trial, the largest randomized trial of coronary disease prevention, shows that advice on risk factor reduction is accepted by middle-aged men and is safe. Interventional measures have been based on life-style changes, apart from control of hypertension. No evidence of adverse effects on noncoronary mortality was obtained in the trial.

▶ It remains difficult to prove in a prospective trial that prevention efforts reduce mortality when the intervention is studied in the general population. Although a trend supporting a decrease in CHD events was evident, it was not statistically significant. Furthermore, there was no impact on total mortality.

I believe prevention is important, particularly for those at high risk. However, extrapolation of data from those with grossly abnormal risk factor profiles to the general population seems inappropriate. A critical analysis of this problem is provided in the article by Oliver, M.F.: *Circulation* 73:1, 1986.—R.L. Frye, M.D.

Cardiovascular Mortality in New Zealand and Australia 1968–1983: How Can the Diverging Trends Be Explained?
Robert Beaglehole, Ruth Bonita, Rodney Jackson, and Alistair Stewart (Univ. of Auckland)
N.Z. Med. J. 99:1–3, Jan. 22, 1986   4–44

Cardiovascular disease causes nearly half of all deaths in New Zealand and Australia. Rates of coronary heart disease (CHD) are higher than in other western nations, but mortality from cardiovascular disease is declining in both countries. Mortality trends for all causes, all cardiovascular diseases, CHD, and cerebrovascular disease were reviewed for 1968–1983 in persons aged 40–69 years.

Initial mortality rates in all categories were higher in Australia than in New Zealand. Mortality rates declined in both countries during the review period, but significantly more in Australia. By 1983, rates of death from all causes considered were higher in New Zealand. The decline in cardiovascular disease accounted for about 90% of the decrease in all deaths in New Zealand and 70% in Australia. Life expectancy for persons aged 40 years has improved in both countries since the mid-1960s, but the rate of improvement has been greater in Australia.

The reasons for the differential rates of improvement in cardiovascular mortality in Australia and New Zealand are unclear. Comprehensive studies monitoring changes in diet, smoking, and exercise are needed, as are surveys of patterns of medical and surgical practices.

▶ The decline in cardiovascular mortality observed in many countries throughout the world is most gratifying. The basis for the decline remains unexplained to this editor, although one can find strong proponents of various arguments. Even more intriguing are the differences in cardiovascular mortality between countries, as noted in this paper, and differences within countries, including the United States. Further epidemiologic studies to explain these phenomena are awaited eagerly. Those interested in this problem may wish to review an analysis of the impact of medical interventions versus changes in life-style on cardiovascular mortality by Goldman L. and Cook, E.: *Annals of Internal Medicine* 101:825, 1984.—R.L. Frye, M.D.

Patterns of Coronary Heart Disease Morbidity and Mortality in the Sexes: A 26-Year Follow-Up of the Framingham Population
Debra J. Lerner and William B. Kannel (Boston Univ. and Boston City Hosp.)
Am. Heart J. 111:383–390, February 1986   4–45

Gender patterns of coronary morbidity and mortality were examined in the Framingham cohort that initially included 5,127 persons free from clinical coronary heart disease (CHD). In 26 years of observation, 1,240 coronary events were recorded.

Men accounted for 60% of all coronary events. Acute myocardial infarction accounted for 43% of events in men, and angina did so in 39%. More than half of events in women consisted of angina. Myocardial infarction contributed 30% of events in women. Women had half the CHD of men, and their rate began to approximate male rates closely only in old age. The increase in coronary morbidity with age was much more evident in women than in men. Women exhibited no survival advantage over men once disease became overt. Myocardial infarction became progressively more frequent with age in both sexes, and unrecognized infarction was clinically significant in both men and women. Angina was uncomplicated more often in women than in men. Differences in risk factors did not totally explain the lower incidence of coronary morbidity in women. No abrupt change in cardiovascular incidence or mortality was found in women at menopausal ages.

Coronary disease is a major cause of morbidity and mortality in both men and women. Female CHD is considerably more age dependent than is male disease. Women are more likely than men to have uncomplicated angina and silent myocardial infarction. Unrecognized infarction is a particular problem in women who would benefit from more attention to atypical symptoms and closer ECG surveillance. Coronary heart disease can be expected to become an increasing public health problem as the aging population enlarges.

▶ This analysis of morbidity and mortality in the Framingham Study provides an important perspective of coronary artery disease in a defined United States population. The predominance of angina in females, and its remarkable acceleration in incidence after age 55, is intriguing. Clinicians aware of the frequency of angina with normal coronary arteries in females may question this observation. However, the upturn in coronary mortality rates for women around ages 45–55 is clear, and the basis for this is uncertain at this time. What actually happens at the time of menopause to explain these epidemiologic observations is unclear. Fascinating data on sex differences in animals in relation to arterial thrombosis and cardiovascular responses have been reported (Uzunova, A., et al.: *Nature* 261:712, 1976; Baker, P.J., et al.: *Am. J. Physiol.* 235(2):H242–H246, 1978).—R.L. Frye, M.D.

Blacks in the Coronary Artery Surgery Study: Risk Factors and Coronary Artery Disease
Charles Maynard, Lloyd D. Fisher, Eugene R. Passamani, and Thomas Pullum (Univ. of Washington and Natl. Heart, Lung, and Blood Inst., NIH, Bethesda)
Circulation 74:64–71, July 1986   4–46

The distribution of risk factors by race was examined in the population of the Coronary Artery Surgery Study (CASS). Data on 23,581 of the 24,959 persons enrolled in the CASS at 15 centers in the United States and Canada were available for analysis. The study group included 573 blacks. These were younger and the group included more women than did the white group in the study population. Two thirds of black men and only 40% of white men performed manual labor. The same was true for 27% of black women and 11% of white women.

Higher proportions of blacks of both sexes were current smokers and had elevated blood pressure. No significant racial differences in the serum cholesterol concentration were evident. Fewer blacks reported an early family history of angina or myocardial infarction, but a high proportion reported a history of hypertension. Diabetes was more prevalent in blacks, as were higher body weight and congestive heart failure. White men had a higher rate of past myocardial infarction. Blacks of both sexes had considerably less coronary artery disease than did whites. Multivariate analysis showed that being black was associated with less coronary disease after control for other important risk factors, e.g., age, sex, cholesterol elevation, and smoking.

Further efforts are needed to reduce smoking and control hypertension in blacks. Many blacks have chest pain but normal coronary arteries; further understanding of the causes of chest pain in blacks is needed. Studies of predominantly black populations from different parts of the United States would be of interest.

▶ Access to health care for minorities is an important societal issue. This analysis of the CASS registry demonstrates the small percentage of blacks in this important international multicenter trial. The findings of less frequent and less severe coronary artery disease in the blacks studied raises important questions for further research.—R.L. Frye, M.D.

High Density Lipoprotein Cholesterol Is Not a Major Risk Factor for Ischemic Heart Disease in British Men

S.J. Pocock, A.G. Shaper, A.N. Phillips, M. Walker, and T.P. Whitehead (Royal Free Hosp., London, and Queen Elizabeth Med. Ctr., Birmingham, England)
Br. Med. J. 292:515–519, Feb. 22, 1986   4–47

Considerable interest has arisen concerning high-density lipoprotein (HDL) cholesterol as a protective factor against ischemic heart disease, but some believe that there is no sound biologic basis for regarding HDL cholesterol as protective. Serum concentrations of HDL cholesterol were estimated in a prospective series of men aged 40–59 years in 24 British towns. Of 7,415 men in whom both HDL cholesterol and total cholesterol concentrations were determined, major ischemic heart disease developed in 193 after an average follow-up of about 4 years.

The mean HDL cholesterol concentration was lower in men with ischemic heart disease than in others, but the difference was insignificant after adjustment for age, body mass index, blood pressure, cigarette smoking, and the concentration of non-HDL cholesterol. The higher mean non-HDL cholesterol value in these patients remained highly significant after adjustment for other factors. Men with non-HDL cholesterol concentrations in the highest quintile had more than three times the risk of major ischemic heart disease than did those with values in the lowest quintile. The non-HDL cholesterol concentration was a better predictor of risk than the HDL to total cholesterol ratio on multivariate analysis.

The serum concentration of HDL cholesterol does not appear to be an important risk factor for major ischemic heart disease in middle-aged

British men. It is possible that HDL cholesterol has a larger role in communities having lower total cholesterol concentrations and different diets.

▶ This provocative paper casts doubt on HDL cholesterol as an independent risk factor for coronary artery disease. We need to maintain a critical attitude toward accepted "dogma." Anyone who practices medicine must frequently answer the question, "Why do I have coronary artery disease with a normal cholesterol (or HDL cholesterol) level?"—R.L. Frye, M.D.

The Risk of Myocardial Infarction After Quitting Smoking in Men Under 55 Years of Age
Lynn Rosenberg, David W. Kaufman, Susan P. Helmrich, and Samuel Shapiro
(Boston Univ.)
N. Engl. J. Med. 313:1511–1514, Dec. 12, 1985   4–48

Cigarette smoking is a major cause of myocardial infarction; smokers have been encouraged to quit, and many have done so. Previous studies have suggested that exsmokers eventually have an incidence of myocardial infarction similar to that of persons who have never smoked, but generally they have not taken into account predisposing factors, nor have they established how soon the risk declines, particularly among those predisposed to infarction for other reasons.

The effect of quitting cigarette smoking on the incidence of nonfatal myocardial infarction in men younger than age 55 was assessed in a case-control study of 1,873 men with first episodes of myocardial infarction and 2,775 controls. For current smokers (men who had smoked in the previous year), compared with those who had never smoked, the estimated relative risk of myocardial infarction adjusted for age was 2.9. Among exsmokers (those who had last smoked at least 1 year previously), the relative risk estimate declined to a value close to unity for those who had abstained for at least 2 years; estimates were 2.0 for men who had abstained for 12–23 months and about 1.0 for men who had abstained longer. The results were unchanged by allowance for multiple confounding factors. A similar pattern was apparent among exsmokers who had smoked heavily for many years, among those predisposed to myocardial infarction because of family history, hypertension, or other risk factors, and among those with no apparent predisposition. The results suggest that the risk of myocardial infarction in cigarette smokers decreases within a few years of quitting to a value similar to that in men who have never smoked.

▶ An innovative study design is described that provides further support for the importance of cessation of tobacco smoking as a preventive measure in cardiology. Physicians may find the apparently rapid decline in risk after stopping cigarettes useful in convincing patients that benefits may occur even after a long history of cigarette smoking. Vlietstra et al. (*JAMA* 255:1023, 1986) reported interesting data from the Coronary Artery Surgery Study that also support efforts to convince patients to stop smoking cigarettes.—R.L. Frye, M.D.

Noninvasive Prediction of CAD and Prognosis

Noninvasive Identification of Left Main and Triple Vessel Coronary Artery Disease: Improved Accuracy Using Quantitative Analysis of Regional Myocardial Stress Distribution and Washout of Thallium-201

Jamshid Maddahi, Alnoor Abdulla, Ernest V. Garcia, H.J.C. Swan, and Daniel S. Berman (Cedars-Sinai Med. Ctr., Los Angeles, and Univ. of California at Los Angeles)

J. Am. Coll. Cardiol. 7:53–60, January 1986   4–49

Visual analysis of thallium stress redistribution scintigrams has low sensitivity for identifying extensive coronary artery disease (CAD) (triple-vessel and/or left main coronary disease). The value of quantitative analysis of the perfusion defect and washout rate of myocardial activity was studied in 105 consecutive patients who also underwent coronary angiography and exercise ECG study. Patients had scintigraphy in conjunction with multistage treadmill exercise, and the findings were analyzed visually and by computer processing. Fifty-six patients had angiographic findings of extensive CAD, including 13 with left main coronary disease.

Of the 56 patients with extensive CAD, visual thallium analysis identified only 9 (sensitivity, 16%), but with quantitative analysis 35 were correctly classified (sensitivity, 63%). Combining quantitative analysis of thallium images with exercise ECG and blood pressure response increased sensitivity to 86% for identification of patients with extensive CAD, with a decline in specificity from 86% to 76%. Improvement in the test result with quantitative analysis resulted from a slow regional myocardial washout rate.

Quantitative analysis of myocardial thallium stress distribution and washout substantially increases the sensitivity of the method for identifying triple-vessel coronary disease and left main coronary disease. The results are usefully combined with those of the ECG and blood pressure responses to exercise.

▶ Noninvasive identification of patients with triple-vessel and/or left main coronary disease with mild or no angina is an important objective. This study shows the ability of quantitative analysis of thallium washout to enhance the sensitivity of this type of scintigraphy in identifying patients with triple-vessel and/or left main disease.

It should be emphasized that quality control of these studies is extremely important, and a considerable commitment is required by anyone hoping to match the results obtained by this outstanding laboratory.—R.L. Frye, M.D.

Relative Value of Clinical Variables, Bicycle Ergometry, Rest Radionuclide Ventriculography and 24-Hour Ambulatory Electrocardiographic Monitoring at Discharge to Predict 1 Year Survival After Myocardial Infarction

Paolo Fioretti, Ronald W. Brower, Maarten L. Simoons, Harald ten Katen, Anita Beelen, Taco Baardman, Jacobus Lubsen, and Paul G. Hugenholtz

(Erasmus Univ., Academic Hosp. Dijkzigt, and Interuniv. Cardiology Inst., Rotterdam)
J. Am. Coll. Cardiol. 8:40–49, July 1986   4–50

Bicycle ergometric testing slightly improves predictions of survival in the first year after myocardial infarction beyond routine clinical variables. An attempt was made to determine whether more expensive tests (e.g., 24-hour ambulatory ECG monitoring and radionuclide ventriculography) are of further prognostic value. Discriminant function analysis was used to compare these tests with predischarge clinical variables in predicting 1-year survival in 351 hospital survivors of acute infarction.

The extent of blood pressure rise with exercise slightly improved predictive accuracy beyond the use of simple clinical variables. The latter included a history of past infarction, persistent heart failure, and the use of digitalis at discharge. Radionuclide ventriculography and 24-hour ECG monitoring did not improve prediction of survival. The predictive value for mortality of clinical variables alone was 12% and with stress testing added, 15%. These tests were slightly additive to clinical data, independent of eligibility for stress testing.

Symptom-limited stress ECG testing is recommended as a routine discharge procedure after acute myocardial infarction. Further tests (e.g., radionuclide angiography and 24-hour ambulatory ECG monitoring) are indicated only if there are contraindications to stress testing or an equivocal risk profile. Noninvasive tests can guide the use of coronary angiography.

▶ This study again confirms the importance of clinical variables in identifying high-risk patients after myocardial infarction. It is important in analyzing all of these studies, in making judgments in terms of one's own practice, to look carefully and in detail at how the patients are selected for study. In this particular study it is important to note the conclusions about the lack of value of additional indices of left ventricular function with radionuclide ventriculography or 24-hour ambulatory monitoring; these investigations apply only to patients who are able to complete a stress test, a group with a better prognosis anyway. All studies that have attempted to provide better information on this important topic have their own set of biases in terms of selection of patients, and these must be taken into account as one analyzes these data. However, the point of this study is well taken, and it should be a challenge for any proposed test for any purpose, namely: What does it add to the recognized pretest likelihood of a given outcome over and above what is obvious from simple clinical variables?—R.L. Frye, M.D.

Prediction of Multivessel Coronary Artery Disease and Prognosis Early After Acute Myocardial Infarction by Exercise Electrocardiography and Thallium-201 Myocardial Perfusion Scanning

Robert D. Abraham, S. Benedict Freedman, Richard F. Dunn, Henry Newman, Gary S. Roubin, Phillip J. Harris, and David T. Kelly (Royal Prince Alfred Hosp., Sydney)
Am. J. Cardiol. 58:423–427, Sept. 1, 1986   4–51

The value of both exercise thallium perfusion scintigraphy and exercise ECG study, performed early after acute myocardial infarction, for identifying patients with multivessel coronary disease was examined in a series of 103 patients with uncomplicated infarction who also underwent coronary angiography. The noninvasive studies were performed a mean of 24 days after infarction. Multivessel coronary disease was present in 44 patients. No patient had more than 50% stenosis of the left main coronary artery.

There were three deaths and four recurrent infarctions. One patient was resuscitated from cardiac arrest. Four patients were hospitalized with unstable angina. The combined rate of medical events and bypass grafting was 23%. The combined noninvasive tests were 42% sensitive and 96% specific in predicting multivessel coronary disease, with a predictive accuracy of 88%. Only 13% of the patients with two negative results had multivessel coronary disease. Medical events were not predicted to a significant degree by an abnormal exercise ECG, a remote thallium defect, or the presence of multivessel coronary disease.

A combination of exercise ECG testing and thallium scanning shortly after uncomplicated acute myocardial infarction can identify patients with a high probability of having multivessel coronary artery disease. The combined tests are especially useful in a population with a low prevalence of multivessel coronary disease, to avoid angiography in patients likely to have single-vessel disease. Angiography may be indicated in patients in whom both test results are positive.

▶ This is an interesting and helpful review of experience in identifying multivessel disease early after myocardial infarction by the excellent group at the Royal Prince Alfred Hospital in Sydney. We still have a problem in defining high-risk subsets of patients after myocardial infarction. This study and that of Gibson et al. (*Am. J. Cardiol.* 47:1010, 1981) report rather disappointing sensitivity data on detecting the presence of multivessel disease with exercise ECGs and thallium scintigraphy. The data concerning prognosis certainly show a trend toward more events with more positive tests, but the event rate in this selected sample is low, which compromises the statistical power of the observation. We rely more on radionuclide measurement of left ventricular function at rest and with exercise in selecting patients for coronary arteriography who otherwise do not have clear indications for invasive study.—R.L. Frye, M.D.

Prognostic Value of Exercise Electrocardiogram in Men at High Risk of Future Coronary Heart Disease: Multiple Risk Factor Intervention Trial Experience
Pentti M. Rautaharju, Ronald J. Prineas, William J. Eifler, Curt D. Furberg, James D. Neaton, Richard S. Crow, Jeremiah Stamler, and Jeffrey A. Cutler for the Multiple Risk Factor Intervention Trial Research Group (Dalhousie Univ., Halifax, Nova Scotia)
J. Am. Coll. Cardiol. 8:1–10, July 1986   4–52

The prognostic value of the exercise ECG was studied in a series of 6,438 men assigned to usual care in the Multiple Risk Factor Intervention Trial, a primary prevention trial designed to test the effects of multifactor intervention on mortality from coronary heart disease (CHD). The total trial population included 12,866 men aged 35–57 years. The usual care group was referred to customary sources of health care in the community. An abnormal response to exercise was defined as an ST depression integral of at least 16 µV-s.

The exercise response was abnormal in 12% of the group. A nearly fourfold increase in 7-year CHD mortality was observed in these men, for a risk ratio of 3.8 with 95% confidence limits of 2.5–5.5. The risk ratio for death from CHD, adjusted for age, diastolic blood pressure, serum cholesterol level, and smoking status, was 3.5, and the risk ratio for death from all causes was 1.6. A similar trend was seen for angina, but no significant relationship with nonfatal myocardial infarction was evident. On multivariate analysis, the exercise response was a strong independent predictor of CHD death. Men with both an abnormal resting ECG and an abnormal exercise response had a more than sixfold relative risk of CHD death compared with those who had abnormal results on the resting ECG but a normal ST response to exercise.

An abnormal ST depression integral in a submaximal exercise test is an independent predictor of future coronary death in men at high risk of future myocardial infarction. Excessive risk is evident among men with a normal resting ECG. Computer-analyzed exercise ECGs may be especially useful in clinically asymptomatic middle-aged men who have increased risk factors.

▶ This paper is an important contribution to our knowledge regarding the screening of asymptomatic patients, because it clearly documents the relatively poor prognosis of men with abnormal exercise ECGs. It is important to note here, however, that the ECG analysis was not done on the basis of visual interpretation in the usual way, but involved computer analysis that included upsloping J-point depression as an abnormal response based on a derivation of an ST interval. The Multiple Risk Factor Intervention Trial has received considerable criticism, but I believe that the work is extremely important and helpful, both in a theoretical and a practical sense, and this study confirms that. The fact is that those patients in the trial who had, on the basis of exercise testing, a high-risk factor profile for death actually benefited the most in reduction of their expected mortality as a result of the special intervention program.—R.L. Frye, M.D.

Sudden Death

Out-of-Hospital Cardiac Arrest: Significance of Symptoms in Patients Collapsing Before and After Arrival of Paramedics
Mickey S. Eisenberg, Richard O. Cummins, Paul E. Litwin, and Alfred P. Hallstrom (Univ. of Washington and King County Dept., Seattle)
Am. J. Emerg. Med. 4:116–120, March 1986   4–53

Experience suggests that patients who collapse in cardiac arrest after the arrival of paramedics are no more likely to be resuscitated than those entering cardiac arrest shortly before their arrival. Experience was reviewed with 265 arrest-after-arrival (AAA) patients and 414 arrest-before-arrival (ABA) patients, seen in Seattle between 1976 and 1983. The AAA group included 70% males and had an average age of 67 years; the ABA group included 78% males and had an average age of 65 years. Symptoms were reported by 182 patients in the AAA group; 146 others reported no symptoms before collapse.

Overall, 61% of the patients with symptoms were in ventricular fibrillation or ventricular tachycardia, compared with 93% of the patients without symptoms. Of the latter, 57% were discharged, compared with 32% of those with symptoms. The most prominent symptom was chest pain. Heavy exercise or activity at or shortly before collapse was recorded in 2% of symptomatic patients and in 17% of those without symptoms. Ventricular fibrillation was found in 10 of 11 symptomatic patients who exercised; 7 were discharged. Fibrillation was present in 23 of 25 nonexercising patients without symptoms, and 17 were discharged.

Sudden cardiac arrest may be associated with symptomatic thrombosis-ischemia, or may reflect an asymptomatic electric event. Patients with symptoms of myocardial ischemia or infarction should be treated aggressively. Those with indications of infarction should be taken rapidly to a facility where intracoronary thrombolysis can be carried out. Thrombolytic therapy should also be considered in patients with electric failure. Intravenous thrombolytic therapy in the emergency department, and even in the prehospital setting by paramedics, is worth consideration.

▶ I share the surprise of the authors that cardiac arrest after the arrival of trained personnel was not associated with a better prognosis than when arrest occurred in the absence of such personnel. It seems that arrests related to an ischemic-thrombotic episode are those with the worst prognosis and need aggressive anti-ischemic therapy as promptly as possible. I suspect, as do the authors of this paper, that a procedure for prompt on-the-site administration of thrombolytic agents will evolve. The concepts expressed on this clinical model fit with the evolving knowledge of instability of patients with coronary disease, as noted in another segment of this chapter.—R.L. Frye, M.D.

Sudden Death and Vigorous Exercise: A Study of 60 Deaths Associated With Squash

Robin J. Northcote, Clare Flannigan, and David Ballantyne (Victoria Infirmary, Glasgow)
Br. Heart J. 55:198–203, February 1986   4–54

The popularity of squash in the United Kingdom means that many middle-aged men at risk are exposed to the possible hazards of physically exhausting activity. The circumstances surrounding 60 sudden deaths, occurring between 1976 and 1984, were reviewed. These deaths occurred within 1–24 hours after onset of symptoms. The 59 men and 1 woman had a mean age of 46 years. Autopsy records were available for 51 patients.

All had played squash for at least a year, and most had begun playing after age 30 years. Many patients had professional or executive jobs. The certified cause of death was coronary artery disease in 51 patients, valvular heart disease in 4, cardiac arrhythmia in 2, and hypertrophic cardiomyopathy in 1. Only two deaths resulted from noncardiac causes. In patients with coronary disease, the left anterior descending artery was the single vessel most often diseased. Twelve patients had severe triple-vessel disease. In nine, fresh thrombus occluded a coronary artery. Forty-five patients had reported at least one prodromal symptom within a week before dying; many had clearly ignored such symptoms. Thirty-two patients dying of coronary disease had at least one risk factor. Fourteen had documented hypertension, but only two had been taking medication. None was considered by relatives to be unfit. Psychological or emotional stress may have contributed to four deaths.

Coronary artery disease causes most sudden deaths associated with vigorous sports activities. Further reports may increase the awareness of both the public and physicians of the dangers of exhausting exercise in unsuitable individuals.

▶ This is a fascinating paper for those interested in exercise. It seems clear from a number of studies now that, almost certainly, patients who die suddenly during sport activities of whatever kind have probably not been asymptomatic. In particular, in this study, there was a rather extraordinary degree of obvious cardiac pathology even before the event. I believe we all have to be careful in advising patients with known coronary disease in terms of their heavy physical activity and should certainly try to document the safe levels of exercise that might be appropriate for the individual patient.—R.L. Frye, M.D.

The Effect of Medical and Surgical Treatment on Subsequent Sudden Cardiac Death in Patients With Coronary Artery Disease: A Report From the Coronary Artery Surgery Study

David R. Holmes, Jr., Kathryn B. Davis, Michael B. Mock, Lloyd D. Fisher, Bernard J. Gersh, Thomas Killip, III, Mary Pettinger, and participants in the Coronary Artery Surgery Study (Mayo Clinic and Found.)
Circulation 73:1254–1263, June 1986   4–55

Past studies of coronary bypass grafting for prevention of sudden cardiac death have suggested benefit, but they have been limited by small sample size, variable patient selection, or retrospective design. The effects of operation and medical management on sudden cardiac death were examined in 13,476 patients with significant coronary artery disease and operable vessels. Patients were assigned to treatment on the basis of clinical judgment rather than by randomization.

There were 452 sudden deaths (3.4%) during a mean follow-up of 4.6 years. The 5-year survival rates without sudden death were 94% in the medically treated group and 98% in the surgical group, a significant difference. Sudden death occurred in 4.9% of the medical group and 1.6% of the surgical group. Among high-risk patients with triple-vessel disease and a history of congestive heart failure, 91% of those operated on did not die suddenly, compared with 69% of those managed medically. Operation had an independent effect on the occurrence of sudden death after correction for baseline variables; the effect was most evident in high-risk patients.

Coronary bypass grafting was associated with a significant reduction in sudden cardiac deaths in this large population. For all the patients the relative risk of sudden death in the medical group compared with the surgical group was 2.9. The relative risk of nonsudden cardiac death was less, at 1.9, in the medical than in the surgical group. The difference in sudden deaths was most marked in patients with extensive coronary disease and past congestive heart failure. The role of operation in preventing sudden cardiac death remains to be determined, and efforts should continue to identify patients at increased risk, for whom operation may offer considerable promise.

▶ This is an extremely important study that documents in the Coronary Artery Surgery Study the beneficial effect of coronary bypass surgery in reducing the frequency of sudden death in patients with coronary disease. Again, the patients at highest risk can usually be identified based on the known variables that influence survival, in particular, the status of the left ventricle, extent of coronary disease, and the clinical manifestation of impaired left ventricular function, namely, heart failure. Coronary bypass surgery seems to be the most extensively studied procedure, and I think the information is quite solid that, in patients with triple-vessel disease who have high risk characteristics, revascularization has a definite impact on survival.—R.L. Frye, M.D.

Miscellaneous Topics

The Role of Exercise Testing in Identifying Patients With Improved Survival After Coronary Artery Bypass Surgery

Donald A. Weiner, Thomas J. Ryan, Carolyn H. McCabe, Bernard R. Chaitman, L. Thomas Sheffield, Lloyd D. Fisher, and Felix Tristani (Univ. Hosp., Boston)

J. Am. Coll. Cardiol. 8:741–748, October 1986   4–56

An attempt was made to determine whether exercise testing can identify patients who may survive longer after coronary artery bypass surgery by comparing the surgical results with those of medical management in a series of 5,303 nonrandomized patients from 15 centers in the Coronary Artery Surgery Study (CASS) registry. The 3,660 medically treated patients and 1,643 who had operation differed substantially in baseline variables.

Analysis of 32 variables with the use of the Cox regression model for survival demonstrated an independent beneficial effect of bypass surgery. The surgical benefit was greatest in 789 patients who had at least 1 mm of ST segment depression and were able to exercise only to stage 1 or less.

Among 398 such patients who had triple vessel coronary artery disease, survival at 7 years was 81% for patients who had operation and 58% for patients who were treated medically. Patients with more severe left ventricular dysfunction had a 7-year survival of 67% when they had surgery and of 49% when they were treated medically. No significant difference in survival was found in relation to treatment among patients without ischemic ST segment depression who were able to exercise to stage 3 or higher.

Based on findings in the CASS group, exercise testing appears to be a useful means of classifying patients with coronary artery disease and identifying those whose survival will probably be promoted by coronary artery bypass surgery. Other patients can be expected to do well with medical management.

▶ This analysis of the CASS registry for determining the importance of exercise testing in identifying those patients who may have improved survival with surgery as compared with medical therapy is an important contribution. Exercise testing identifies patients at high risk based on ST segment depression consistent with ischemia and the duration of exercise on the Bruce protocol. The data show a positive impact of surgery on improving survival in patients with triple-vessel disease and evidence of early exercise-induced ischemia. It is interesting that these data are in contrast to the report of the randomized patients in the CASS trial regarding exercise testing reported by Ryan et al. [*Circulation* 72(Suppl V):V31–V38, 1985]. In a review of the randomized trial of CASS, the only variable that identified those patients with triple-vessel disease and moderate impairment of left ventricular function in whom survival was enhanced with surgery was the occurrence of exercise-induced angina; ST segment shifts did not have this prognostic significance.

Actually, as one analyzes the prospective randomized trials (e.g., the European Trial and the VA Trial) in addition to CASS, as well as other observational studies, it seems clear that coronary bypass surgery is of most benefit in terms of prolonging survival in patients with triple-vessel disease who are identified as being at high risk on the basis of not only exercise testing but of other variables noted previously in the literature. Such studies should help to focus the decision making of physicians and surgeons in terms of advising invasive intervention in patients with multivessel disease and mild symptoms. Thus, if patients are in a relatively low risk group based on left ventricular function and exercise performance, medical therapy may be entirely satisfactory, and an invasive approach can be delayed.—R.L. Frye, M.D.

Application of Clinically Valid Cardiac Risk Factors to Aortic Aneurysm Surgery

Richard A. Yeager, Ronald M. Weigel, Edward S. Murphy, Donald B. McConnell, Truman M. Sasaki, and R. Mark Vetto (VA Med. Ctr., Portland, and Oregon Health Sciences Univ.)
Arch Surg. 121:278–281, March 1986   4–57

Cardiac complications are the chief cause of mortality associated with abdominal aortic aneurysm operations. Such aneurysms were repaired in 107 consecutive patients between 1979 and 1984. There were 97 unruptured and 8 ruptured infrarenal aneurysms and 2 suprarenal aneurysms in the series. Clinical coronary artery disease was present in 45 of the 97 patients with unruptured infrarenal aneurysm. Twenty-six of these patients had a convincing history of past myocardial infarction.

All four operative cardiac deaths were among the patients with clinical coronary artery disease. Operative mortality in this group was 9%. Increased risk was associated with angina, congestive heart failure, a history of myocardial infarction, and an abnormal ECG. Only a history of myocardial infarction contributed independently and significantly to an unfavorable 30-day outcome. No risk factor significantly influenced the outcome at 1 year. Hypertension, however, increased the risk of death when survival to 2 years was analyzed. The mean follow-up was 25 months. Patients with a previous coronary bypass graft tended to survive longer.

Patients without clinical coronary artery disease generally require no further cardiac workup before abdominal aortic aneurysm operations. Stress testing should be limited to sedentary patients or those with clinical coronary disease. Coronary angiography and revascularization may be considered in patients who are suitable candidates for heart surgery and have either poorly controlled angina or an abnormal cardiac stress test.

▶ This deals with the important problem of the preoperative assessment of patients undergoing noncardiac vascular surgery. With the increasing age of our population, we are all confronted with more patients in the elderly age groups with diffuse vascular disease. It is clear that the major mortality in operations for carotid endarterectomy, abdominal aortic aneurysms, and other revascularization procedures of the lower extremities relate to cardiac disease. How, then, are we to evaluate these patients appropriately, and in whom should coronary bypass surgery be accomplished prior to the other vascular surgery? We do not have absolute answers to these questions. Highly symptomatic patients with angina are not a problem in the sense that they clearly require cardiac revascularization before any other procedures. However, if cardiac symptoms are mild, some type of stress evaluation needs consideration, as suggested in this paper. We really need a well-organized prospective study of diagnostic strategies in this group of patients, as it not only is important from a quality of care point of view but also to provide critically needed advice in terms of the most cost-effective approach of evaluating such patients. The use of intravenous dypyridamole to assess preoperative risk in patients unable to exercise is undergoing investigation in a number of centers.—R.L. Frye, M.D.

Improvement of Left Ventricular Contractile Function by Exercise Training in Patients With Coronary Artery Disease
Ali A. Ehsani, Daniel R. Biello, Joan Schultz, Burton E. Sobel, and John O. Holloszy (Washington Univ.)
Circulation 74:350–358, August 1986

4–58

Previous studies indicated that exercise training does not improve myocardial blood supply and ventricular contractility at the same oxygen requirement in patients with coronary artery disease, but an inadequate training stimulus may have been responsible. Long-term training of progressive intensity has now led to adaptations suggesting improved myocardial ischemia and contractile function. Twenty-five patients with coronary disease who had an abnormal left ventricular response to exercise completed a year of endurance training. The 24 men and 1 woman had an average age of 52 years. All but three had had myocardial infarction, and four had undergone coronary revascularization. Training, which involved running or bicycle exercise, progressed to 70% to 90% of maximal attainable oxygen consumption. Fourteen comparable patients, 11 with past infarction, did not exercise.

Peak attainable oxygen consumption increased by 37% during training. Five of the ten patients with effort angina became asymptomatic, and three others improved. Ejection fraction during maximal supine exercise increased from 52% to 58% after training, whereas the resting ejection fraction was essentially unchanged. Exercise systolic blood pressure and the rate-pressure product was higher after training, and the systolic pressure to end-systolic volume relationship shifted up and to the left, with a smaller end-systolic volume. No such changes were seen in the patients who did not train. Exercise-induced contraction abnormalities improved in eight of ten patients after training. Training was associated with weight loss and with a 13% increase in the high-density lipoprotein cholesterol concentration.

Progressive endurance exercise training is able to improve left ventricular contractile function in many patients with coronary artery disease. This apparently reflects improved oxygenation of some underperfused regions of myocardium.

▶ This is an important study clearly documenting that patients with coronary disease and depressed left ventricular function can experience improvement in left ventricular function with a progressive exercise program that ultimately becomes quite intense. As the authors point out, prior studies suggesting that it is not possible to improve the performance of the ischemic left ventricle with exercise did not achieve an adequate training stimulus, as was targeted in this study. The problem from a practical point of view, of course, is to be able safely to exercise patients to these levels. It should be noted that all exercise sessions were supervised by a physician.—R.L. Frye, M.D.

Prognostic Significance of Severe Narrowing of the Proximal Portion of the Left Anterior Descending Coronary Artery
Lloyd W. Klein, William S. Weintraub, Jai B. Agarwal, Ricky M. Schneider, Paul A. Seelaus, Robert I. Katz, and Richard H. Helfant (Presbyterian-Univ. of Pennsylvania Med. Ctr. and Univ. of Pennsylvania)
Am. J. Cardiol. 58:42–46, July 1, 1986   4–59

It is generally assumed that proximal narrowing of the left anterior descending (LAD) coronary artery carries a poorer prognosis than disease elsewhere in the coronary system. An attempt was made to confirm this impression by reviewing data on 866 medically managed patients with significant coronary disease who were followed for a mean of 17 months. The group included 116 patients who were considered to be poor surgical risks.

Mortality was 7% during follow-up. Mortalities were 4% in single-vessel disease, 7% in double-vessel disease, and 13% in triple-vessel disease. The prognosis was best predicted by at least 70% narrowing in the LAD artery before the first two large branches. Cumulative survivals at 3 years were 94% in patients with less than 70% narrowing at this site and 82% in others. Proximal LAD artery narrowing did not predict survival in patients with a normal ejection fraction, who had an excellent overall prognosis. The poor prognosis of patients with proximal LAD artery narrowing and a low ejection fraction was independent of preservation of systolic function in the anterior myocardial wall.

The presence and severity of significant stenosis in the proximal LAD coronary artery are better predictors of prognosis in patients with coronary artery disease than are stenoses at other coronary sites. Obstruction of the LAD artery is a cause of decreased left ventricular function. In patients with a normal global ejection fraction, survival may be long and variable enough so that the untoward effects of any given lesion cannot be demonstrated even over several years of observation.

▶ This is an interesting observational study, and the authors correctly emphasize in their discussion that this is the case. However, the results are of interest, and demonstrate that proximal stenosis of the LAD artery is associated with a higher mortality risk than proximal stenoses in other single coronary arteries. The authors have carefully analyzed these data in relation to left ventricular function. As in other studies, it becomes apparent that the single most important predictor of survival is an index of global function. The authors have observed that LAD narrowing was not the best predictor of prognosis in patients with normal ejection fractions. In fact, it seems that the basis for the strength of a proximal LAD lesion in predicting outcome was its association with an abnormal ejection fraction. These data are of importance as we consider the appropriateness of balloon dilatation in patients with single vessel and proximal LAD disease who have only mild symptoms and normal left ventricles. In fact, this study, in my opinion, contributes to the large body of evidence suggesting that the simple presence of such a lesion with a normal left ventricle is not an indication for balloon dilatation (or bypass surgery), but that other factors in the overall profile of the patient should influence the decision to intervene, particularly evidence of early and profound exercise-induced ischemia or limiting symptoms.—R.L. Frye, M.D.

Potential Errors in the Estimation of Coronary Arterial Stenosis From Clinical Arteriography With Reference to the Shape of the Coronary Arterial Lumen

A.C. Thomas, M.J. Davies, S. Dilly, N. Dilly, and F. Franc (St. George's Hosp. Med. School, London, Royal Marsden Hosp., Sutton, England, and Czechoslovak Academy of Science, Prague)
Br. Heart J. 55:129–139, February 1986   4–60

Coronary angiographic measurements of coronary artery stenosis may underestimate the degree of narrowing if only one plane is available for examination. The effects of coronary luminal shape on estimates of stenosis were studied in nine hearts obtained from patients dying of ischemic heart disease. The hearts were perfused fixed with formol-saline for 24–48 hours before angiography was performed with 5% gelatin-barium sulfate suspension at a pressure corresponding with the perfusion-fixation pressure. The epicardial coronary arterial tree was then dissected en bloc and sectioned at 3-mm intervals.

No variation in the observed degree of stenosis was found in different rotational x-ray planes for vessels with circular lumina. Ovoid lumina, however, exhibited substantial variation in observed stenosis depending on the plane. Calculation by area of observed stenosis could both overestimate and underestimate the true stenosis (Fig 4–4). Underestimation occurred by a greater amount and for a wider range of incident x-ray beam angles. Most stenotic lesions resulted in circular, elliptical, or D-

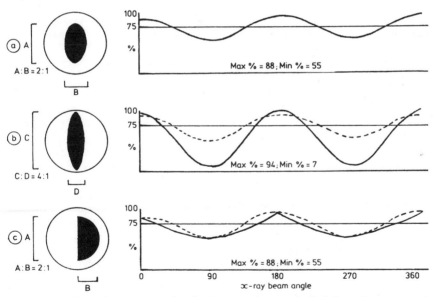

Fig 4–4.—Calculated stenotic area plotted against x-ray beam angle. Each lumen has true stenotic area of 75% of maximum vessel area as indicated by horizontal line on graph. **a,** Ratio of principal diameters (and therefore radii) A to B is 2:1 of central elliptical lumen. **b,** Ratio C to D is now 4:1. This greatly increases maximum and minimum estimation error and also increases range of beam angles at which stenosis is underestimated. **c,** Principal diameters A and B are same as in **a.** This illustrates effect of lumen shape on range of beam angles at which stenosis is underestimated. Broken line in **b** and **c** indicates superimposed graph from **a.** (Courtesy of Thomas, A.C., et al.: Br. Heart J. 55:129–139, February 1986.)

shaped lumina. Both elliptical and D-shaped lumina accounted for certain stenotic lesions being evident in only one x-ray plane.

The coronary lumen need deviate only slightly from circular for error to be introduced into estimates of stenosis by current methods. The elliptical or D-shaped lumen may result in either underestimation or overestimation of the degree of stenosis. Calculations of percent stenosis from densitometric measurements or computerized reconstructions of the lumen are more accurate. Reconstructions may help to detect lesions complicated by thrombosis, plaque fissuring, or both, that are therefore most likely to lead to myocardial infarction or sudden death.

▶ This is a critical paper for all cardiologists to review. The "gold" standard of coronary arteriography is "bronze" at best. These studies provide a clear perspective of the limitations of coronary arteriography, particularly with subjective interpretation of images alone. Others have documented the limitations of coronary arteriography as currently practiced, using other techniques. Obviously, work on new approaches to quantitation of myocardial perfusion are extremely important. The bottom line for clinicians is to critically analyze all arteriograms, which must include multiple angles of view, and to be as certain as possible that it all fits with the individual patient.—R.L. Frye, M.D.

Active Transient Myocardial Ischemia During Daily Life in Asymptomatic Patients With Positive Exercise Tests and Coronary Artery Disease

Stephen Campbell, Joan Barry, George S. Rebecca, Michael B. Rocco, Elizabeth G. Nabel, Richard R. Wayne, and Andrew P. Selwyn (Brigham and Women's Hosp., Boston, and Harvard Univ.)
Am. J. Cardiol. 57:1010–1016, May 1, 1986   4–61

In the management of symptomatic patients with coronary artery disease (CAD), severity of chest pain, exercise tolerance test response, coronary anatomy, and left ventricular function are used for diagnosis, treatment, and prognosis. Although it is more difficult to manage patients with no symptoms, the exercise test is widely used. Positive tests for myocardial ischemia even in the absence of symptoms suggest obstructive CAD and indicate an adverse prognosis. Although it would be desirable to protect asymptomatic patients from the potentially damaging effects of myocardial ischemia, little is known about the activity of their CAD during daily life, which may be of importance. The activity of transient myocardial ischemia during daily life was assessed in seven patients with CAD who had no symptoms but were found to have an exercise test response indicative of myocardial ischemia. All had angiographically proved CAD, and all underwent ambulatory Holter monitoring of ST segments outside of the hospital.

During a total of 384 hours of monitoring, 37 asymptomatic episodes of ST depression (1 mm or greater and lasting for at least 30 seconds) were recorded in five patients. Most episodes (68%) were 10 minutes or less in duration, but they ranged from 1 minute to 253 minutes, and most

(70%) had maximal ST depression of 1–2 mm. A small increase in heart rate, ranging from 1 beat per minute to 34 beats per minute, preceded 65% of the episodes, but 35% were associated with no change or even a decline before the onset of ischemia. Overall, 54% of the episodes occurred during rest or usual light physical activity, 8% during sleep, and only 38% during exercise, including a prolonged bout while the patient was jogging. During 78% of the episodes, the patients rated their mental activity as usual, and only 14% of the episodes occurred during mental stress. A distinct diurnal variation was found; 57% of the ischemic events occurred between 6 A.M. and noon.

Most of these patients had active myocardial ischemia outside of the hospital, during normal activities, and with many of the characteristics previously observed in symptomatic patients. This evidence may explain why some asymptomatic patients have an adverse prognosis and raises the question whether all myocardial ischemia needs to be controlled to improve morbidity and mortality.

▶ The concept of silent ischemia is receiving increasing attention. Selwyn and his colleagues have had a major role in contributing to our knowledge about this entity. The current study expands our knowledge regarding *asymptomatic* patients with well-documented coronary artery disease. It seems likely that silent ischemia implies an adverse prognosis in the asymptomatic patient with coronary artery disease, but more quantitative data in larger numbers of patients are required before its significance in terms of prognosis can be assessed.—R.L. Frye, M.D.

5 Cardiac Surgery

Introduction

The staggering volume of cardiac surgical publications continues unabated. Dividing the various publications into categories with some meaningful order is not always simple. The following selections should certainly not be regarded as the only significant publications, or even necessarily the best, of their class, although considerable effort has been expended to select high-quality, pertinent, and exemplary manuscripts for abstracting.

In the general area of cardiopulmonary bypass and myocardial protection there has emerged no clearly superior technique or combination of ingredients for achieving optimal myocardial protection. Most surgeons use some variety of cold cardioplegia. Topical hypothermia is used by many. A few persist with only moderate systemic hypothermia and intermittent aortic cross-clamping for coronary bypass surgery with quite excellent results. An area of enormous complexity seems to be the relationship between protamine and heparin, and the adverse physiologic effects that sometimes accompany the post-bypass administration of protamine. Every surgeon is familiar with the syndrome of hypotension, diminished cardiac output, reduced systemic vascular resistance, and increased pulmonary vascular resistance characteristic of a "protamine reaction." The nature of this untoward event, mercifully uncommon in its severe form, has never been perfectly explained, nor has there emerged an entirely effective treatment. New techniques for the autotransfusion of shed mediastinal blood have and will continue to reduce blood transfusion associated with cardiac surgery.

In congenital cardiac disease it finally appears that the arterial switch operation has surpassed the atrial switch operation in management of transposition of the great arteries. Both operations should be part of the armamentarium of every congenital cardiac surgeon, but the procedure of choice seems to be arterial switch for most patients.

In valve replacement surgery there has been a gradual return to prosthetic valves after a relatively short era of increasing popularity for tissue valves. The virtual certainty of tissue valve failure between 5 and 15 years after operation has given pause for reconsideration. For those patients with a particular reason for avoiding anticoagulants, tissue valves certainly provide an alternative, albeit at the cost of earlier mechanical failure. Although there is still some effort to discover a management program for prosthetic valves that does not involve warfarin anticoagulation, there does not seem to be any widespread reliance on antiplatelet agents alone.

In coronary surgery, utilization of balloon angioplasty has made a substantial impact. Extension of angioplasty to include individuals with complex three-vessel coronary obstruction has reduced the volume of patients referred for surgery in some centers. An additional effect has been the more serious coronary obstruction seen in the average patient undergoing open operation. The use of one or both internal mammary arteries for coronary bypass is enjoying increasing popularity. But cautionary notes from certain large centers with a wide experience in internal mammary artery coronary bypass indicate that some patients (diabetics, the elderly) may have a higher than average risk for postoperative complications. Publicity surrounding the publication of improved patency in internal mammary artery grafts has led many patients to inquire specifically about the availability of such grafts from their surgeons. There also is increasing concern about the progression of atherosclerotic disease, even without angiographic evidence in vein grafts beyond 5 years after implantation. Whether all such late vein grafts should be removed in the event of reoperation is an open question, but it has been asked.

It is interesting that the place of left ventricular aneurysm resection in the management of patients with compromised left ventricular function secondary to myocardial infarction has not yet been defined. Although some patients have improved left ventricular function in the short term, it seems extremely difficult to demonstrate convincingly that ventricular aneurysmectomy has a substantial impact on longevity.

The trend in aortic aneurysm surgery is toward more frequent replacement of the ascending aorta when it is dilated, or in the presence of Marfan's syndrome. In some centers patients with Marfan's syndrome are being advised to undergo elective ascending aortic replacement in the absence of symptoms or aortic insufficiency when the ascending aorta is seen to be moderately dilated. This reflects the increasing safety of composite graft replacement for the ascending aorta in elective procedures and the hazard of such operations under emergency circumstances. Surgical repair and replacement of the transverse arch are gradually becoming safer with techniques for operative management being published from several centers.

More and more frequently, cardiac surgeons are asked to assist genitourinary surgeons in the surgical management of renal and adrenal tumors extending into the vena cava and even into the right atrium. Some remarkably good results have been achieved with such extended operations, and this trend will surely continue.

In the area of cardiac and cardiopulmonary transplantation there continues to be a tendency to expand the criteria for acceptance of candidates for treatment. Unfortunately, the pool of donors has not kept pace. It appears certain that waiting lists will become longer, perhaps favoring more seriously ill patients, particularly those needing mechanical cardiac assist devices. If this occurs, the overall results of cardiac transplantation may eventually be compromised.

As the level of skill and technological capability in cardiac surgery advances, so the population of patients with increasing severity of illness expands and increases. We will undoubtedly see some rise in the mortality associated with coronary bypass and valve replacement surgery as older and sicker patients are treated. We will also see, and have already begun to see, manipulation of surgical statistics by some institutions in an attempt to appear superior when surgical results are published in the lay press. It is incumbent upon surgeons to define categories of risk so that published statistics may bear some relation to the skill of those reporting such data. Otherwise, this inclination toward surgical "glasnost" will be misdirected.

John J. Collins, Jr., M.D.

Cardiopulmonary Bypass and Myocardial Protection

Myocardial Energy Depletion During Profound Hypothermic Cardioplegia for Cardiac Operations

L. Kaijser, E. Jansson, W. Schmidt, and V. Bomfim (Karolinska Hosp., Stockholm)

J. Thorac. Cardiovasc. Surg. 90:896–900, December 1985   5–1

Hypothermic cardioplegia has become standard procedure for reducing the cardiac metabolic rate and preserving energy stores. Nonetheless, studies still show the presence of advanced anaerobic metabolism under these conditions. Debate continues about the optimal myocardial temperature during blood cardioplegia. An extremely low temperature reduces myocardial oxygen requirements, but it also impedes release of oxygen from hemoglobin. To minimize myocardial energy decline, even greater reductions in myocardial temperature than previously used were tried, and the effects on myocardial energy metabolism were assessed in ten patients whose mean age was 63 years. All ten had aortic valve replacement during which continuous perfusion blood cardioplegia at a temperature of 10 C was used.

Cardioplegia lasted from 55 to 89 minutes. The myocardial lactate concentration increased markedly in the first 10 minutes of cardioplegia. Further but slower increases occurred in the next hour. The myocardial adenosine triphosphate (ATP) concentration decreased in the first 10 minutes and fell further during the next hour of cardioplegia. By 60 minutes the heart was almost depleted of creatine phosphate, and creatine values fell during the 60-minute period. In the 30 minutes immediately after cardioplegia, there were problems with bradyarrhythmia in four patients and atrial fibrillation in three. Three patients required inotropic treatment.

Some depletion of energy stores had occurred before cardioplegia, because creatine phosphate concentrations were already low at this time. This was probably because of the manipulations that preceded establishment of extracorporeal circulation. There was great interpersonal variation in this finding, possibly caused by varying reductions in myocardial perfusion. In contrast, the myocardial lactate concentration was near normal at the start of cardioplegia. The accumulation of lactate and depletion of ATP in the early stages of cardioplegia were greater than those seen in the next 60 minutes, in contrast with results of skeletal muscle and animal experiments. In previous experiments at slightly higher temperatures, the ATP decrease was less pronounced, but the lactate increase was more so, suggesting that the lower temperature decreases energy-rich phosphates, by decreasing the rate of ATP regeneration, more than it decreases myocardial energy requirements. Alternatively, there may be a direct injurious effect of the low temperature on cell membrane function, leading to leakage. In addition to creatine, significant amounts of adenine nucleotide metabolites appear to be lost from myocardial cells during profound hypothermic continuous blood cardioplegia at the temperature used in this study. A low ATP concentration, of itself, leads to depressed cell membrane function and, ultimately, to irreversible damage. That such profound changes occur in such a short time during cardioplegia under these conditions points to the importance of rapidly stopping and cooling the heart during induction of cardioplegia. However, the decline of total creatine concentration, which may result from the very low temperature, is probably of greater consequence in postoperative recovery of myocardial metabolism and function. Continuous perfusion could also aggravate total creatine loss. Substrate depletion, rather than uneven perfusion, could explain why a subnormal arterial-coronary sinus oxygen difference persists for up to 1 hour after the end of cardioplegia. This could seriously delay reestablishment of normal myocardial metabolism and function. Although these observations are based on only a small number of patients, they suggest that extremely low myocardial temperatures should be avoided during cardioplegia.

▶ As the only example of the great multitude of papers published (and reviewed) on various permutations of hypothermia and cardioplegia, this one stands out principally for pointing out the possible deleterious effect of continuous cold blood cardioplegia, which has been touted as more complex but the most effective of cardioplegic regimens. After many hours of study and considerable contemplation of the results of published research, there is still no clearly superior technique for intraoperative myocardial protection (de Jong, J. W., et al.: *Ann. Thorac. Surg.* 42:593–598, 1986). There continues to be no substitute for expeditious operations with rapid restoration of adequate myocardial blood flow accompanied by intermittent cardiac contractions.—J.J. Collins, Jr., M.D.

Rate of Protamine Administration: Its Effect on Heparin Reversal and Antithrombin Recovery After Coronary Artery Surgery
James R. Zaidan, Steve Johnson, Russell Brynes, Sandra Monroe, and Anita V. Guffin (Emory Univ., CCAA Inc., Las Vegas, Nev., and Mount Sinai Med. Ctr., New York)
Anesth. Analg. 65:377–380, April 1986   5–2

The appropriate heparin-reversing dose of protamine remains a controversy. After elective coronary artery surgery, 20 patients received a calculated dose of protamine as a bolus over a 5-minute period (group 1), or as a constant infusion over a 30-minute period (group 2) to determine the relationship between the rate of protamine administration and the adequacy of heparin reversal and rate of return of antithrombin III (AT III) activity. Plasma heparin concentrations and AT III activities were measured at specific times both during and 3 days after cardiac surgery. All patients received fentanyl-diazepam-relaxant anesthesia and 400 units of heparin per kg. The postoperative blood loss was similar in both groups.

Clinically acceptable clotting, return of the activated coagulation time to normal, and zero heparin concentrations after 24 hours were achieved with both rates of protamine administration. Plasma heparin concentrations did not differ between groups, but a prolonged coagulation profile, as evidenced by a prolonged partial thromboplastin time (47.3 seconds vs. 33.7 seconds), Lee-White coagulation time (13.8 minutes vs. 4.0 minutes), and activated coagulation time (135 seconds vs. 123 seconds), was observed in group 1 compared with group 2 patients. Normal AT III activity returned on the second postoperative day, not immediately after protamine administration.

Slowly administered protamine results in clinically acceptable coagulation. Because protamine treatment does not restore AT III activity, blood is potentially hypercoagulable immediately after heparin reversal. The importance of preoperative antiplatelet therapy should be emphasized.

Effects of Protamine Administration After Cardiopulmonary Bypass on Complement, Blood Elements, and the Hemodynamic State
J.K. Kirklin, D.E. Chenoweth, D.C. Naftel, E.H. Blackstone, J.W. Kirklin, D.D. Bitran, J.G. Curd, J.G. Reves, and P.N. Samuelson (Univ. of Alabama, Birmingham, VA Med. Ctr., Birmingham, Ala., VA Med. Ctr., San Diego, Brigham and Women's Hosp., Boston, and Scripps Clinic and Res. Found., La Jolla, Calif.)
Ann. Thorac. Surg. 41:193–199, February 1986   5–3

Administration of protamine sulfate for reversing the anticoagulating effect of heparin during cardiopulmonary bypass (CPB) may occasionally be associated with severe hemodynamic derangement. A clinical and in vitro study was undertaken to determine the effects of protamine administration after CPB on complement, blood elements, and the hemodynamic state. Nineteen patients undergoing isolated coronary artery bypass procedures were evaluated prospectively. The protamine dose ranged from 270 mg to 600 mg (mean, 410 mg). Complement activation by heparin alone, protamine alone, and combined heparin and protamine were evaluated in the in vitro study.

Overall, administration of protamine sulfate after CPB was associated with increased C3a, C4a, and C4d. Peak levels of C3a and C4a were observed in samples obtained 10 minutes after protamine administration, whereas levels of C4d were noted in samples obtained after 5 hours. Only C3a was elevated after CPB and before protamine administration. Addition of a protamine sulfate-heparin mixture in vitro, but not heparin or protamine alone, resulted in increased levels of C3a, C4a, and C5a. In both in vivo and in vitro studies after protamine administration the C4d:C4 ratio exceeded 1. Small but transient decreases in white blood cells, granulocytes, and platelets were observed 5 minutes after protamine administration. The decrease in granulocyte counts correlated with the change in C3a. Protamine administration caused a small but transient reduction in systemic and pulmonary arterial and left and right atrial pressures. The systemic vascular resistance fell and pulmonary vascular resistance rose after protamine administration, although these changes could be due to chance.

Similar to other reports, these data indicate that complement activation occurs during CPB by the alternative pathway and again during protamine administration by the classic pathway. Complement activation is associated with a systemic inflammatory reaction and hemodynamic changes that, if extreme, may result in a severe hemodynamic alteration.

▶ The biochemistry of protamine-heparin relationships is both complex and potentially productive of harmful or fatal side effects. It seems remarkable that our understanding remains so superficial in this important area of pathophysiology common to all of open-heart surgery.—J.J. Collins, Jr., M.D.

Superoxide Generation During Cardiopulmonary Bypass: Is There a Role for Vitamin E?
Nicholas C. Cavarocchi, Michael D. England, John F. O'Brien, Eduardo Solis, Pierantonio Russo, Hartzell V. Schaff, Thomas A. Orszulak, James R. Pluth, and Michael P. Kaye (Mayo Clinic and Found.)
J. Surg. Res. 40:519–526, June 1986   5–4

The generation of oxygen free radicals (OFR) has been implicated in the pathophysiology of many diseases, including arthritis and myocardial infarction, as well as, most recently, those associated with cardiopulmonary bypass (CPB). Cytotoxic oxygen radicals (e.g., superoxide, hydrogen peroxide, or the hydroxyl radical) can play a role in complement-directed, leukocyte-mediated endothelial damage that results in increased vascular permeability. This cascade of events can be curtailed by free radical scavengers and antioxidants such as ascorbate and vitamin E, which interrupt lipid peroxidation by OFR. The effects of CPB on the generation of free radicals, lipid peroxidation, and pulmonary leukosequestration were examined with respect to the role played by ascorbate and vitamin E. Twenty controls and ten patients pretreated with vitamin E were examined to determine whether such pretreatment would combat the generation of OFR. Twelve hours prior to CPB, 2,000 international units of vitamin E were given orally to the treated patients.

Plasma peroxide levels doubled during CPB in the controls, whereas in the patients treated with vitamin E, there was no significant change. Treated patients had reduced peroxide levels at all sampling intervals after initiation of CPB, compared with controls. Both groups of patients had significant sequestration of leukocytes after bypass; the sequestration was mainly polymorphonuclear leukocytes. Serum vitamin E levels were reduced to half of the prebypass levels in untreated controls. In contrast, there was no significant change in the serum vitamin E concentration in pretreated patients. Vitamin C levels rose in the untreated controls, but did not change in the treated group.

Pulmonary vascular changes after CPB can be caused by toxic quantities of OFR generated by sequestered polymorphonuclear neutrophil leukocytes in the lungs. The single unpaired electron in OFRs renders the radical chemically reactive; such OFRs are potent oxidizing and reducing agents. One target for these compounds is the lipid-rich core of biomembranes. Another is nucleic acids. Oxygen radicals can generate other radicals, and more damage can result from these secondary radicals. Oxidation by OFR of polyunsaturated fatty acids in membranes yields lipid peroxides, which decompose to form aldehydes. Proteins, lipids, and nucleic acids can be cross-linked by aldehydes, resulting in a reduction in cellular integrity. Cells have several mechanisms to prevent this kind of damage, including various enzymes that degrade OFR. These enzymes are usually intracellular and may not be able to protect the membrane, or their capacities can be overwhelmed by great excesses of OFRs. Vitamin E is probably the most important OFR scavenger because of its lipid solubility. Its presence in cell membranes interrupts the chain-propagating peroxyl radicals. Ascorbate also suppresses lipid peroxidation. The two vitamins may act synergistically, with vitamin E acting as the primary antioxidant and ascorbate regenerating vitamin E.

Pretreatment with vitamin E lowered the level of peroxides after CPB despite leukocyte sequestration. Vitamin E levels were maintained in the pretreated patients during and after CPB, in contrast to controls. Large amounts of ascorbate are found in the fluid lining of the respiratory epithelium. The rise in ascorbate levels immediately after CPB and their subsequent return to normal at 24 hours suggest an interaction with vitamin E in untreated controls. Pretreatment of CPB patients with vitamin E can trap OFR generated during the operation and break the chain of lipid peroxidation leading to endothelial injury and capillary leakage.

▶ This is another of several fascinating papers on the physiology of the post-cardiopulmonary bypass state. Is it possible that there may be some relationship between generation of OFRs and the activation of complement by the protamine-heparin interaction? It seems reasonable, in the face of these similar investigations, to investigate the variety of changes from the several studies in a single group of patients to discover whether any relationship exists, and, if so, what association there is between these, at present, isolated observations.—J.J. Collins, Jr., M.D.

Treatment With Desmopressin Acetate to Reduce Blood Loss After Cardiac Surgery: A Double-Blind Randomized Trial

E.W. Salzman, M.J. Weinstein, R.M. Weintraub, J.A. Ware, R.L. Thurer, L. Robertson, A. Donovan, T. Gaffney, V. Bertele, J. Troll, M. Smith, and L.E. Chute (Beth Israel Hosp., Boston, Harvard Univ., Boston City Hosp., and Boston Univ.)
N. Engl. J. Med. 314:1402–1406, May 29, 1986   5–5

Bleeding after cardiopulmonary bypass (CPB) results in reoperation for 3% of patients. This hemorrhagic tendency reflects complex hemostatic dysfunction, including mild thrombocytopenia, platelet function defects, unneutralized heparin, excessive protamine, and other factors. Desmopressin acetate (DDAVP) is a synthetic vasopressin analogue that lacks vasoconstrictor activity but improves hemostasis, possibly by inducing release of factor VIII:Willebrand factor, particularly the larger multimers. Because the defect in platelet function is thought to make a large contribution to the hemorrhagic tendencies after CPB, the effects of DDAVP were studied in 70 patients who had operations requiring CPB. Desmopressin was given in a dose of 0.3 µg/kg. Half the patients received DDAVP and half were given placebo, in double-blind fashion.

The group given DDAVP had less total blood loss than the placebo group, the means being 1,317 ml and 2,210 ml, respectively. Blood loss was less both in the operating room and for 24 hours afterward. Three patients in the placebo group had hemorrhage requiring resumption of CPB or a return to the operating room. One DDAVP patient underwent repeat exploration because of postoperative cardiac arrest. Eleven of 14 patients who lost more than 2 L of blood were in the placebo group. Subsequent blood loss after operation was related to preoperative concentrations of factor VIII:Willebrand factor. Larger amounts of blood loss in the placebo group were associated with Willebrand factor concentrations of less than 1.8 units per ml. This was true for 1 patient of 15 in the DDAVP group, compared with 10 of 22 in the placebo group. Although plasma concentrations of Willebrand factor were similar in the two groups before operation, patients receiving DDAVP had higher values 90 minutes after its administration. Patients who had low Willebrand factor values before operation were at a hemostatic disadvantage, which appeared to be offset by administration of DDAVP. One patient in each treatment group died in the early postoperative period. Two DDAVP-treated patients and one given placebo had strokes from which they recovered. Desmopressin had no obvious effect on blood pressure.

Desmopressin acetate appears to reduce blood loss during and in the first 24 hours after CPB. This would represent a considerable savings in blood and a benefit to the patient of reduced risk from transfusion. Warfarin or aspirin therapy could be started earlier after operation if DDAVP were used. There was no evidence to support any early concerns about the existence of a thrombotic state with DDAVP. The exact mechanism by which DDAVP exerts its effects is unknown, but it is probably related to the Willebrand factor elevation and possibly to a change in the distribution of Willebrand factor multimers. This drug can be recommended as a therapeutic adjunct for patients undergoing complex cardiac operations with CPB. Preoperative Willebrand factor concentrations may have predictive value in identifying patients most at risk of bleeding after CPB. Such information could be used to select those who would gain the most from DDAVP.

▶ This very interesting paper showed a significant effect of DDAVP on blood loss with a suggestion that platelet function was substantially improved, probably by stimulation of release of von Willebrand factor. If this conclusion is warranted, perhaps the extra blood loss seen in patients treated preoperatively with aspirin may be reduced by treatment with DDAVP.—J.J. Collins, Jr., M.D.

An Improved Technique for Autotransfusion of Shed Mediastinal Blood
Delos M. Cosgrove, Daniel M. Amiot, and John J. Meserko (The Cleveland Clinic Found.)
Ann. Thorac. Surg. 40:519–520, November 1985   5–6

The technique for reinfusing shed mediastinal blood during cardiac surgery has reduced the need for transfusions and resulted in less risk to the patient. Application of the concept has been slow because of problems with the means presently available; devices are costly, inconvenient, and prone to obstruction by clots or contamination by bacteria. A method was developed of using the cardiotomy reservoir as a receptacle for the patient's blood so that autotransfusion can be performed. Use of the reservoir alleviates many of the problems that occur with other devices. Thus far, more than 2,000 patients seen at the Cleveland Clinic have undergone this procedure.

METHOD.—After the reservoir has served its initial purpose in cardiopulmonary bypass, it is reconfigured for use as a receptacle for shed mediastinal blood as shown in Figure 5–1. The bypass tubing is removed from the inlet ports, which are then sealed with sterile caps. Eventually, the ports will be connected to tubing that drains the mediastinum. The cardiotomy outlet tubing is replaced by an adapter that converts the 9.5-mm port to standard intravenous tubing size. At the end of the operation, the chest tubes are attached to the inlet ports of the reservoir, allowing chest tube drainage to pass through a 20-μm filter. Filtered blood collects in the bottom of the reservoir, ready for reinfusion. The desired amount of negative pressure is applied to the reservoir, and the blood is reinfused with a standard infusion pump. Mediastinal drainage is measured every hour, and the infusion pump flow is adjusted to deliver this amount of blood during the next hour. Reinfusion continues as long as there is substantial chest tube drainage. Hemodynamic stability is thus maintained by immediate reinfusion of lost blood; the potential for bacterial contamination is reduced by minimizing extracorporeal time and maintaining a closed system. In about 1% of the patients a clot will obstruct the cardiotomy filter. To alleviate this problem, a shunt is placed between the nonfiltered rapid prime port and the filtered portion of the cardiotomy. This shunt maintains a constant negative pressure on the chest tube even when the filter becomes obstructed with a clot.

The cost of this procedure is about $35.50 for any amount of blood; costs for the other available procedures increase as the number of transfusions increases. The reservoir offers the advantages of being a closed system, thereby reducing the chance of contamination. The integral filter provides improved filtration of the mediastinal drainage, and the continuous reinfusion of blood gives greater hemodynamic stability. The system

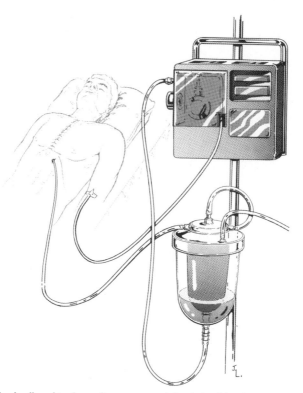

Fig 5–1.—Blood collected in the cardiotomy reservoir is reinfused hourly using a standard infusion pump. (Courtesy of Cosgrove, D.M., et al.: Ann. Thorac. Surg. 40:519–520, November 1985.)

is cost effective and is readily accepted by nursing personnel because it is easy to use and only minimal labor is required. The system is also acceptable to Jehovah's Witnesses.

▶ This ingenious method for using the cardiotomy reservoir in salvaging shed mediastinal blood for postoperative reinfusion seems to have the rare combination of practicality, safety, efficacy, and economy. Perhaps cardiotomy reservoirs should be specifically designed to be converted to reservoirs for shed blood eliminating the added expense of a more complex suction system.—J.J. Collins, Jr., M.D.

Congenital

Transthoracic Intracardiac Monitoring Lines in Pediatric Surgical Patients: A Ten-Year Experience
Jeffrey P. Gold, Richard A. Jonas, Peter Lang, E. Marsha Elixson, John E. Mayer, and Aldo R. Castaneda (Children's Hosp., Boston, and Harvard Univ.)
Ann. Thorac. Surg. 42:185–191, August 1986   5–7

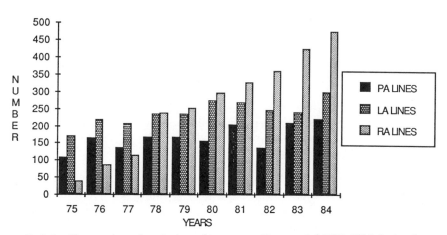

Fig 5–2.—The annual use of monitoring catheters over a 10-year period (1975–1984), broken down by anatomical location of the catheter employed. (PA = pulmonary artery; LA = left atrial; RA = right atrial.) (Courtesy of Gold, J.P., et al.: Ann. Thorac. Surg. 42:285–191, August 1986.)

Transthoracic intracardiac monitoring has become nearly routine in patients having surgery for congenital or acquired cardiac disease. In all, 6,690 monitoring catheters were placed in 5,666 children undergoing cardiac surgery in 1975–1984. Polyethylene 19G Deseret catheters were used. Right atrial catheters were placed in 39% of the patients and left atrial catheters in 36% (Fig 5–2). Pulmonary artery catheters were used in one fourth of the procedures. They were usually inserted through needle holes in the appropriate ventricular outflow tract. Most catheters were removed on the first or second postoperative day.

Forty patients had complications related to catheter monitoring, for a rate of 0.6%. There was one death. Bleeding occurred in only 0.1% of left atrial procedures and in none of the right atrial procedures. Retention complications developed in 0.6% and 0.15% of the patients, respectively. Hemodynamic compromise occurred in about 0.5% of those in whom a pulmonary artery catheter was inserted through the right ventricular infundibulum. Fewer complications occurred when pulmonary artery catheters were placed through the atrial wall.

Intraoperative confirmation of catheter position and mobility should limit complications associated with monitoring. Hemostasis at the insertion site also is important. Pulmonary artery catheters produced the greatest number and the most serious complications. Monitoring is especially useful in patients having a modified Fontan procedure, those with tetralogy of Fallot, and those with a reactive pulmonary vascular bed.

▶ Transthoracic monitoring catheters are commonly used in cardiac surgery, but complications must be expected. The number and seriousness of complications may be reduced by a variety of measures to avoid hemorrhage, retained catheters and wires, and position aberrations that may result in arrhythmias or hemodynamic complications. In this article the authors have reviewed a very large group of pediatric patients with the finding that complications are unusual (0.6%), but they may be serious (one death). The message is clear: Even "routine monitoring" has a cost in complications. The need for information should be reviewed in every institution from time to time so that nonutilitarian measurements are deleted.—J.J. Collins, Jr., M.D.

Surgical Management of Patients With Pulmonary Valve Dysplasia

Walter H. Merrill, James R. Stewart, John W. Hammon, Jr., Robert J. Boucek, Jr., and Harvey W. Bender, Jr. (Vanderbilt Univ.)
Ann. Thorac. Surg. 42:264–268, September 1986   5–8

Pulmonary valve dysplasia is a distinct deformity occurring in 10% to 20% of patients with pulmonary valve stenosis. The anatomical abnormality consists of markedly thickened, deformed, and largely immobile pulmonary valve leaflets, with little or no commissural fusion. Valvotomy has been associated with a high operative mortality and incomplete relief of obstruction. A review was made of a 10-year surgical experience with pulmonary valvectomy in 21 consecutive patients with pulmonary valve dysplasia. The mean age at operation was 26.7 months. Right ventriculography performed in the lateral or steep oblique projection demonstrated a severely thickened valve with little if any motion between diastole and systole, and no doming at systole.

Definitive surgical repair consisted of partial valvectomy in 2 patients and total valvectomy in 19. In addition, a transannular outflow tract patch was performed in nine patients with a hypoplastic pulmonary annulus. There were no operative or late deaths, and all patients were asymptomatic at a mean follow-up of 37.9 months. Repeat cardiac catheterization in five patients who underwent total valvectomy showed a mean systolic right ventricular-to-pulmonary artery gradient of 25 mm Hg.

Total pulmonary valvectomy appears to be a safe, effective procedure for the surgical management of pulmonary valve dysplasia. It provides an excellent long-term clinical course without symptoms or limitations. A simultaneous transannular right ventricular outflow tract patch should be performed in patients with associated hypoplastic annulus. The accurate preoperative diagnosis of pulmonary valve dysplasia depends on the results of right ventriculography in the lateral projection.

▶ The authors emphasize the importance of recognizing pulmonary valve dysplasia among patients with valvular pulmonary outflow tract obstruction. The relatively short follow-up (mean, 37.9 months) suggests the need for caution in interpreting the excellent functional status of patients after total pulmonary valvectomy.—J.J. Collins, Jr., M.D.

Aortic Aneurysm After Patch Angioplasty for Aortic Isthmic Coarctation in Childhood

Karen S. Rheuban, Howard P. Gutgesell, Martha A. Carpenter, Joy Jedeikin,

J. Francis Damman, Irving L. Kron, Jeanette Wellons, and Stanley P. Nolan
(Univ. of Virginia)
Am. J. Cardiol. 58:178–180, July 1, 1986   5–9

Repair of aortic coarctation is associated with relatively low morbidity and mortality. Newer techniques (e.g., patch angioplasty and subclavian flap angioplasty) avoid the complications of stricture at the anastomotic site and allow for future growth of the aorta. However, reports of formation of aneurysms in the region of the patch angioplasty have generated concern about the long-term safety of this procedure. Aneurysms developed in patients who had primary repair of coarctation of the aorta with patch angioplasty. The incidence and possible predictive factors were analyzed in 174 patients.

Patch repair was done as described by Vossschulte. A large, elliptical patch graft of knitted Dacron and a continuous nonabsorbable suture of Prolene were used. If there was a significant coarctation ridge noted on the juxtaductal aorta, it was excised before placement of the patch. Two-dimensional echocardiography was used for imaging of patients who had an abnormal aortic contour on chest radiograph. Of the 79 patients available for follow-up, 45 had patch aortoplasty, 26 had end-to-end anastomosis, 5 had subclavian flap angioplasty, and 3 had insertion of a tubular graft. Progressive dilatation of the aorta occurred in 8 of the 45 patients who had patch angioplasty, but it did not occur in any patient who had another procedure. The mean age at operation was lower in patients with aneurysms, but who underwent resection of an intimal ridge had no higher incidence of aneurysm.

The mechanisms involved in development of aneurysm are uncertain. The difference in tensile strength between the graft and the aorta may transmit turbulence to the elastic part of the aorta opposite and adjacent to the graft, causing progressive weakening and dilatation of the aortic wall. In addition, the surgical technique of patch angioplasty leaves abnormal residual juxtaductal tissue behind, and it is this tissue that is exposed to the abnormal pulse wave opposite the patch.

Previous reports have been limited to patients older than age 17 years; in this study, all patients were younger than age 17 years at the time of surgery. Thus, age, per se, does not seem to be an important causative factor. Some have suggested that underlying structural abnormalities may be responsible, but this was not confirmed pathologically in the two patients who underwent resection. This mechanism is unlikely because there have been no aneurysmal changes in any patient except for those who had patch angioplasty.

Taking these results into account, the morbidity and mortality involved in patch angioplasty must be considered in the choice of operative procedures. In infancy and childhood, aortic coarctation should be repaired by subclavian flap angioplasty; older children should have end-to-end anastomosis. Patients who have had patch angioplasty should be evaluated periodically by chest radiography or two-dimensional echocardiography for aneurysmal changes. The appearance of an aneurysm is an indication for careful surveillance with surgical resection tailored to the size and growth rate of the lesion.

Incidence and Pathogenesis of Late Aneurysms After Patch Graft Aortoplasty for Coarctation

F.W. Hehrlein, J. Mulch, H.W. Rautenburg, M. Schlepper, and H.H. Scheld (Justus-Liebig Univ., Giessen, and Kerckhoff Clinic, Bad Nauheim, FRG)
J. Thorac. Cardiovasc. Surg. 92:226–230, August 1986   5–10

Several techniques are used to manage coarctation of the aorta. The choice depends on the patient's age and extent of the defect. In 1955, Vossschulte described direct and indirect isthmoplasty, procedures that have become the methods of choice in many departments. Despite early encouraging results, an increasing incidence of postoperative aneurysm has been observed. This prompted review and analysis of data on 317 patients treated by this technique to evaluate the incidence of such aneurysms at the operative site. Of these, 54 were younger than age 12 months. Indirect repair was performed on 285 patients and direct repair on 32.

A primary operative risk of 3% was found for patients older than age 1 year. Eighteen patients had late aneurysms occurring 4–18 years after operation. There were three deaths. Thirteen patients underwent reoperation for late aneurysm and are symptom free. All had undergone indirect isthmoplasty with lateral implantation of a patch. Twelve of 14 patients underwent extensive resection of the fibrous membrane, and in 10 a woven Dacron patch was used. The aneurysms generally developed in the periphery of the patch or in the direction of the aortic wall facing the transplant. The area of the previously resected membrane was therefore mostly involved. Degeneration of the media was seen in more than half of the patients on histologic examination. Advanced fibrosis and calcification at the suture line were found in five. In five other patients, elastic fibers were diminished in number or were absent. None of the patients had evidence of an infective origin.

The reported incidence of aneurysms after patch implantation ranges from 1% to 25%. This is a serious late complication, and its pathogenesis may be manifold. A congenital abnormality may be an important consideration and may be the reason that aneurysms occur in patients who have not had surgical treatment. It is not rare for one or more true aneurysms to be found in the vicinity of the stenotic area at the first surgical correction. Lacerations of the intima caused by too extensive excision of the intimal membrane may be a factor. Until evidence to the contrary is established, it must be assumed that resection of the intimal fibrous ridge is an important reason for the development of late aneurysms. The development of an aneurysm in the aortic wall facing the graft may be caused by the rigidity of the patch, which leads to increased wall stress in the opposite wall.

After age 4 years direct isthmoplasty should be used, or if this is impossible, resection should be performed. Excision of the posterior fibrous ridge should definitely be avoided. Subclavian flap aortoplasty is an alternative when indirect plastic repair must be avoided. If there is extensive damage to the wall, with potential risk for late aneurysm, resection and end-to-end anastomosis should be preferred.

▶ In this large series of patients followed after repair of coarctation, the occurrence of an aneurysm at the site of repair is a formidable complication. The conclusion that excision of the posterior fibrous ridge may contribute to late degeneration is probably quite correct. Subclavian flap aortoplasty appears to be a reasonable choice for most patients. The hazard of rigid prosthetic repairs is emphasized. Patch aortoplasty using a segment of internal mammary artery is an ingenious technique that may obviate the need for a rigid prosthetic patch (Campalani, G., et al.: *J. Thorac. Cardiovasc. Surg.* 90:928–931, 1985).—J.J. Collins, Jr., M.D.

Balloon Dilation Angioplasty for Coarctation of the Aorta
Hugh D. Allen, Gerald R. Marx, Theron W. Ovitt, and Stanley J. Goldberg (Univ. of Arizona)
Am. J. Cardiol. 57:828–832, Apr. 1, 1986   5–11

Balloon dilation angioplasty has been considered an alternative to surgery in patients with coarctation of the aorta. A review was made of prospective experience with 11 patients with coarctation of the aorta un-

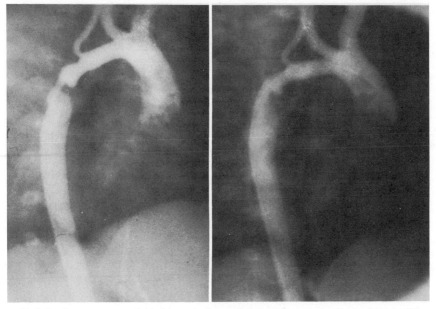

Fig 5–3.—Aortograms recorded before angioplasty and during follow-up. An abnormality resembling an aneurysm was present before the angioplasty procedure. It was unchanged 6 months after the angioplasty. (Courtesy of Allen, H.D., et al.: Am. J. Cardiol. 57:828–832, Apr. 1, 1986.)

dergoing balloon dilation angioplasty from November 1983 to January 1985. Eight had previous surgery, including end-to-end anastomoses in five, subclavian flap angioplasty in two, and an interpositioned Dacron tube graft between a narrow aortic isthmus and the descending aorta in one; the remaining three patients had native coarctation of the aorta.

Two balloon angioplasty procedures were unsuccessful: one in a patient who had tube graft-descending aortic anastomosis narrowing and the other in a patient with a native wedge type of coarctation. Immediately after angioplasty, the mean pressure gradient fell from 47 mm Hg to 13 mm Hg in all patients. One day after angioplasty, a transient increase in gradient was noted in five patients; it was fairly pronounced in three, possibly as result of aortic spasm. These values returned to levels similar to the immediate postprocedure gradient. At a mean of 8 months after angioplasty, repeat catheterization showed a mean gradient of 6 mm Hg in seven patients. Angiography showed a significant increase in the mean aortic coarctation to ascending aortic diameter ratio from 0.44 to 0.80 immediately after the procedure and a mean ratio of 0.76 at follow-up catheterization. No aneurysms were noted in seven patients, including two with native coarctation of the aorta. One patient had an aortic deformity that resembled an aneurysm after subclavian flap coarctectomy, but it remained unchanged after angioplasty (Fig 5–3).

These early longitudinal results suggest that balloon dilation angioplasty may be effective in patients with postoperative recoarctation and native membrane types of aortic coarctation. However, the duration of follow-up in this series is limited, and because other studies report the presence of aortic aneurysms in patients with native wedge type coarctation, further longitudinal studies are necessary before reaching conclusions about the advantage of this procedure over surgery.

▶ Virtually every type of vascular narrowing has now been dilated with some type of balloon catheter. These early results in coarctation of the aorta suggest that some patients with postoperative residual gradients may be dilated successfully, and that certain patients with a membrane deformity may be dilated as a primary procedure. Long-term studies are awaited with interest.—J.J. Collins, Jr., M.D.

Persistent Ventricular Adaptations in Postoperative Coarctation of the Aorta

Brian P. Kimball, Bette L. Shurvell, Sylvain Houle, John C. Fulop, Harry Rakowski, and Peter R. McLaughlin (Toronto Gen. Hosp.)
J. Am. Coll. Cardiol. 8:172–178, July 1986   5–12

During chronic, acquired pressure overload, the myocardium normalizes ventricular wall stress by compensatory myocyte hypertrophy. The recent recognition of supranormal ventricular performance in congenital outflow tract obstruction, however, suggests a basically different response to congenital hemodynamic burden, possibly as a result of fundamental alterations in contractile organization and preservation of myocyte hyperplasia in the prenatal and early postnatal period. To determine whether a fundamental alteration in ventricular performance and myocardial contractility exists after surgical correction of congenital cardiac pressure overload, 25 asymptomatic adults who underwent surgical repair of congenital coarctation of the aorta a mean 10.6 years before the study was evaluated. Quantitative rest and exercise radionuclide ventriculography and computer-assisted two-dimensional echocardiography were performed, and the data were compared with those of age-matched and sex-matched normal controls.

Baseline and exercise hemodynamics were identical in both groups. However, the global left ventricular ejection fraction and maximal ejection velocity, both at rest and exercise, were significantly accentuated among postoperative coarctation patients. Time-activity curves revealed an intrinsic delay in the activation/contraction sequence, as shown by a significantly prolonged time to peak ejection rate and total systolic time. Left ventricular meridional wall stress did not differ between groups, but intrinsic myocardial contractility, as assessed by the peak systolic pressure/volume ratio, was significantly increased in the postoperative coarctation group.

This study demonstrates the presence of enhanced ventricular performance and intrinsic myocardial contractility after surgical correction of congenital coarctation of the aorta. Fetal cardiac growth is predominantly a function of cellular hyperplasia independent of hemodynamic factors. At birth, the ventricular growth rate is dependent on hemodynamic factors related to the institution of parallel circulations and the involution-reduction in pulmonary vascular resistance. This period is particularly critical in patients with congenital coarctation of the aorta, during which functional closure and regression of the ductus arteriosus may create progressive aortic obstruction. The relative ventricular overcompensation may result from primary changes in the cardiac ultrastructure induced during the imposition of congenital pressure overload, with residual characteristics suggesting incomplete resolution after surgical correction.

▶ This very interesting paper confirms the presence of a hypercontractile state persisting indefinitely in the myocardium of patients with congenital aortic coarctation. Although the precise mechanism is not explained, the fact appears clear.—J.J. Collins, Jr., M.D.

The Arterial Switch Operation: An Eight-Year Experience

Jan M. Quaegebeur, John Rohmer, Jaap Ottenkamp, Tjik Buis, John W. Kirklin, Eugene H. Blackstone, and A.G. Brom (Univ. Hosp., Leiden, The Netherlands)
J. Thorac. Cardiovasc. Surg. 92:361–384, September 1986   5–13

Since 1977, 66 patients have had arterial switch repair. Twenty-three neonates had transposition with intact ventricular septum; 33 infants and children had transposition and a large ventricular septal defect (VSD); and 10 patients had a double-outlet right ventricle with a subpulmonary VSD. The actuarial survival at 11 months, including hospital and later deaths, was 81%. Lower birth weight and a patent ductus arteriosus of any size increased the risk of death, as did an earlier date of operation. Systolic left ventricular function was normal late after operation in all but 1 of 36 patients who underwent two-dimensional echocardiography. Three survivors had evidence of mild semilunar valve incompetence. Sinus rhythm was present at last follow-up in 96% of the patients. Most patients gained weight relative to normal for age after operation. All but 2 of 55 were in New York Heart Association class I at last follow-up, the exceptions being in class II. Two patients had reoperations for complications related to the arterial switch procedure. Three patients had repair of a residual VSD.

The arterial switch operation is anatomically applicable to nearly all patients who have transposition with a VSD or an intact septum, or double-outlet right ventricle with subpulmonary VSD. Hospital mortality is low. The results are superior to those of the atrial switch operation. Operation is indicated in the first 2 weeks of life in patients with transposition and intact ventricular septum, with or without patent ductus. Patients with transposition and a large VSD should have closure of the defect and arterial switch repair at about age 3 months, or earlier if congestive failure or rapidly progressive pulmonary vascular disease develops. Preliminary pulmonary artery banding is not indicated, but it does not contraindicate an arterial switch operation if performed previously.

▶ Emerging data confirm that the arterial switch operation for patients with transposition of the great arteries or double-outlet right ventricle is superior to atrial switch repair. The operation can be done in the first few days or weeks of life if necessary (for those with transposition of the great arteries and intact ventricular septum, with or without patent ductus) or palliative balloon septostomy may be performed. The major contraindication to arterial switch operations occurs in patients with a small left ventricle. In these instances, atrial switch remains the more successful repair. (Ashraf et al. reported that late results of atrial switch operations in the series from Children's Hospital of Buffalo were also excellent, with survival of about 92% at age 18 years. *Ann. Thorac. Surg.* 42:385–389, 1986).—J.J. Collins, Jr., M.D.

Membranous Supravalvular Mitral Stenosis: A Treatable Form of Congenital Heart Disease
Ian D. Sullivan, Peter J. Robinson, Marc de Leval, and Thomas P. Graham, Jr. (Hosp. for Sick Children, London)
J. Am. Coll. Cardiol. 8:159–164, July 1986   5–14

Preoperative diagnosis of supravalvular mitral stenosis may be possible with two-dimensional echocardiography. Without such diagnosis, there is usually a delay from onset of symptoms to operation to allow as much growth as possible for the child and for the mitral anulus. The likelihood of valve replacement is high in this condition, and with delay there can be clinical and cardiopulmonary deterioration. A review was made of experience with 14 patients who had operative intervention for supravalvular mitral stenosis. Clinical, operative, and follow-up data were evaluated, and an attempt was made to clarify specific echocardiographic findings that might facilitate early diagnosis. Patients were aged 6 weeks to 13 years at operation. All had signs and symptoms of mild to severe left ventricular inflow obstruction.

A correct preoperative diagnosis was made in 45% of the patients who had echocardiography. Preoperative angiograms showed a mitral valve abnormality in 10 patients and an additional suspected supravalvular membrane in 3. Twelve of the 14 patients had resection of the membranous supravalvular mitral stenosis. On retrospective echocardiographic analysis, a membrane was delineated in 10 of 11 patients, but it was difficult to detect and was seen only on a few video frames in 4 patients. At times the membrane could be seen only by stop-framing the mitral valve motion. When the 11 echocardiograms from the study patients plus those from 7 other patients with isolated valvular mitral stenosis were examined blind, membranous supravalvular mitral stenosis was correctly identified in 10 of the 11 patients with this condition. However, it was incorrectly diagnosed in three of the seven with isolated valvular mitral stenosis. When measurements of the valves and great arteries were obtained, there was obvious left atrial enlargement in all patients. Most also had right ventricular and right atrial enlargement. The aorta was normal to slightly decreased in size, whereas the pulmonary artery was normal to mildly enlarged.

A paucity of data have been reported on membranous supravalvular mitral stenosis. The preoperative echocardiographic diagnosis is difficult. In this study, the nature of patient selection may have biased the results in favor of those in whom a membrane could have been more easily recognized on echocardiography. Recognition was easier when there was clear separation between the membrane and the mitral valve leaflets, but it was more difficult when the membrane was apparently adherent to the mitral leaflets in systole and diastole. Diagnosis can probably be improved with better recognition of the echocardiographic features of supravalvular mitral stenosis, but there are technical limitations to visualizing a membrane that is usually less than 1 mm thick and that lies close, or is adherent, to the mitral valve. There was an association between a left superior vena cava draining into the coronary sinus and membranous supravalvular mitral stenosis in 6 of 14 patients, a finding that may be related to abnormal fetal flow patterns into the left ventricle in patients with a prominent coronary sinus. Only two patients required mitral valve replacement in addition to resection of the membrane, although more than half of the patients overall had an abnormal mitral valve. Thus, this entity is a potentially treatable cause of left ventricular inflow obstruction and should be diagnosed early. Operation should be performed without delay in patients with clinical findings of pulmonary edema and pulmonary hypertension. The tendency to delay operation because of the common need for valve replacement may be unjustified, because the data indicate that a significant number of patients have predominantly or solely membranous supravalvular mitral stenosis that can be treated effectively with early operation. Follow-up showed excellent relief from left ventricular inflow obstruction.

Any patient with suspected left ventricular inflow obstruction and without an obvious anatomical cause should undergo extensive echocardiographic evaluation with multiple subcostal and precordial views. Doppler echocardiography may also be helpful, but it is unlikely that invasive examination will further clarify the nature of the mitral obstruction. Angiocardiography may suggest, but does not prove, the diagnosis of supravalvular mitral stenosis. Exploration may be warranted in some patients. The authors' policy of early operation when the appearances suggest supravalvular mitral stenosis assumes that the possible benefit of such an operation outweighs the risk.

▶ Differentiation between supravalvular membranous left atrial outflow stenosis and mitral valvular stenosis may be difficult. The authors' recommendation that exploratory surgery is warranted in some patients without a definitive diagnosis brings up the possibility that occasional patients may be encountered in whom severe mitral valve disease necessitates mitral valve replacement at an inopportune time. The contention that this risk is worthwhile seems defensible only if cardiac function is declining significantly and neither echocardiographic nor angiocardiographic investigations have yielded a certain diagnosis. Spevak et al. report that valve replacement in young children continues to carry a significant, albeit improving, operative risk (*J. Am. Coll. Cardiol.* 8:901–908, 1986).—J.J. Collins, Jr., M.D.

Coronary Artery Surgery

Antiplatelet Drugs in the Management of Patients With Thrombotic Disorders

Laurence A. Harker (Scripps Clinic and Res. Found., La Jolla, Calif.)
Sem. Thromb. Hemost. 12:134–155, April 1986   5–15

The ideal antiplatelet agent should be nontoxic, orally effective, and have sustained action and good antithrombotic potency without excessive risk of abnormal bleeding. None of the currently available agents satisfies all of these requirements. Agents evaluated to date include aspirin, sulfinpyrazone, dipyridamole, suloctidil, and ticlopidine. The effects of each drug may be different in each clinical disorder. Therapy is hampered by the fact that it is not known which aspects of platelet function require inhibition for an antithrombotic effect to occur.

In cerebrovascular disease, recurrent transient ischemic attacks have a particularly poor prognosis. Some studies have shown effective prophylaxis with aspirin, but not with dipyridamole. A double-blind, randomized, multicenter study of 585 patients found that aspirin reduced the risk of stroke or death by 31%, but sulfinpyrazone was ineffective; also, the benefit was seen only in men. Suloctidil had some effect in blunting the progressive neurologic deficit that occurs after stroke. Sulfinpyrazone, but not aspirin, reduced total mortality in institutionalized geriatric patients in some studies but not in others. Thus, aspirin offers some benefit in reducing stroke or death in men, and possibly in women, but no additional benefit is gained from combining aspirin with sulfinpyrazone or dipyridamole. Results with ticlopidine are pending. Dipyridamole, sulfinpyrazone, or suloctidil alone gave no protection. The optimal dosing schedule for aspirin remains unknown.

In acute myocardial infarction (MI), the possibility of primary prevention with antithrombotic drugs must be considered along with the question of drug safety. Three agents have been evaluated: aspirin, aspirin plus dipyridamole, and sulfinpyrazone. Aspirin produced a significant reduction in mortality in men with a recent infarction; mortality was halved with 300 mg of aspirin per day. Other studies have shown some effects, but they did not reach significance. Some studies that found no effect with aspirin had a greater preponderance of patients with risk factors in the aspirin groups, which could have biased the results. Good results with aspirin were seen in one study if the infarction was less than 6 months old; mortality was 51% less in the aspirin group. Six studies of aspirin alone showed trends in favor of the drug, but other results were less conclusive. A reduction of up to 75% in sudden cardiac death was found in one study of sulfinpyrazone, but the study methods and end points were criticized. Reanalysis of the results showed no significant effect of sulfinpyrazone. A trend in favor of greater efficacy was observed with a combination of aspirin and dipyridamole, but aspirin alone produced similar effects.

In angina, thromboxanes may play a role in the complications that may accompany this condition. Platelet activation and release of thromboxanes may trigger vasospasm. However, studies using thromboxane synthesis inhibitors do not support a role for this compound. The precipitating event in unstable angina is now known, but thromboxane may be involved. Aspirin can reduce the frequency of death or acute MI by 51% in such patients, an effect that has been corroborated by other workers. Sulfinpyrazone showed no effect. Benefits were similar for both sexes.

The mechanism of effectiveness for aspirin is unknown; it could involve inhibition of thromboxane-induced vasospasm or a decrease of platelet thrombus formation on exposed surfaces of the atherosclerotic plaque. Again, the optimal dose of aspirin remains an unresolved issue. These results parallel those seen in transient ischemic attacks and suggest the possibility of similar mechanisms for the complications produced by these two disorders.

Platelet-modifying drugs may increase graft patency in saphenous coronary artery bypass grafts by reducing platelet deposition and intimal lesion formation. Aspirin, dipyridamole, and sulfinpyrazone are effective when given after surgery. A double-blind trial of these three agents is underway to resolve the question of relative efficacy. Platelets do not appear to play a central role in venous thrombosis, but they may take part in its initiation. Both aspirin and dipyridamole were ineffective in preventing venous thrombosis. At present, the routine use of antiplatelet drugs in prevention of venous thromboembolism cannot be recommended. The natural course of peripheral occlusive arteriosclerosis can be slowed by long-term treatment with an aspirin/dipyridamole combination. The most benefit was shown by smokers and hypertensives. Prostaglandins E_1 and prostacyclin have been used in the management of chronic peripheral vascular disease. The promising results require confirmation, however.

Thromboembolism is a significant complication for patients with prosthetic heart valves. Antiplatelet therapy can inhibit the development of thrombi in such patients. Aspirin, in combination with anticoagulants, appears to be more effective than aspirin alone. A combination of dipyridamole and anticoagulants is recommended because of the high frequency of gastrointestinal tract bleeding with aspirin. Complications associated with cardiopulmonary bypass and prosthetic vascular grafts can be alleviated somewhat with prostaglandin I_2 therapy. This agent may produce significant hypotension, however.

Aspirin has promise in stroke prevention, management of transient ischemic attacks, thrombotic occlusion of hemodialysis cannulas, and prevention of acute MI. Side effects are frequent because of gastrointestinal tract irritation, however. The efficacy of sulfinpyrazone is less well established, but it may inhibit venous graft occlusion. Dipyridamole can decrease thromboembolism with prosthetic heart valves, and may be more effective than aspirin alone in reducing the progression of peripheral vascular disease. Ticlopidine, a chemically distinct agent, has an unknown mechanism of action. It may alter platelet membrane reactivity and inhibit platelet aggregation induced by thromboxane. Suloctidil can normalize platelet function in patients with prosthetic heart valves, but it does not reduce the frequency of stroke and death. Results in venous thrombosis are controversial.

▶ This excellent review summarizes the results of numerous studies of various agents that have been used to alter platelet activity in the hopes of preventing thrombotic complications of both venous and arterial disease. The various studies that purport to have shown a favorable result of the use of antiplatelet agents in the management of patients with atherosclerotic disease are cited, with the principal conclusions highlighted. The review does not critically evaluate the quality of data, but it does provide a succinct summary of the data on which current practice in the use of antiplatelet agents is based. The bibliography is excellent.—J.J. Collins, Jr., M.D.

Perioperative Risk of Bilateral Internal Mammary Artery Grafting: Analysis of 500 Cases From 1971 to 1984
Bruce W. Lytle, Delos M. Cosgrove, Floyd D. Loop, Judith Borsh, Marlene Goormastic, and Paul C. Taylor (Cleveland Clinic)
Circulation 74:III-37–III-41, November 1986   5–16

Bilateral internal mammary artery (IMA) grafting was carried out in 500 patients starting in 1971. In 1984, about one fourth of all patients having primary isolated myocardial revascularization received bilateral IMA grafts.

The hospital mortality was 1.4%, but two of the seven deaths occurred in patients having noncoronary procedures at the same time. A significant elevation in the serum glutamic oxaloacetic transaminase level occurred after surgery in 15% of the patients. Reoperation for bleeding was necessary in 7%. One patient had phrenic nerve paralysis. Major complications occurred in 16% of the patients in all; they were less frequent later in the series. Nearly 30% of patients aged 70 years or more had major complications. Major complications also were more frequent in patients undergoing reoperation.

Perioperative risks of bilateral IMA grafting have declined, as for most cardiac operations. Wound complications are a prominent problem in diabetics. The long-term advantages of IMA grafting are evident. Bilateral IMA grafting increases the difficulty of myocardial revascularization, but the short-term risks appear to be acceptable. Caution is needed in performing bilateral IMA grafting in patients more than 70 years of age.

▶ The benefits of internal mammary artery conduits for coronary bypass have been extolled in many publications: Bashour, T. T., et al.: *Am. Heart J.* 111:143–151, 1986; Loop, F. D., et al.: *N. Engl. J. Med.* 314:1–6, 1986; Sauvage, L. R., et al.: *Ann. Thorac. Surg.* 42:449–465, 1986; Spencer, F. C.: *N. Engl. J. Med.* 314:50–51, 1986 (editorial). It has been incontrovertibly demonstrated that internal mammary artery conduits remain patent significantly longer than vein grafts, but there is no evidence that coronary vessels grafted with internal mammary arteries are less likely to have progressive atherosclerosis than those grafted with vein segments. Lytle et al. here point out the increased rate of perioperative complications, even in expert hands, associated with bilateral internal mammary artery utilization. The deleterious influence of diabetes mellitus and advanced age on patients undergoing bilateral internal mammary artery grafting has been observed in many centers. Unfortunately, the inadequacy of peripheral veins may still make bilateral internal mammary artery grafting the procedure of choice in some such patients.—J.J. Collins, Jr., M.D.

Long-Term Follow-up of Survivors of Prehospital Sudden Cardiac Death Treated With Coronary Bypass Surgery
Donald D. Tresch, Jule N. Wetherbee, Ronald Siegel, Paul J. Troup, Michael H. Keeland, Jr., Gordon N. Olinger, and Harold L. Brooks (Med. College of Wisconsin, Milwaukee)
Am. Heart J. 110:1139–1145, December 1985   5–17

Recurrences of sudden death are common among survivors. The possible value of coronary bypass surgery in this setting is uncertain. Forty-nine survivors of prehospital cardiac arrest were followed for up to 102 months after coronary bypass surgery. The 42 men and 7 women had a mean age of 56 years. About two thirds were known to have heart disease before cardiac arrest, and nearly 40% had prior myocardial infarction. Seven patients had had unstable angina. About one third had evidence of acute infarction at the time of prehospital arrest. All but three patients had multivessel coronary artery disease.

An average of 3.2 bypass grafts were placed. Actuarial survival was 92% 1 year after bypass surgery and 72% at 5 years. Four patients died postoperatively. Thirty-five of 45 patients discharged from the hospital have been asymptomatic. Four of five patients who experienced heart failure after discharge died. More than two thirds of 32 previously employed patients returned to their work after bypass surgery.

These results are encouraging compared with the outcome in previous series of medically treated survivors of prehospital cardiac arrest. Bypass surgery alone would not be expected to help patients having severe diffuse left ventricular dysfunction or aneurysm. However, bypass surgery may benefit survivors who have a substantially viable ischemic myocardium supplied by coronary arteries with high-grade stenosis.

▶ Cardiac arrest in patients with multivessel coronary obstructive disease is almost invariably related to ischemia. Correction of ischemia by coronary bypass surgery reduces the risk of cardiac arrest resulting from arrhythmias, although the arrhythmias themselves may be altered only slightly or not at all after revascularization surgery. Many, if not most, patients after revascularization for ischemic events associated with cardiac arrest may have a continuing need for antiarrhythmic medication. This decision must be based on results of electrophysiologic investigation of ventricular irritability under controlled conditions.—J.J. Collins, Jr., M.D.

Graft Patency Evaluation in Coronary Artery Bypass Grafting: Clips Versus No-Clips
P. Blysma (Gemini Hospital, The Netherlands)
Ann. Radiol. 29:249–251, 1986   5–18

Graft patency was evaluated in 303 patients having coronary bypass graft surgery to compare closure of the side branches of the venous bypass with clips and closure with a suture technique. Clips were used in 159 grafts and the no-clip technique in 179 grafts. The operations, done in 1979–1981, all were performed by surgeons having experience with the techniques.

The graft patency rate after clip procedures was 61% and after no-clip procedures, 79%. There was no significant difference in the degree of graft occlusion using flow rate as a criterion, in those having clip procedures. In the no-clip group, however, grafts with a flow rate of less than 40 cc/min were associated with occlusion. Autopsy studies showed fibrous tissue near the clips that caused contraction and luminal narrowing of the graft. The tissue reaction probably was caused by the metallic clips.

Lower graft patency was found in patients having clip procedures in this series. Low graft flow probably is not directly responsible for occlusion in these cases, but when suturing is carried out the flow rate had a definite effect on occlusion. It would appear that metallic clips should not be used in coronary bypass graft surgery.

▶ This interesting paper suggests that the use of metal clips is specifically detrimental to venous coronary bypass conduits. I rather suspect that the problem lies in distortion of the conduit lumen by the technique of clip application rather than the presence of the clip itself. Great care must be taken to avoid constriction bands at the site of either ligation or clipping of venous side branches. The use of clips may invite undue traction on venous branches, resulting in adventitial distortion.—J.J. Collins, Jr., M.D.

Management During Reoperation of Aortocoronary Saphenous Vein Grafts With Minimal Atherosclerosis by Angiography

William G. Marshall, Jr., Jeffrey Saffitz, and Nicholas K. Kouchoukos (Washington Univ.)
Ann. Thorac. Surg. 42:163–167, August 1986   5–19

Atherosclerotic changes occur in a substantial number of saphenous vein coronary bypass grafts. After two patients were found to have occluded single-vein grafts 7 years and 12 years postoperatively, but only 2 years after negative angiographic findings, a policy of elective replacement of all vein grafts was instituted for patients having repeat surgery 5 years or more after the initial operation. Sixteen patients with at least one vein graft with less than 30% luminal compromise had repeated bypass surgery in 1984–1985. The patients, whose mean age was 63 years, had vein grafts in place for a mean of 9 years. An average of 2.3 grafts were placed initially. Fifteen patients had recurrent angina and one had failure of an aortic bioprosthesis.

One patient died in the hospital and one had perioperative infarction. None of five grafts with normal angiographic appearances were free of

COMPARISON OF ANGIOGRAPHIC AND
PATHOLOGICAL FINDINGS

	Pathological				
Angiographic	Normal	Minimal	Moderate	Severe	Total
Normal	0	2	2	1	5
Minimal	0	1	1	6	8
Moderate	0	0	2	1	3
Total	0	3	5	8	16

(Courtesy of Marshall, W.G. Jr., et al.: Ann. Thorac. Surg. 42:163–167, August 1986.)

atherosclerotic change, and angiography underestimated the severity of disease in 81% of instances (table). Disease was substantially underestimated in more than half of the patients. The severity of atherosclerosis was not related to the time the grafts were in place.

Angiography may seriously underestimate the degree of atherosclerotic disease present in vein bypass grafts, as in the native coronary circulation. This fact, and the tendency of disease to progress unpredictably, suggest that all vein grafts present for at least 5 years be replaced at the time of reoperation. The additional surgery has not caused more morbidity.

▶ The authors point out that a normal coronary arteriogram does not mean an anatomically normal graft is well taken. However, the contention that all previous vein grafts should be replaced is open to some argument. Although in the small series reported here no additional morbidity was detected, there seems little question that some additional risk will be encountered in many patients, particularly because of the occurrence of atherosclerotic changes at the distal point of anastomosis. Nevertheless, this suggestion requires careful consideration.—J.J. Collins, Jr., M.D.

Why Small Caliber Vascular Grafts Fail: A Review of Clinical and Experimental Experience and the Significance of the Interaction of Blood at the Interface
Carlos O. Esquivel and F. William Blaisdell (Univ. of California at Davis)
J. Surg. Res. 41:1–15, July 1986   5–20

As the number of vascular reconstructive procedures increases, so does interest in the materials from which prostheses are constructed. Results are generally more favorable for large-bore prostheses than for small-bore ones, less than 6 mm in diameter, in which thrombosis often occurs. The interaction of blood with foreign surfaces was examined in an attempt to understand the mechanisms responsible for graft failure in small vessels.

Endothelium is the only blood-compatible surface known thus far; others tend to attract or alter cellular elements. Most prostheses are composed of hydrophobic materials that are nonthrombogenic. Adsorption of plasma proteins and blood factors may alter this, however. Platelet survival is decreased when synthetic graft materials are used, but platelets may not be the only factor involved in graft failure. Prostheses may be made of bovine arterial material, Dacron, human umbilical cord vein, or expanded polytetrafluoroethylene. Each has advantages and disadvantages, but none is as satisfactory as autologous vein grafts.

Graft failure is multifactorial, involving the characteristics of the lining, changes in the constituents of the blood after surgery, and the interaction of blood flow velocity with the graft. Increased fibrinogen and decreased fibrinolytic activity increase the tendency for thrombosis. Obesity, advanced age, malignancy, recent trauma, oral contraceptive use, smoking, and hereditary factors that cause decreased plasminogen activators and antithrombin III levels are also risk factors for great failure. Graft patency depends on the relationship between blood velocity and activation of co-agulation factors; if blood velocity is too slow, thrombus formation increases, causing occlusion. Improvement of graft patency lies in improving the surface, compliance, flexibility, and durability of graft materials. Anticoagulation therapy may also be effective.

Current prostheses are far from ideal. Other materials are under investigation, including the modified Mandril-grown graft, the polyglactin 910 suture mesh graft, and heparin-bonded grafts, as is the use of prior seeding with endothelial cells to enhance graft performance. However, investigations are hampered by the lack of an adequate in vivo test for predicting graft patency. Results from animal studies should be extrapolated carefully to human beings because considerable differences may exist. An appropriate testing method would facilitate selection of new materials. Regardless of material, the concomitant administration of anticoagulant or antiplatelet drugs improves graft patency. Heparin bonding and endothelial seeding appear to be the most promising new avenues of investigation.

▶ Efforts to develop prosthetic or bioprosthetic small-caliber vascular grafts continue. In this article the authors review the multitude of complex factors related to thrombosis of such conduits. The problem is well stated, but the solution is elusive.—J.J. Collins, Jr., M.D.

The Cost of Simultaneous Surgical Standby for Percutaneous Transluminal Coronary Angioplasty

James M. Wilson, Edward J. Dunn, Creighton B. Wright, Warren W. Bailey, George M. Callard, David B. Melvin, Donald L. Mitts, Raymond J. Will, and John B. Flege, Jr. (The Christ Hosp., Cincinnati, The Jewish Hosp. of Cincinnati, and Univ. Hosp., Univ. of Cincinnati)
J. Thorac. Cardiovasc. Surg. 91:362–370, March 1986   5–21

A review was made of experience with 699 patients (average age, 56 years) who underwent percutaneous transluminal coronary angioplasty (PTCA), with simultaneous surgical standby available for all operations. The use of PTCA is preferred at some institutions. The method is cost effective compared with coronary bypass grafting. It is generally accepted that cardiac surgical facilities are an on-site prerequisite of PTCA, although the nature of such support has not been defined. The monetary and personnel requirements of using simultaneous surgical standby for all PTCA operations were evaluated. The average of lesions was 1.2 per patient.

Overall, 124 patients underwent immediate operation after PTCA, either because the lesion could not be dilated or because intervention was needed to manage a complication of PTCA. Complications included coronary occlusion, dissection, coronary perforation, or atrial perforation. The left anterior descending artery was most frequently involved. Of the 79 patients with complications, 18% needed cardiopulmonary resuscitation en route to the operating room. The most common ECG finding was ventricular irritability. The average time from onset of a complication to reperfusion of the coronary artery was 87 minutes (range, 40–165 minutes). The average number of grafts per patient was 2.0 (range, 1–5). In this set of patients with complications, ventricular discoloration or dyskinesis was noted in 81%.

There was only one operative death. The average stay in the intensive care unit was 2.5 days, which was no longer than that for patients having elective coronary bypass. By enzyme criteria, 39% of the patients had a myocardial infarction. Patients spent 8–29 days in the hospital, which was longer than the time spent by standard bypass patients. For those who had complications and required operation, 86% returned to full employment. The low mortality in this series was probably because of expeditious reestablishment of flow to the ischemic myocardium, a consequence of having immediate access to surgical facilities.

The standby team consisted of an average of 2.5 nurses, 1.5 cardiovascular nurses, 2 surgical assistants, and 1 perfusionist. Each PTCA attempt required 2.6 hours, plus 0.3 hours to set up and additional time in the cardiac catheterization laboratory, as well as cleanup time. The cost of surgical standby was $632.00 per angioplasty attempt in patient charges, but the actual cost was $1,700 per attempt. Surgeon man hours averaged 3.6 per attempt; only a small portion of this time could be used productively by assisting on other procedures or making ward rounds.

Underestimation of the cost of simultaneous surgical standby is a common occurrence in many reports, because frequently it is not included in the cost of the PTCA procedure. The procedure requires a sizeable time commitment by the surgeon. These impressive time and monetary demands should be considered when a PTCA facility is planned. Nonetheless, the ability to limit the time that the myocardium is ischemic after a PTCA complication occurs is important, and the availability of surgical standby led to reduced mortality and morbidity in this series.

▶ The authors emphasize an often neglected point. The cost of an operating room with necessary personnel including nurses, technicians, and surgeons "standing by" while a catheterization laboratory procedure is performed has a very substantial impact on the total cost of the procedure. Whereas "simultaneous standby" in this sense is now not often used in busy cardiac surgical centers, many angioplasties are performed in community hospitals and the cost of standby facilities must be considered.—J.J. Collins, Jr., M.D.

Risk of Noncardiac Operation in Patients With Defined Coronary Disease: The Coronary Artery Surgery Study (CASS) Registry Experience
Eric D. Foster, Kathryn B. Davis, Joyce A. Carpenter, Sally Abele, and David Fray and other members of the CASS group.
Ann. Thorac. Surg. 41:42–50, January 1986   5–22

Controversy exists over whether ischemic heart disease constitutes a risk factor for noncardiac surgery. Several previous studies have noted an increased risk of cardiac complications in such patients, but, in most cases, the precise cardiac status was not defined. An attempt was made to assess the overall risk of operative mortality and cardiac morbidity after noncardiac operations in a well-characterized patient population in which coronary status was documented by cardiac catheterization. The influence of coronary artery bypass grafting (CABG) prior to the noncardiac operation was evaluated. It was hoped that factors correlating with increased risk from noncardiac operation could be identified in patients with and without major coronary artery disease (CAD), and that the risks of such operations could be compared in patients with and without CAD. The risks to patients with CAD treated medically were compared with those patients who had undergone CABG.

Of the 1,600 patients included, 399 had no evidence of major CAD, 743 had CAD that had been treated with CABG prior to the noncardiac operation, and 458 had CAD but were not treated with CABG prior to the noncardiac operation. The end points were operative mortality and cardiac morbidity after the noncardiac procedure. The three most common operations were cholecystectomy, prostatectomy, and hysterectomy. Patients with CAD tended to be older, male, more symptomatic, and cigarette smokers. Patients with major CAD had higher left ventricular scores and end-diastolic pressures, more roentgenographic evidence of cardiac enlargement, and a higher incidence of myocardial infarction (MI) prior to surgery.

The incidence of MI within 6 months of the noncardiac procedure was similar in all groups. Patients who had prior CABG had more angina symptoms than did non-CABG patients, and they had more triple-vessel disease. Patients given medical treatment for CAD were taking more nitrates prior to the noncardiac operation. The operative mortality overall was 1.3%. The group without CABG prior to noncardiac operation had a higher mortality (2.4%) than those who had prior CABG (0.9%). Mortality in the CABG group was statistically similar to that in the patients without CAD. Deaths resulting directly from a cardiac event occurred in one patient in the group without CAD, in three in the CABG group, and in six in the non-CABG group. The overall incidence of nonfatal cardiovascular complications was 10.3%. The non-CABG group had a higher incidence of chest pain after surgery compared with other groups of patients. When data on the morbidity and mortality from specific operations were reviewed, there were no differences among the three patient groups. Among persons who had a history of MI and documented CAD, there were no differences in operative mortality between CABG and non-CABG patients. Variables that correlated independently with operative mortality or cardiovascular morbidity, or both, were high left ventricular score, preoperative use of nitrates, male sex, diabetes, age, dyspnea on exertion, and left ventricular hypertrophy on the ECG.

This study did not substantiate the assumption that a history of MI, particularly within 6 months of a noncardiac procedure, has a statistically significant independent association with operative mortality or cardiac morbidity. It appears to be the degree of myocardial damage and ventricular impairment that is significant, rather than simply the history of MI.

In addition, the results show a clear reduction in operative mortality among individuals with major obstructive CAD who had prior CABG. It is the patient with major CAD associated with the risk variables defined in this review who should be particularly considered for CABG prior to a noncardiac operation in an effort to reduce operative cardiac complications.

▶ This analysis of data from the CASS study attempts to answer the dilemma of whether patients being considered for major noncardiac, nonvascular operations should be considered for preliminary coronary bypass (or perhaps coronary angioplasty) when there is evidence of CAD by history or symptoms. It is interesting to note that the presence of symptoms appears to be an independent risk factor. There is no mention, unfortunately, of the significance of exercise testing. Presumably, a strongly positive exercise test would be at least the equivalent of anginal symptoms.—J.J. Collins, Jr., M.D.

Left Ventricular Aneurysm

The Influence of Surgery on the Natural History of Angiographically Documented Left Ventricular Aneurysm: The Coronary Artery Surgery Study
David P. Faxon, William O. Myers, Carolyn H. McCabe, Kathryn B. Davis, Hartzel V. Schaff, John W. Wilson, and Thomas J. Ryan (Univ. Hosp., Boston, Marshfield Clinic, Wis., Univ. of Washington, and Mayo Clinic and Found.)
Circulation 74:110–118, July 1986   5–23

Surgical treatment is often considered for left ventricular (LV) aneurysm, a complication of myocardial infarction. Several studies have shown a low operative mortality, but they have been uncontrolled. Some have shown that the prognosis for medically treated patients with aneurysm is better than was once thought. Data were reviewed concerning 1,131 patients enrolled in the Coronary Artery Surgery Study to see whether operation benefits patients with angiographically defined LV aneurysm. There were 950 men and 181 women in the group; the mean age was 53 years.

Forty-two percent of the patients were operated on. Medically treated patients were generally older and had less severe angina, and fewer had three-vessel disease than those in the surgically treated group. Results in patients who had bypass grafting alone were compared with those in patients who had LV resection alone or with bypass. A large aneurysm and congestive heart failure were more common in the group that had resection, whereas the bypass group had more severe angina. The overall operative mortality was 7.9%. For bypass alone, mortality was 7%, and for bypass plus resection it was 9% (Fig 5–4). Predictors of operative mortality included duration of chest pain, functional limitation as a result of congestive heart failure, and surgical priority. When baseline differences in selected variables were considered, a significant improvement in survival was associated with operation. Among patients with single-vessel or double-vessel disease, survival rates were similar in those treated medically and surgically; in patients with three-vessel disease, operation improved survival at 6 years. Thus, improvement in survival is apparently restricted

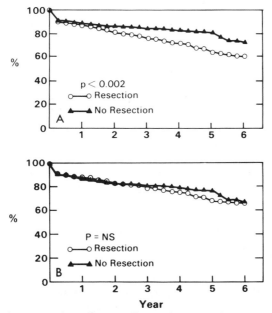

Fig 5–4.—Cumulative survival rates for surgically treated patients with and without concomitant left ventricular resection (**A**). After adjustment for congestive heart failure at entry, no difference in survival was found (**B**). (Courtesy of Faxon, D.P., et al.: Circulation 74:110–118, July 1986. By permission of the American Heart Association, Inc.)

to high-risk patients. The primary cause of death was cardiac in both groups. Angina was more likely to improve in patients who were operated on, although they were more symptomatic at entry. Drug use was more likely to decrease in surgically treated patients. More patients in the group having resection showed improvement of congestive heart failure, compared with patients undergoing only bypass grafting.

Bypass grafting improves long-term survival in certain high-risk subgroups of patients with angiographically defined LV aneurysm. Operation relieves angina, and resection reduces subsequent symptoms of congestive heart failure. Operative risk does not appear to be influenced by resection, nor does survival. Neither the LV score nor residual LV score was related to outcome when all variables were considered. The incidence of stroke was low in both groups, despite infrequent use of anticoagulants. The findings support the use of bypass grafting with and without ventricular resection in patients with LV aneurysm.

▶ The title of this article suggests that the conclusions may be useful in deciding whether LV aneurysm resection is a helpful surgical maneuver. Unfortunately, this is not the case. The definition adopted for LV aneurysm ("a segment of the left ventricular wall protruding from the expected outline of the ventricular chamber and displaying either akinesis or dyskinesis") is unsatisfactory in my view because patients may fulfill this criterion without having significant evidence of LV failure either by symptoms or hemodynamic abnormalities. This is the beginning of the difficulty. Comparison of patients in groups treated medically, with revascularization, with "aneurysm" resection, or with resection plus revascularization is then bravely attempted despite the fact that the authors mention repeatedly that the surgical indications for "aneurysm" resection are unknown. As might be expected, no conclusion can be reached as to whether aneurysm resection is in any way efficacious for any subset of patients studied. It is stated that aneurysm resection caused no discernible harm in terms of complications or long-term survival. This does little to solve the questions of whether resection of LV aneurysms is ever efficacious and, if so, in what patient group it should be done. The study data from the Coronary Artery Surgery Study were simply inadequate, and the adopted definition of LV aneurysm is ill suited for solution of the problem that was addressed. Rankin et al. have discussed the possibility that revascularization may change even akinetic segments diagnosed by ventriculography (*J. Thorac. Cardiovasc. Surg.* 90:818–832, 1985). The difficulties in interpreting wall motion data are well described in this publication and in the discussion that follows.—J.J. Collins, Jr., M.D.

Surgical Management of Postinfarction Ventricular Septal Rupture
Richard Heitmiller, Marshall L. Jacobs, and Willard M. Daggett (Harvard Univ.)
Ann. Thorac. Surg. 41:683–691, June 1986   5–24

Improved surgical methods and prosthetic materials and better myocardial protective techniques have improved the results of surgery for postinfarction ventricular septal defect (VSD). Septal rupture, which occurs in a zone of necrotic myocardium usually within 10–14 days after acute infarction, has a poor prognosis. Prompt right heart catheterization is indicated. Pharmacotherapy should not delay surgery on the critically ill patient; there basically is no effective medical treatment for most patients with postinfarction VSD. Patients in cardiogenic shock represent true surgical emergencies.

Surgery is done under hypothermic total cardiopulmonary bypass and myocardial protection. A transinfarction approach is useful. The ventricular margins of the infarct are removed back to viable muscle, and the right ventricular muscle is trimmed conservatively so that the margins of the defect are visualized completely. The infarctectomy should be closed without tension using as much prosthetic material as necessary. The patch is placed epicardially to the free wall. Suture lines are buttressed with Teflon felt strips or pledgets.

Patients operated on since 1975 have had a hospital mortality of 25%. Eighteen of 28 patients are long-term survivors, and all but three of them are in New York Heart Association functional class I or II. The results justify surgical treatment for postinfarction VSD. Delay is warranted only for a patient whose condition is thoroughly stable.

▶ Although the prognosis associated with emergency surgical repair of postinfarction ventricular septal rupture has improved in the past decade, as reported in this communication, the risk is still formidable. These authors are to be congratulated for their remarkably fine results.—J.J. Collins, Jr., M.D.

Results of Operations for Ventricular Tachycardia in 105 Patients
Charles D. Swerdlow, Jay W. Mason, Edward B. Stinson, Philip E. Oyer, Roger A. Winkle, and Geraldine C. Derby (Stanford Univ.)
J. Thorac. Cardiovasc. Surg. 92:105–113, July 1986   5–25

A review was made of experience with electrical activation sequence mapping during cardiac surgery in the treatment of drug-refractory ventricular tachycardia (VT). At least one of the following four specific map-guided procedures was performed whenever possible: transmural ventriculotomy, endomyocardial resection, cryothermal endomyocardial destruction, and nontransmural endocardial ventriculotomy.

There were 105 patients who met certain selection criteria (e.g., two or more episodes of spontaneous sustained VT or ventricular fibrillation) underwent one or more of the map-guided procedures. An epicardial map of one monomorphic VT was completed in 87 patients (83%), and an endocardial map was completed in 56 of 99 patients (57%) in whom it was attempted. Eighteen patients for whom no useful mapping data could be obtained underwent visually guided antiarrhythmic or conventional cardiac operations. Operative death was defined as any death occurring within the first 30 days postoperatively.

Operative mortality was 16% (17 patients), all deaths occurring in patients with coronary artery disease. The most common cause of death was heart failure (six patients) and VT (four patients). There were three pulmonary deaths, including one patient who was immunosuppressed and died of *Candida* pneumonia. The best univariate predictor of long-term antiarrhythmic efficacy is failure to initiate VT after surgery. In a postoperative electrophysiologic study that was done in 79 patients, VT could not be induced in 75% of those who had undergone map-guided operations or in 36% of those who had visually guided operations.

▶ This interesting paper describes experience with a variety of ablative surgical techniques for the treatment of repetitive VT. The operative mortality of 16% in this series confirms the substantial risk of arrhythmia surgery, particularly in patients with significant coronary heart disease. The exact place for ablative surgery has not yet been established. The authors' conclusion that failure to initiate VT by electrophysiologic studies after operation is the best univariate predictor of operative success is incontrovertible. The question, however, is whether simpler or less risky measures may have been efficacious, at least for some patients in the group. Currently, it does not seem reasonable to favor the expansion of endocardial mapping capability to every cardiac surgical center. The question of which patients may benefit and what operation is best is sufficiently open that such operations should be confined to a relatively small group of centers prepared to investigate not only surgery but alternative methods if useful conclusions are to be reached. Several other papers provide significant further data on surgical arrhythmia therapy (Hammon, J. W., Jr., et al.: *Ann. Surg.* 203:679–684, 1986; Miller, J. M., et al.: *J. Am. Coll. Cardiol.* 6:1280–1287, 1985; Platia, E. V., et al.: *N. Engl. J. Med.* 314:213–216, 1986).—J.J. Collins, Jr., M.D.

Valve Surgery

Balloon Dilatation of Calcific Aortic Stenosis in Elderly Patients: Postmortem, Intraoperative, and Percutaneous Valvuloplasty Studies

Raymond G. McKay, Robert D. Safian, James E. Lock, Valerie S. Mandell, Robert L. Thurer, Stuart J. Schnitt, and William Grossman (Harvard Univ.)
Circulation 74:119–125, July 1986   5–26

Balloon aortic valvuloplasty is a hemodynamically successful procedure in the short term, but the anatomical correlates of successful dilatation are mostly unknown. The efficacy and safety of percutaneous balloon valvuloplasty were examined in five autopsied patients who had critical calcific aortic stenosis. Five others were studied intraoperatively before aortic valve replacement, as were two elderly patients at the time of diagnostic catheterization. Senile calcific degenerative stenosis was diagnosed in nine patients, rheumatic aortic stenosis in two, and congenital bicuspid calcific stenosis in one. Operative valvuloplasty was done using a 15-mm balloon or 18-mm balloon, with maximum inflation to 3 atm for 30 seconds. A 12-mm balloon was used initially for percutaneous valvuloplasty.

The aortic orifice consistently increased after dilatation in patients with increased leaflet mobility. Leaflet fracture was observed in two patients with nodular calcification but not commissural fusion (Fig 5–5). The valve cusps never were torn, and no liberation of calcific or other debris was evident. Aortic gradients declined and cardiac index increased in both

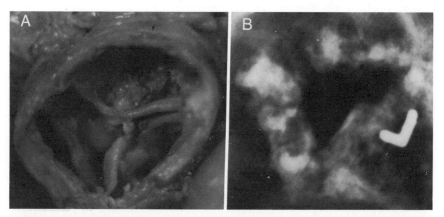

Fig 5–5.—**A**, postmortem specimen after valvuloplasty in an 82-year-old woman with calcific aortic stenosis (aortic valve area 0.5 sq cm), showing leaflet fracture *(arrow)* on gross examination. **B**, the fracture was also evident on radiographic examination of the postmortem specimen. (Courtesy of McKay, R.G., et al.: Circulation 74:119–125, July 1986.)

patients having percutaneous valvuloplasty. Aortic insufficiency increased to a mild degree. There was no evidence of embolism.

This experience suggests that aortic valvuloplasty may be done palliatively in patients with significant stenosis who are not candidates for surgery. Moderate aortic insufficiency contraindicates the procedure. Seven additional elderly patients have had percutaneous balloon valvuloplasty with hemodynamic benefit and no evidence of systemic embolization or significantly worse aortic insufficiency.

▶ This report of initial experience with balloon valvuloplasty for calcific aortic stenosis represents a courageous application of the concept of balloon dilatation that is now being widely used to treat virtually any intravascular stenosis. For patients with extremely critical aortic stenosis, particularly in the older age groups, this technique with its promise of instantaneous alleviation without the stress of major surgery may be lifesaving, either as a definitive therapy (which remains to be seen) or as a bridge to elective aortic valve replacement under better controlled conditions than would otherwise be possible. We await with interest data to substantiate the optimism attendant upon early results.—J.J. Collins, Jr., M.D.

Mechanical Decalcification of the Aortic Valve
R. Michael King, James R. Pluth, Emilio R. Giuliani, and Jeffrey M. Piehler (Mayo Clinic and Found.)
Ann. Thorac. Surg. 42:269–272, September 1986   5–27

The results of mechanical decalcification of aortic valves were reviewed in 92 patients treated during a 25-year period. Ages ranged from 14 to 74 years. Most patients had aortic stenosis or insufficiency and were New York Heart Association class III or IV. Calcification was caused by rheumatic fever in 54% of the patients, bicuspid aortic valves in 35%, and senile calcification in 10%. Early in the series, mechanical decalcification was almost always done because of the lack of a suitable alternative. Later, the procedure was reserved for patients with senile aortic stenosis with leaflet architecture preserved and calcium originating in the area of the anulus, with encroachment on the cusp tissue.

TECHNIQUE.—The calcium is removed by carefully caressing the intimal surface of the leaflet at the edge of the calcified plaques with a scalpel to prevent tearing into normal leaflet tissue. The calcium is grasped with a forceps while the leaflet tissue is teased from the undersurface of the calcium with a small dental curet spatula. Care must be taken to prevent calcium pieces from falling into the ventricle or embolizing into the coronary ostia.

There were 12 operative deaths, all occurring in class IV patients operated on prior to 1969. All 12 died of cardiac failure; calcium emboli were found in three. The overall survival at 1 year was 96%; at 5 years, 69%; and at 20 years, 38%. Patients in whom the calcification was secondary to rheumatic involvement had a slightly lower survival rate, as did patients with senile calcification. Overall, 30% of patients died of valve-related complications. Reoperation was needed slightly more often in patients with a rheumatic etiology for calcification.

Many patients in this series had calcified valves of rheumatic origin or that were bicuspid, and in whom a poor result might have been predicted. Results were generally dismal in patients who had poorly preserved architecture. However, valve replacement also has risks. Results obtained in patients with senile calcification were especially encouraging in this series. Although the incidence of reoperation was high, it is perhaps not out of line with what might be expected. Indications for mechanical decalcification include senile calcification, age older than 75 years, calcification of the aorta or anulus, poor left ventricular function, presence of severe coronary artery disease, and an ejection fraction of less than 25%. Patients who cannot tolerate anticoagulant therapy should also be considered for this procedure. The procedure seems ideally suited for patients with concomitant coronary artery disease and mild-to-moderate aortic stenosis. Extensive calcification and aortic incompetence are best treated by valve replacement.

▶ This report of a relatively small series of patients seen over a 25-year interval makes one important point. Patients with calcification of an otherwise anatomically acceptable trileaflet aortic valve probably have a greater than 50% chance of acceptable rehabilitation for at least 5 years. This is not the ideal solution to the problem of calcific aortic stenosis, but it does represent an option, particularly for patients in the older age group with significant aortic calcification or a small aortic anulus in whom aortic valve replacement would be either difficult or require a prosthetic device necessitating continuing anticoagulation. Although the indication for mechanical débridement may well be limited, it does not seem to be nonexistent, and such an operation should be part of the surgical armamentarium.—J.J. Collins, Jr., M.D.

Survival and Functional Results After Valve Replacement for Aortic Regurgitation From 1976 to 1983: Impact of Preoperative Left Ventricular Function
Robert O. Bonow, Anthony L. Picone, Charles L. McIntosh, Michael Jones, Douglas R. Rosing, Barry J. Maron, Edward Lakatos, Richard E. Clark, and Stephen E. Epstein (NIH, Bethesda)
Circulation 72:1244–1256, December 1985   5–28

Left ventricular systolic function is an important determinant of prognosis in patients with chronic aortic regurgitation. Numerous hemodynamic, angiographic, and echocardiographic studies indicate that indices of preoperative left ventricular (LV) function identify patients at low risk and at high risk of death or persistent LV dysfunction after aortic valve replacement. However, a few recent reports suggest that survival after valve replacement for aortic regurgitation is no longer influenced by preoperative LV function. These studies suggest that improved operative techniques have negated the influence of preoperative LV function on post-

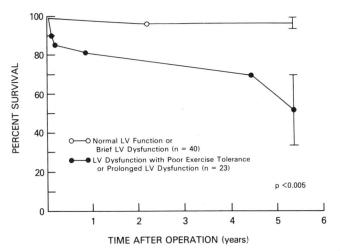

Fig 5–6.—Survival after aortic valve replacement in high-risk and low-risk subgroups of patients. (Courtesy of Bonow, R.O., et al.: Circulation 72:1244–1256, December 1985. By permission of the American Heart Association, Inc.)

operative prognosis. The importance of preoperative LV function in aortic regurgitation was evaluated.

Echocardiographic and radionuclide angiographic studies were performed on 80 consecutive patients undergoing valve replacement from 1976 to 1983. None had associated coronary artery disease. For all patients, the mean 5-year survival was 83%, significantly better than the 62% for patients operated on between 1972 and 1976. The preoperative resting LV ejection fraction, fractional shortening, and end-systolic dimension were the most significant predictors of survival (univariate life-table analysis). The mean 5-year survival was 63% for 50 patients with a subnormal ejection fraction, compared with 96% for 30 with a normal ejection fraction. Patients with a subnormal LV ejection fraction and poor exercise tolerance, or long duration of LV dysfunction (longer than 18 months), comprised the high-risk subgroup (mean 5-year survival, 52%) (Fig 5–6). Patients in this subgroup also had persistent LV dysfunction after operation, with greater LV end-diastolic dimension and reduced ejection fraction compared with patients who had a normal preoperative LV ejection fraction or only a brief duration of LV dysfunction (less than 14 months). Cold hyperkalemic cardioplegia was used for myocardial preservation in 46 patients. Survival was not influenced by cardioplegia. Nor did cardioplegia alter the influence of LV function on postoperative prognosis.

Despite improved operative techniques and better long-term survival, compared with earlier experience, preoperative resting LV dysfunction continues to identify patients with aortic regurgitation at risk of death or persistent LV dysfunction after aortic valve replacement. Early operation in such patients may result in further improvement in survival and functional results.

Have the Results of Mitral Valve Replacement Improved?

Paolo Ferrazzi, David C. McGiffin, John W. Kirklin, Eugene H. Blackstone, and Robert C. Bourge (Univ. of Alabama at Birmingham and Birmingham VA Hosp.)

J. Thorac. Cardiovasc. Surg. 92:186–197, August 1986   5–29

It is conventional wisdom that the results of cardiac surgery are better now than in earlier years because of scientific progress and better technique. This belief was examined by comparing data on 478 patients treated during 1975–1979 and 341 treated during 1979–1983. All operations used cardiopulmonary bypass, with temperatures of 25–28 C. Beginning in 1977, operations were performed with cold cardioplegia.

All patients underwent isolated or combined mitral valve replacement. Patients from the later era were older and had higher left ventricular end-diastolic pressures, differences unlikely to be random. In the later group there were fewer lesions caused by rheumatic fever but more that were ischemic. Patients in the later era generally had more complex operations and received fewer mechanical valves and more bioprostheses. Hospital mortality in the earlier era was 5.4%, compared with 8.5% later. Actuarial survivals 2 weeks after operation were 96.0% in the earlier era and 94.7% in the later. Survivals at 4.5 years were 71% in the earlier group and 67% in the later. The hazard function for death and the parametric survivorships were not different for the two periods. Most patients in both groups died of heart failure, with a higher percentage of such deaths in the later period. Deaths from other causes were similar in both groups. Neither the era nor the specific year in which the patient was operated on had an effect on survival.

This experience is consistent with that from other cardiac surgical centers. Because the patients who underwent valve replacement in the later period were older and had less satisfactory cardiac function, this might have obscured a true improvement in results. However, the analysis used in this study took such factors into account. Therefore, scientific progress did not appear to have a favorable impact on the outcomes for this type of surgery. Survival of patients who have valve replacement has always been considerably less than that of the general population. The operation is palliative, not curative. Thus, efforts to improve results must continue. Chronic heart failure, which caused death in more patients in the later than the earlier era, is probably related to advanced, and possibly irreversible, cardiomyopathy present at operation. This emphasizes the disadvantage of delaying mitral valve replacement until late-stage disease. Earlier operation is needed to improve the long-term result. The continuing occurrence of cardiac failure also indicates the need for improved methods of cardiac protection during operation, particularly for patients with advanced symptoms. Consideration should be given to induction of cardioplegia with a warm, glutamate-enriched blood cardioplegic solution, the addition of verapamil to the solution, initial reperfusion with a warm blood cardioplegic solution, or continuous retrograde infusion of the solution through the coronary sinus. Perhaps these precedures would improve survival after mitral valve replacement.

▶ These two papers (5–28 and 5–29) deal with the general question of whether modern techniques and myocardial preservation have substantially altered the early and late clinical results of valve replacement operations. In both studies care was taken to identify incremental risk factors and to compare these for the earlier and later eras. The authors in each instance are well aware of the inherent difficulties in such a metachronous comparison. It is interesting that the authors of both papers conclude that advances in the modern era have not been as important a factor in improving results of valve replacement surgery in the aortic or mitral position as deterioration of the left ventricular contractile capability has been as a detrimental factor. It remains impossible to make a silk purse from a sow's ear. The question is how to recognize the early stages of left ventricular contractile deterioration so as to intervene before it becomes irreversible. The present reliance on dimensional changes, whether determined by angiography or echocardiography, is unsatisfactory. Some other gauge of functional deterioration before dimensions change may well be more important than minute variations in cardioplegic technique for determining improvement in survival. It is also possible that certain technical changes in response to better understanding of postoperative physiology may be necessary to significantly improve valve replacement results. (See Kreindel, M. S., et al.: *Am. J. Cardiol.* 57:408–412, 1986; Spence, P. A., et al.: *Ann. Thorac. Surg.* 41:363–371, 1986.)—J.J. Collins, Jr., M.D.

Fourteen Years' Experience With the Björk-Shiley Tilting Disc Prosthesis
B. Sethia, M. A. Turner, S. Lewis, R. A. Rodger, and W. H. Bain (Western Infirmary, Glasgow)
J. Thorac. Cardiovasc. Surg. 91:350–361, March 1986   5–30

Between 1970 and 1984, 1,574 Björk-Shiley valve prostheses were implanted in 1,171 patients. In the first 10 years, 1,023 standard disk prostheses were placed, and 551 convexoconcave valves were placed subsequently. There were 222 multiple valve replacements in the earlier series and 89 in the later one. Coronary bypass grafting was done in 3% of the earlier and 9% of the later patients.

Hospital mortality was 10% in the standard prosthesis series and 7% in the group given convexoconcave prostheses. The survival rate was 88.5% at 4 years and 69% at 12 years. More than 90% of patients were in New York Heart Association class I or II at last follow-up. Systemic embolism was comparably frequent in both groups. Anticoagulant-related bleeding requiring hospital admission occurred at a rate of 0.2% per patient-year. The rate of prosthetic valve endocarditis was 0.3% per patient-year. Mechanical valve failure occurred at a rate of 0.6%, and periprosthetic leakage at a rate of 2% per patient-year or less. Fifty-two patients underwent reoperation. The rate of freedom from all valve-related complications was 89% at 4 years and 66% at 12 years for the entire group.

Long-term experience with both the standard and convexoconcave Björk-Shiley valve prostheses has been satisfactory. Thrombotic mechanical failure is less frequent with the convexoconcave prosthesis, but there is a problem of outlet strut fracture. Systemic embolism and periprosthetic leakage may be minimized by careful anticoagulation and optimal implantation technique.

A Prospective Evaluation of the Björk-Shiley, Hancock, and Carpentier-Edwards Heart Valve Prostheses
Peter Bloomfield, Arthur H. Kitchin, David J. Wheatley, Philip R. Walbaum, Walter Lutz, and Hugh C. Miller (Univ. of Edinburgh)
Circulation 73:1213–1222, June 1986   5–31

The 540 patients having cardiac valve replacement in 1975–1979 were randomized to receive a Björk-Shiley tilting-disk prosthesis or a porcine heterograft valve. A Hancock valve was used in 107 of the latter patients and a Carpentier-Edwards valve in 160 patients treated subsequently. Sixty patients had both mitral and aortic replacements, and eight also required tricuspid valve replacement. The groups were clinically similar at the outset.

In those given mitral prostheses, hospital mortality was highest at 15.5% in patients given a Carpentier-Edwards prosthesis. The overall rate was nearly 9%. Highly significant functional improvement was noted in survivors as a whole, with no significant decline at later follow-up. The late mortality was 21%. Thirty-seven patients had reoperation for valve failure and four for bacterial endocarditis. Eighteen embolic events occurred in patients having aortic replacement, with no deaths (Fig 5–7). In the mitral group thromboembolism was more frequent, and three patients died as a

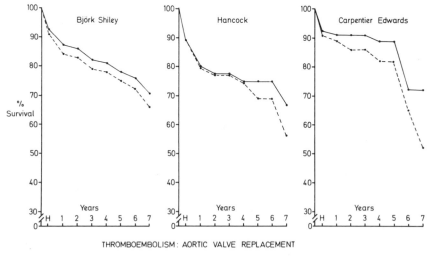

THROMBOEMBOLISM: AORTIC VALVE REPLACEMENT

——— Survival   - - - - - Survival Free from Embolism

Fig 5–7.—Actuarial survival and survival free from embolism for patients undergoing aortic valve replacement with the three prostheses. (Courtesy of Bloomfield, P., et al.: Circulation 73:1213–1222, June 1986.)

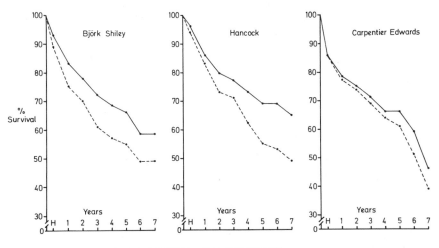

THROMBOEMBOLISM : MITRAL VALVE REPLACEMENT

——— Survival   ------- Survival Free from Embolism

Fig 5–8.—Actuarial survival and survival free from embolism for patients undergoing mitral valve replacement with the three prostheses. (Courtesy of Bloomfield, P., et al.: Circulation 73:1213–1222, June 1986.)

result (Fig 5–8). Embolism was associated with atrial fibrillation in the group given mitral prostheses, and with rheumatic disease and age under 65 years in the aortic group. The risks of anticoagulation were low.

No significant advantage of any of these prostheses is apparent, but longer follow-up is essential. The median follow-up in the present series is less than 6 years. It appears reasonable to use anticoagulants in all patients undergoing aortic replacement who have coexisting mitral valve disease and patients undergoing mitral replacement who are in atrial fibrillation.

▶ Continuing analysis of large groups of patients late after cardiac valve replacement confirms the potentially excellent rehabilitation possible with various types of prosthetic devices. (Kinsley, R. H., et al.: *J. Thorac. Cardiovasc. Surg.* 92:349–360, 1986; Harlan, B. J., et al.: *J. Thorac. Cardiovasc. Surg.* 91:86–91, 1986; Grunkemeier, G. L., et al.: *J. Thorac. Cardiovasc. Surg.* 91:918–923, 1986; Best, J. F., et al.: *Am. Heart. J.* 111:136–142, 1986.) There does not seem to be any significant difference between the various types of porcine valves available, and the difference between porcine valves and other tissue prostheses is probably not particularly great either. (Spencer, F. C., et al.: *Ann. Surg.* 203:691–700, 1986; Nistal, F., et al.: *Am. J. Cardiol.* 57:161–164, 1986.) All valves in the tricuspid position have a higher risk of thrombosis than valves in the mitral and aortic position (Boskovic, D., et al.: *J. Thorac. Cardiovasc. Surg.* 91:1–8, 1986). At present, it appears that the hemodynamic performance of all of the leaflet prostheses and tilting disk prostheses is quite satisfactory; their utility is limited principally by thromboembolic potential.—J.J. Collins, Jr., M.D.

Comparative Study of Warfarin Versus Antiplatelet Therapy in Patients With a St. Jude Medical Valve in the Aortic Position

Renee S. Hartz, Joseph LoCicero, III, Vincent Kucich, Arthur DeBoer, Susan O'Mara, Sheridan N. Meyers, and Lawrence L. Michaelis (Northwestern Univ.)
J. Thorac. Cardiovasc. Surg. 92:684–690, October 1986   5–32

The St. Jude Medical valve has excellent hemodynamic characteristics and decreased thrombogenicity. Its bileaflet design permits malfunction of one leaflet without catastrophic valve failure. The valve was implanted in 90 adults in the aortic position; 4 also received a porcine mitral valve. The morbidity and mortality related to the prosthesis itself and to anticoagulant therapy were evaluated. Of the 83 survivors, 41 were treated with conventional long-term warfarin therapy and 42 were given antiplatelet therapy. The mean age of the entire group was 54.2 years. The decision to use warfarin was not randomized; it depended on patient age, reliability, history of thromboembolism, and risk of anticoagulant hemorrhage.

Overall mortality was 7.7%. Six of the seven deaths occurred because of heart failure, persistent sepsis, or arrhythmia. The mean length of follow-up was 29 months. Cardiac mortality in the warfarin group was 2.7% per patient-year. One of the three deaths was immediately preceded by a massive cerebrovascular accident. In the antiplatelet group, the one death was of a patient who had stopped taking warfarin on her own and had started to take aspirin-dipyridamole. Cardiac mortality in this group was 1.1% per patient-year. Eight major complications occurred in the warfarin group, including embolic myocardial infarction, transient ischemic attacks, and serious hemorrhage. Late morbidity was 7.3% per patient-year. There were four complications in the antiplatelet group, for a late morbidity of 3.2% per patient-year. The difference between groups was not significant. Two complications were embolic and two were thrombotic in the antiplatelet group.

There are few reports of structural failure or thrombosis associated with the St. Jude Medical heart valve. Most trials have been in children, however, and some workers have concluded that the coagulation mechanism in children is quite different. Among adults, there have been reports of valve thrombosis in patients not receiving anticoagulants. Unfortunately, no major conclusions can be drawn from these data with respect to anticoagulation. The trials were not randomized, follow-up was not long enough, and maintenance anticoagulant therapy was inadequate. Clearly, factors other than anticoagulation play a role in thrombosis of the St. Jude valve. Orientation of the valve in relation to the interventricular septum may be important. The prosthesis can be obstructed not only by minute amounts of thrombus, but also by hypertrophied septal tissue. In the series reported here, only one leaflet failed. Orientation of the valve should be personalized on the basis of the patient's anatomy. In these two similar groups of patients, no significant differences in late cardiac deaths or embolization could be found. Even the two instances of thrombus do not allow the conclusion that warfarin therapy is mandatory for all patients with aortic St. Jude valves.

Most patients should receive warfarin, unless there is a question of noncompliance or if contraindications to its use exist. In such patients, antiplatelet therapy can be administered after a brief, postoperative period of warfarin therapy. All patients should have baseline cinefluoroscopic studies of the valve before leaving the hospital to assess leaflet mobility. Warfarin has many unwanted side effects; therefore, the search for a better agent must be continued. In the meantime, the dictum that warfarin is required for all patients with mechanical heart valves needs to be reevaluated.

▶ This provocative study again raises the possibility that warfarin therapy may not be necessary for all patients with prosthetic valves. There is no doubt that the use of warfarin therapy made a substantial difference in the incidence of thromboembolic problems with early prosthetic valves, but there has been little organized evaluation of the variation in warfarin dosage or the total elimination of warfarin in patients given prosthetic devices during the past 25 years. Certain baseline studies may provide a profile of thrombotic risk (antithrombin III levels, platelet function studies) that might be used to calculate the risk of discontinuance of warfarin therapy for many patients. It is also arguable whether for most patients the exact level of anticoagulation achieved with warfarin is related to the probability of embolic events. Particularly in patients in whom a combination of antiplatelet and anticoagulant medication is used there is no strong evidence to suggest that hazardous levels of anticoagulation have a reduced probability of thromboembolism.—J.J. Collins, Jr., M.D.

In Vitro Hemodynamic Characteristics of Tissue Bioprostheses in the Aortic Position

Ajit P. Yoganathan, Yi-Ren Woo, Hsing-Wen Sung, Frank P. Williams, Robert H. Franch, and Michael Jones (Emory Univ. and National Heart, Lung, and Blood Inst., NIH, Bethesda)
J. Thorac. Cardiovasc. Surg. 92:198–209, August 1986   5–33

Trileaflet tissue bioprostheses are intended to mimic the natural aortic valve, but present bioprostheses have high pressure drops, narrow jet-type flow characteristics, and unsatisfactory leaflet opening and closing features. In addition, leaflet calcification occurs and material wears and fatigues. The in vitro hemodynamic properties of various older and newer porcine and bovine pericardial bioprostheses were studied under pulsatile saline flow conditions while in the aortic position. The study included models 2625 and 2650 Carpentier-Edwards porcine valves; the Carpentier-Edwards pericardial valve; models 242, 250, and 410 Hancock porcine valves; the Hancock pericardial valve; and the standard and low-profile Ionescu-Shiley bioprostheses.

Pressure fall studies showed that the older valves have performance indices in the range of 0.3–0.4, whereas the newer low-pressure fixed designs have indices of 0.5–0.7. Flow visualization and velocity and turbulent shear stress estimates, made using a two-dimensional laser Doppler anemometer system, showed that all valve designs created jet-type flow fields, but that the intensity of the jets and level of turbulence were less with the new designs. The pericardial valves generally had better hemodynamic characteristics than the porcine bioprostheses had.

Newer tissue bioprostheses have superior pressure drop features and better utilize their stent orifice areas than do the older designs. Turbulent shear stresses remain high enough to damage formed blood elements. The annular region between the outflow surfaces of the leaflets and the channel wall remain relatively stagnant in most of systole, tending toward deposition of thrombotic, calcific, or fibrotic material on the leaflet surfaces.

▶ The superior mechanical properties of newer model tissue bioprostheses are documented by this interesting study. The question of whether this apparent superiority will result in a better clinical outcome remains to be seen. Nevertheless, studies such as this one may well be used in consideration of design modifications and, for that reason, it is important that clinical correlations be established as quickly as possible, whether positive or negative. The general problem and a suggested approach for clinical evaluation of new prosthetic valves for aortic and mitral valve replacement have been well reviewed by Gersh et al. (*J. Thorac. Cardiovasc. Surg.* 91:460–466, 1986).—J.J. Collins, Jr., M.D.

Suture Technique in Preventing Dehiscence of Prosthetic Mitral Valves
Geoffrey M. Stiles, Jules A. Kernen, and Quentin R. Stiles (Univ. of Southern California)
Arch. Surg. 121:1136–1140, October 1986   5–34

Suture dehiscence has complicated 2.5% to 10% of reported mitral valve replacements; no suturing technique has been universally accepted. The holding strength was compared for simple interrupted sutures placed at right angles to the anulus, figure-eight sutures, horizontal mattress sutures placed parallel to the anulus, and horizontal mattress sutures with pledgets. Each technique was used in 15 fresh porcine hearts. Sutures of 2–0 polyester were placed in the anulus, one in the anterior leaflet and each commissure and two in the posterior leaflet.

All suture techniques had poor holding strength in the posterior leaflet. At the commissures, figure-eight sutures and horizontal mattress sutures with pledgets were significantly stronger than the other types. Simple interrupted sutures and figure-eight sutures placed across the "grain" of the anterior leaflet fibers held better than either type of horizontal mattress suture. Dehiscence always occurred in the posterior leaflet with the valve ring sewn in place. Anterior leaflet sutures did not dehisce.

The strongest sutures presumably will lead to the lowest rate of perivalvular leakage after prosthetic mitral valve replacement. Simple interrupted or figure-eight sutures may be used in the anterior leaflet, horizontal mattress sutures with pledgets in the posterior leaflet, and either these or figure-eight sutures at the commissures. It also is acceptable to use horizontal mattress sutures with pledgets in all areas. Because there is little or no tissue growth into the prosthetic ring, all parameters of suturing are important in preventing leakage.

▶ This very interesting study is based upon inherently faulty assumptions, in my view. These are that (1) the security of prosthetic mitral valves is entirely a function of holding strength, and (2) resistance to disruption is necessarily an advantage no matter how it is achieved. The authors have ignored the possible influence of tissue devitalization by suture constriction as a possible mechanism of failure of prosthetic valve attachment. Furthermore, the general premise that resistance to forcible disruption immediately after suture placement is the most important feature of security of placement is highly questionable. It seems to be inadvisable to publish studies of this sort without commentary. They may well resurface in the hands of contentious lawyers as evidence of what constitutes acceptable technique.—J.J. Collins, Jr., M.D.

Aortic Aneurysm Surgery

Computed Tomography: The Investigation of Choice for Aortic Dissection?

H. Singh, E. Fitzgerald, and M.S.T. Ruttley (Univ. of Wales)
Br. Heart J. 56:171–175, August 1986   5–35

Acute dissection of the aorta must be accurately and promptly diagnosed for effective management. Computed tomography (CT) has become established as a complementary and reliable diagnostic method, apart from aortography. The diagnosis is confirmed by CT if contrast medium fills two or more channels in the aorta and if an intimal flap is identified. Computed tomography avoids the need for vascular catheterization, but it is limited by low spatial resolution, so that aortic branches cannot be assessed reliably. Artifacts may complicate the diagnosis, and even high-quality tomograms may occasionally fail to show a dissection. Two patients were seen in whom CT proved to be better than aortography for diagnosis of dissection of the aorta.

Both were elderly persons with sudden onset of interscapular pain. Both were hypertensive, but neither was in cardiac failure or had murmurs, and the ECGs were normal. In the first patient, aortograms were normal, but chest x-ray findings were suspect. Because CT showed a dissecting aneurysm, aortography was repeated. Findings were again normal and the patient was not operated on. Six months later, repeat CT still showed signs of aneurysm, but the patient was well. In the second patient, CT showed a dissecting aneurysm but aortograms were normal. Operation was postponed. When the patient's condition deteriorated, CT was repeated and showed visible leakage. Operation confirmed the aneurysm, although its extent had not been accurately represented on the first tomogram.

In both patients examination of good-quality aortograms failed to show a dissecting aneurysm that was subsequently seen on CT and confirmed, in one case, at operation. This experience suggests that CT should be the preferred initial diagnostic method in a patient in fairly stable condition. If CT shows that dissection is confined to the descending aorta, and that there are no complications (e.g., mediastinal compression and hemorrhage), medical management is appropriate. If dissection affects the ascending aorta, cardiac catheterization is generally regarded as a prerequisite for operation, because it can show the severity of aortic regurgitation and give high-resolution images of the coronary arteries and aortic arch branches. Aortography is generally considered to be the definitive investigation for acute dissection of the aorta, but false negative results have been reported not only by the authors but by others. Computed tomography is a reliable alternative and may be superior to aortography.

▶ As this report points out, neither aortography nor CT yields totally reliable negative diagnostic studies when a dissecting aneurysm is suspected. When clinical implications are strong, both techniques should be used before a diagnosis of no dissection is adopted and, even in these cases, absolute certainty cannot be achieved.—J.J. Collins, Jr., M.D.

Eleven-Year Experience With Composite Graft Replacement of the Ascending Aorta and Aortic Valve
Nicholas T. Kouchoukos, William G. Marshall, Jr., and Therese A. Wedige-Stecher (Washington Univ.)
J. Thorac. Cardiovasc. Surg. 92:691–705, October 1986   5–36

Composite graft replacement of the ascending aorta and aortic valve was performed in 127 patients in 1974–1985. The mean age was 51 years. About one fifth of the patients had signs of Marfan's syndrome. Annuloaortic ectasia was present in 69 patients and aortic dissection in 51. In the last 24 patients a preclotted prosthesis was used and the inclusion technique was abandoned. Concomitant procedures were done in one fourth of the series. Hypothermic potassium cardioplegia is the preferred method of intraoperative myocardial protection. The mean follow-up was 54 months.

Hospital mortality was 5%, and 12% of patients required reoperation for bleeding. The presence of pseudoaneurysms was associated with use of the inclusion technique. Nine of 31 late deaths were related to the graft valve prosthesis. Actuarial survival was 75% at 5 years and 65% at 7 years. Eight patients required surgery for disease elsewhere in the aorta. Two of ten thromboembolic events were fatal, as was one of nine complications related to anticoagulant therapy. Four of seven patients with prosthetic valve endocarditis were reoperated on. The likelihood of having no valve-related complications was 68% at 5 years and 53% at 7 years. Ten survivors were in New York Heart Association class III or IV at last follow-up.

Composite graft replacement of the ascending aorta and aortic valve continues to be indicated for annuloaortic ectasia and for aneurysms of the sinuses of Valsalva after previous surgery. It also is useful in patients with acute or chronic aortic dissection when the aortic valve is incompetent, especially when dissection extends to the aortic annulus. Interposition or bypass grafts to the coronary arteries are used liberally when aortic dissection is present.

▶ This excellent series is indicative of the present tendency toward "more radical" operations for treatment of acute dissections and other aneurysms of the ascending aorta. The series Cabrol et al. (*J. Thorac. Cardiovasc. Surg.* 91:17–25, 1986) and the series of Gott et al. (*N. Engl. J. Med.* 314:1070–1074, 1986) also show excellent results with their particular variations of the composite graft replacement technique. The utilization by Cabrol and his group of a tube graft connecting the coronary orifices to the composite graft seems an unnecessarily complex modification in most cases. However, in the occasional instance in which there is insufficient room for a primary coronary orifice to graft anastomosis, the Cabrol technique may prove lifesaving.—J.J. Collins, Jr., M.D.

Redo Operations for Recurrent Aneurysmal Disease of the Ascending Aorta and Transverse Aortic Arch

E. Stanley Crawford, John L. Crawford, Hazim J. Safi, and Joseph S. Coselli (Baylor College of Medicine, Houston)
Ann. Thorac. Surg. 40:439–455, November 1985   5–37

Problems requiring redo surgery after primary operation for aneurysmal disease of the ascending aorta and aortic arch have been reported in 6% to 14% of patients. Sixty-seven such operations were done in 59 patients in 1973–1984. Thirty-four patients, 12 with Marfan's syndrome, had a fusiform aneurysm secondary to medial degenerative disease, and 23 had aortic dissection in a previously nondilated aorta. Two patients had an aneurysm persisting or occurring after brachiocephalic bypass; one of them had aortitis. Residual pathology in these patients led to aortic insufficiency, dissection, coronary insufficiency, and progressive aneurysmal dilatation.

The patients underwent composite valve graft replacement of the aortic valve and ascending aorta (Fig 5–9) or arch, or both, and suture of the false aneurysm with a viable tissue wrap. Twenty patients had a distal aortic aneurysm. The early survival rate was 83%, and 68% of patients were well at last follow-up. Expected survival rates at 1 year and 2 years were 70% and 66%, respectively. Most early deaths were caused by coronary artery disease or hemorrhage.

Aneurysm replacement at the time of aortic valve replacement and coronary bypass may prevent the need for redo surgery. Marfan's syndrome patients may have total replacement of the ascending aorta and aortic valve. Non-Marfan's disease patients may have the same procedure, or valve replacement and separate graft replacement. Patients with aortic dissection should have ascending aortic replacement combined with valve resuspension, aortic valve replacement, or composite valve graft placement,

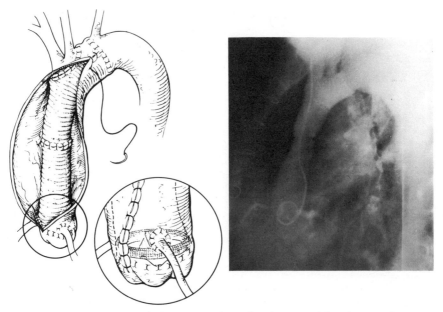

Fig 5–9.—Treatment consisted of composite valve graft replacement of the valve, ascending aorta, and arch. (Courtesy of Crawford, E.S., et al.: Ann. Thorac. Surg. 40:439–455. November 1985.)

depending on whether the aortic sinuses are involved or aortic insufficiency is present.

▶ These authors have perhaps the greatest experience with primary and secondary operations for thoracic aortic aneurysms. Their advice that the most definitive possible repair (including prosthetic graft replacement) on the ascending aorta in patients with medial degenerative disease or other causes of fusiform aortic dilatation is probably wise in patients undergoing aortic valve replacement or coronary bypass surgery. A "conservative" approach with preservation of the native aorta may well lead to the necessity for a very high risk reoperation at a later date. This review of various procedures available for secondary operations may also provide valuable clues for possible techniques in primary procedures.—J.J. Collins, Jr., M.D.

Surgical Repair of Aneurysms Involving the Distal Aortic Arch
Gregory L. Kay, Denton A. Cooley, James J. Livesay, Michael J. Reardon, and J. Michael Duncan (Texas Heart Inst., Houston)
J. Thorac. Cardiovasc. Surg. 91:397–404, March 1986   5–38

A simplified approach to aneurysms involving the aortic arch may be feasible when the process begins in the distal arch and spares the innominate artery. Thirty-two patients, 22 men and 10 women with a median age of 61 years, had repair of such lesions in 1975–1984. The aneurysms arose distal to the innominate artery and involved the arch at the origin of the left subclavian or left common carotid artery. The diseased segment of aorta was cross-clamped between the innominate and left carotid vessels, with no shunt or extracorporeal bypass. Proximal hypertension was managed with nitroprusside. The mean cross-clamp time was 27 minutes for Dacron graft replacement in 28 patients and patch repair in three.

Two patients died postoperatively. None had a stroke, but paraplegia occurred in 9% of the patients. Two required dialysis for renal failure. Both paraplegia and renal failure were related to cross-clamp time. Four patients had respiratory failure, and two patients required reoperation for bleeding. The average postoperative stay was 18 days.

Simple aortic cross-clamping may be used to repair aneurysms of the distal aortic arch. Spinal cord complications are minimized if the duration of ischemia is less than 30 minutes. A similar ischemic period is critical for the kidneys. Vocal cord paralysis is a possibility that must be accepted. Present 2-year survival rates in patients with thoracic aneurysm approach 70%, and 5-year rates exceed 50%.

▶ Clamping the aortic arch between the innominate and left carotid arteries is a useful technique that may often allow application of the clamp at a comfortable level proximal to the onset of aneurysmal dilatation. The 9% incidence of paraplegia is distressingly high, and, for most surgeons, an arterial shunt or femorofemoral bypass is a reasonable alternative.—J.J. Collins, Jr., M.D.

A Reconsideration of Cerebral Perfusion in Aortic Arch Replacement
William H. Frist, John C. Baldwin, Vaughn A. Starnes, Edward B. Stinson, Philip E. Oyer, Craig Miller, Stuard W. Jamieson, R. Scott Mitchell, and Normal E. Shumway (Stanford Univ.)
Ann. Thorac. Surg. 42:273–281, September 1986   5–39

Intraoperative protection of the CNS during operations on the aortic arch is a principal technical problem. Profound hypothermia with total circulatory arrest has been widely adopted, but possible neurologic and hemorrhagic sequelae have tempered enthusiasm for the procedure. A simplified technique of cardiopulmonary bypass (CPB) and selective brachiocephalic perfusion with moderate hypothermia was used in ten selected patients with aortic arch aneurysms. The circuit used is shown in Figure 5–10.

TECHNIQUE.—During surgery, the arch vessels and proximal descending aorta are carefully mobilized. Arterial access is achieved with two cannulas joined to a Y connector attached to a single head on the arterial roller pump. Cannulas are inserted into the femoral and distal innominate arteries. If the innominate artery is unsuitable, the left carotid artery can be used. (The innominate artery was used in six of the ten patients.) Venous drainage cannulas are placed through the right atrium into the superior and inferior venae cavae. The patient is placed on CPB with total bypass flow from the single pump head maintained in the range of 30–50 ml/kg/minute. Moderate hypothermia in the range of 26–28 degrees is used.

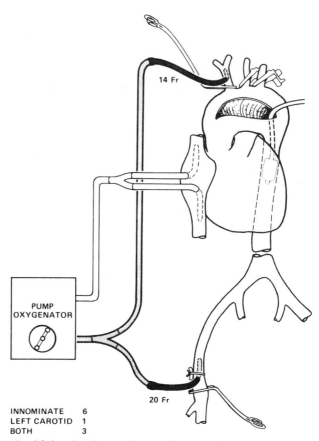

Fig 5–10.—Simplified cardiopulmonary bypass technique with a Y connection between the 14F innominate cannula and the 20F femoral cannula. The arteries and numbers in the left lower corner indicate the number of patients having selective perfusion of that artery. (Courtesy of Frist, W.H., et al.: Ann. Thorac. Surg. 42:273–281, September 1986.)

The proximal aorta is cross-clamped, and the heart is arrested with cold crystalloid cardioplegia. Continuous topical hypothermia is maintained throughout the procedure. The proximal innominate, left carotid, and subclavian arteries are occluded; bypass flow is transiently reduced to 400 ml/minute, and the aneurysm is opened; the clot is then removed. An occlusion balloon placed through a preclotted, low-porosity, woven Dacron graft is inserted into the proximal descending aorta to prevent backflow of blood. A vascular clamp may also be used. Bypass flow is then returned to baseline levels. After aortic reconstruction, the patient is placed in a steep Trendelenburg position, the balloon is partially deflated, the graft is allowed to backfill with blood, and the great vessels proximal to the clamps are massaged and aspirated to evacuate air and debris. When the innominate artery has been used for perfusion, the left subclavian and carotid arteries are first unclamped, and then the innominate artery. The balloon catheter is removed, the graft is clamped proximally, and blood flow from the femoral artery cannula to the brachiocephalic vessels is restored. The brachiocephalic cannula is removed and the defect is secured by a full-thickness, diamond-shaped, purse-string suture. Any associated procedures are done after reinstitution of blood flow during rewarming on CPB. The proximal anastomosis is then performed, air is evacuated from the heart, the heart is resuscitated, and CPB is discontinued.

Eight of the ten patients survived the operation, but one died 3 weeks afterward, for a total mortality of 30%. The mean CPB time was shorter for the survivors, averaging 119 minutes. The cross-clamp time averaged 79 minutes, reflecting the complexity of the procedures in these patients. The range of cerebral perfusion was 20–82 minutes. An average of 5.9 units of whole blood was required during operation and an additional 6.6 units during the subsequent hospitalization. Platelets and plasma were also given. There were no cerebrovascular accidents. Neurologic complications occurred in two patients, but were probably unrelated to the perfusion technique. One patient had vocal cord paresis that resolved in 5 days, and the other had an isolated miosis and transient ulnar nerve paresthesias. The mean length of stay after operation was 8.6 days.

Prevention of myocardial damage during extracorporeal circulation, avoidance of coagulopathy and hemorrhage, and protection of the brain and spinal cord are the most important issues in successful aortic arch operations. Two approaches have been used: profound systemic hypothermia and circulatory arrest, and simplified CPB cerebral perfusion and moderate hypothermia. The incidence of cerebrovascular accidents associated with the first method is high, and the occurrence of coagulopathies, excessive bleeding, diffuse capillary injury, and pulmonary complications have led to exploration of other alternatives. Also, total arrest of the cerebral circulation places time constraints on the surgeon; when difficult or time-consuming repairs are needed, the quality of repair may be compromised. The simplified method described has the advantage of longer working time available, shorter total perfusion time, an unobstructed operating field, and a potentially higher margin of safety when unexpected complications ensue during the operation. Preoperative evaluation of patients can aid in determining which patients will tolerate perfusion through a single brachiocephalic vessel. The two approaches to aortic arch operation can be used in a complementary fashion with the simplified technique used on patients having elective operation on atherosclerotic and degenerative arch aneurysms, and deep hypothermia with arrest used for emergencies and in patients with aneurysms caused by trauma, rupture, infection, or aortic dissection, which preclude safe cannulation of the brachiocephalic vessels.

▶ This excellent paper presents in detail a simple, potentially safer operative approach to aortic arch resection than is provided with deep hypothermia and total cerebral ischemia. The illustrations are excellent, and experienced surgeons should have no difficulty in adapting this technique to their own needs.—J.J. Collins, Jr., M.D.

Transplantation

Donor Availability as the Primary Determinant of the Future of Heart Transplantation

Roger W. Evans, Diane L. Manninen, Louis P. Garrison, Jr., and Anthony M. Maier (Battelle Human Affairs Res. Ctrs., Seattle, and Ctr. for Health Affairs, Project Hope, Millwood, Va.)
JAMA 255:1892–1898, Apr. 11, 1986   5–40

The therapeutic status of heart transplantation is controversial. Of all heart transplant recipients, 80% now survive for at least 1 year, and 50% live for 5 years. The authors project that 25% of all heart transplant recipients will live for 10 years or longer, making heart transplantation competitive with cadaver renal transplantation. The quality of life in heart

POTENTIAL HEART DONORS WITH VARIOUS CONTRAINDICATIONS TO HEART DONATION*

	% of Potential Donors†
Associated disease	
Congenital cardiac disease	0.6
Valvular cardiac disease	0.5
Atherosclerotic cardiac disease	0.2
Peripheral arteriosclerosis	0.2
Diabetes	0.2
Hypertension	0.7
Sepsis	0.8
Malignancy	0.1
Chronic lung disease	0.4
Infections	
Systemic	1.2
Pulmonary	5.7
Central nervous system	0.2
Abdominal	0.5
Genitourinary	1.5
Subcutaneous	0.2
Chest x-ray film results‡	
Widened mediastinum	0.3
Pneumothorax	5.2
Rib fractures	4.2
Pneumonia	3.6
Other contraindications	
Sustained cardiac arrest	8.0
Intracardiac injections	1.8
Transient hypotension	5.8
Mediastinal trauma	2.2
Murmurs on physical examination	0.5
Electrocardiographic abnormalities	3.0
Other reason specified	6.1

*Donors who met age criterion for heart donation.
†Donors may have had more than one reported contraindication.
‡Chest x-ray films were not obtained specifically for the study. Results were reported only if x-ray films were obtained.
(Courtesy of Evans, R.W., et al.: JAMA 255:1892–1898, Apr. 11, 1986. Copyright 1986, American Medical Association.)

transplant recipients also compares favorably with that of patients undergoing dialysis and kidney transplantation. For these reasons, most private insurers now extend transplant insurance coverage to their beneficiaries. Depending on patient selection, it is estimated that as many as 15,000 persons per year could benefit from a heart transplant; however, the actual number who might benefit is constrained by the availability of donor hearts.

The availability of donor hearts was estimated on the basis of data obtained on 1,955 organ donors in the United States. Because of age and other contraindications, only 400–1,100 viable donor hearts may be available each year (table). This finding argues that donor supply is the most critical determinant of the future of heart transplantation, as it will dictate the number of transplantations performed, the survival of transplant recipients, the total program expenditures associated with heart transplantation, the nature of the legal and ethical issues involved, the number of cardiac transplantation programs required to make optimal use of the available donor hearts, and the future role of mechanical circulatory support systems.

▶ This analysis documents the theoretical basis for the observed phenomenon of the shortage of donor hearts. Whether it may be possible to increase the donor pool substantially by education remains to be seen. But, influenced by a multitude of factors, donors selected by the present strict criteria will continue to be in extremely short supply. It seems reasonable to expand the criteria for donor selection to include older age groups who may be screened with the assistance of coronary angiography.—J.J. Collins, Jr., M.D.

Cardiac Transplantation in Patients Over 50 Years of Age
Michael Carrier, Robert W. Emery, Judith E. Riley, Mark M. Levinson, and Jack G. Copeland (Univ. of Arizona)
J. Am. Coll. Cardiol. 8:285–288, August 1986   5–41

The results of cardiac transplantation have improved steadily in the past two decades, in part because of establishment of rigid criteria for acceptance of patients as candidates for transplantation. The patient's age has been considered an important predictor of survival. Whether individuals older than age 50 years can be considered good candidates for transplantation was examined in 62 patients, 13 of whom were more than age 50

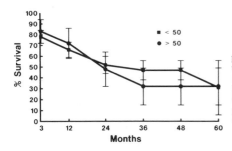

Fig 5–11.—Actuarial survival of 62 transplant patients. One-year survival was 66 ± 7% for those patients younger than age 50 years and 72 ± 14% for those older than age 50 years. (Courtesy of Carrier, M., et al.: J. Am. Coll. Cardiol. 8:285–288, August 1986. Reprinted with permission from the American College of Cardiology.)

at the time of transplantation. The main groups of cardiac disease were ischemic, idiopathic, and viral cardiomyopathies. More of the older patients had ischemic heart disease than the younger patients. All patients were in New York Heart Association functional class IV and were receiving maximal medical treatment before transplantation.

For patients with ischemic heart disease, actuarial survival curves were similar in both age groups. The actuarial survival for all 62 patients is shown in Figure 5–11. None of the older patients needed inhospital care prior to operation, whereas 24% of the younger patients did. Neither early nor late mortality rates were significantly different in the two age groups. Early mortality was 18% among younger patients and 16% among older patients; late mortality was 36% in the older group and 33% in the younger group. Rejection and infection were the principal causes of death in both age groups. The mean length of survival for older patients was 20 months compared with 17 months for the younger group.

Other studies have reported increased mortality as patient age increased. The most significant predictors of survival were patient age, the expertise of the center, and the use of cyclosporine. In the authors' experience, the type of immunosuppressive regimen used did not affect survival. Of patients older than age 50 years, 18% were accepted for transplantation and 11% underwent the operation. Older patients have been rejected mainly on grounds of advanced physiologic age, characterized by advanced chronological age and decreased function of secondary organ systems unrelated to cardiac function. Although the primary objective of cardiac transplantation is survival, the quality of life is important as well. Rehabilitation in both age groups has been excellent in the authors' experience. Because the results of cardiac transplantation were not significantly different in patients older or younger than age 50 years, the former rigid criteria may be unacceptable. Many patients older than age 50 years with severe, nonsurgical ischemic heart disease may be considered candidates for cardiac transplantation if physiologic age is not advanced by disease of other organ systems. Every potential recipient must be evaluated individually in terms of the risk and benefit from cardiac transplantation.

▶ This publication, similar to those documenting successful extension of cardiac transplantation to critically ill patients, serves to increase further the potential pool of cardiac recipients. Whereas there is no doubt that patients over 50 years of age may successfully undergo cardiac transplantation, the need to exclude other threatening systemic illnesses or critical organ dysfunctions becomes even greater lest so many patients be considered potential cardiac recipients that waiting lists become impossibly inflated.—J.J. Collins, Jr., M.D.

Mortally Ill Patients and Excellent Survival Following Cardiac Transplantation

Robert L. Hardesty, Bartley P. Griffith, Alfredo Trento, Mark E. Thompson, Peter F. Ferson, and Henry T. Bahnson (Univ. of Pittsburgh)
Ann. Thorac. Surg. 41:126–129, February 1986   5–42

Cardiac transplantation was resumed at the University of Pittsburgh in 1980 when patients expected to survive for less than 6 months were selected. All 77 orthotopic transplant recipients initially were in New York Heart Association functional class IV, although many were ambulatory. Success with terminally ill patients with arterial hypotension and evidence of reduced blood flow prompted the selection of less markedly ill patients. Nearly half of the patients required intravenous inotropic support or diastolic augmentation until a donor heart became available. Cyclosporine was used for immunosuppression.

The actuarial survival rate at 30 months was 75% in terminally ill patients and 67% in those less ill; the overall rate was 67%. Twenty-nine of 33 mortally ill patients were alive and active at last follow-up. One of three deaths of terminally ill patients in the early postoperative period resulted from hyperacute rejection.

Many very seriously ill patients have survived and become active after orthotopic heart transplantation. All but four of 33 terminally ill recipients in the present series did well.

▶ This remarkable series of terminally ill patients illustrates what can be accomplished with cardiac transplantation even in spite of the necessity for mechanical circulatory augmentation. The constant extension of cardiac transplantation to older and more seriously ill patients expands the potential recipient pool without corresponding expansion of the donor pool. If all centers follow in like manner, the average degree of illness of recipients will increase and eventually the results of cardiac transplantation will suffer.—J.J. Collins, Jr., M.D.

Acute Reversible Cardiogenic Shock: Immune-Mediated With Mild Histologic Change

Lynne Warner Stevenson, William Lewis, Rex N. MacAlpin, and Suzanne Clark (Univ. of California at Los Angeles)
Am. Heart J. 111:611–613, March 1986   5–43

Both primary myocarditis and cardiac transplant rejection are evident histologically by lymphocytic infiltration with myocyte necrosis. Serial biopsy specimens in transplant recipients often show changes prior to cardiac dysfunction; it is thought that life-threatening hemodynamic compromise resulting from rejection is preceded by severe myocardial necrosis that is generally irreversible.

Man, 21, had only mild histologic changes but was in acute cardiac shock. After aggressive therapy, normal cardiac function was regained. An endomyocardial biopsy specimen obtained 9 months after transplantation showed fibrosis without acute rejection. When serum cyclosporine levels decreased because of noncompliance with therapy, the patient collapsed and was hospitalized with low blood pressure and a 40% drop in summed QRS voltage. Histopathology showed persistent fibrosis with increased lymphocytic infiltrates and edema, but many zones appeared normal. There was no myocyte necrosis. Diffuse hypokinesis, increased left ventricular mass, and a left ventricular ejection fraction of 36% were present.

Immunosuppressive therapy was given in the coronary care unit for 4 days and function rapidly improved. By day 12, the infiltrate had decreased and the patient was discharged. By 3 months, ECG voltage and left ventricular mass were normal, and the patient was doing well.

This patient with immune-mediated cardiogenic shock responded well to aggressive therapeutic intervention. The case is remarkable for the absence of strict histopathologic criteria for myocarditis resulting from cardiac rejection. This suggests the possibility of overlooking clinical immune injury by relying heavily on histopathology. This patient deteriorated with mild histologic findings because of the rapid decrease of immunosuppression. This possibility should be recognized in cardiac transplant outpatients who have primary myocarditis.

▶ Everyone with experience in the care of patients after cardiac transplantation is familiar with the syndrome of acute cardiogenic shock as a manifestation of transplant rejection even when a recent biopsy has shown no histologic evidence to suggest that a hemodynamically significant episode was imminent. This publication confirms that complacency is never appropriate with regard to these patients, even when the histology is reassuring.—J.J. Collins, Jr., M.D.

Infections in Heart-Lung Transplant Recipients
J. Stephen Dummer, Carlos G. Montero, Bartley P. Griffith, Robert L. Hardesty, Irvin L. Paradis, and Monto Ho (Univ. of Pittsburgh)
Transplantation 41:725–729, June 1986   5–44

Infectious complications remain important in heart-lung transplantation. Data on 14 of 18 transplant recipients (mean age, 31 years) who survived for more than 30 days were analyzed for such complications. The patients were followed for 265 days on average. Pulmonary hypertension was the most frequent indication for heart-lung transplantation. Immunosuppression was with cyclosporine, methylprednisolone, and antithymocyte globulin. Azathioprine was used in a few cases.

Forty-two infections occurred in these transplant recipients. Bacterial isolates, usually Enterobacteriaceae, accounted for half of all infections. Symptomatic viral infections did not occur in patients treated later in the series. Cytomegalovirus infection was documented in about two thirds of the patients. Two patients had definite symptomatic Epstein-Barr virus infection. The higher incidence of symptomatic viral infection in early patients appeared related to the large number having primary viral infections. Three patients had invasive *Candida* infection. Protozoal infections occurred in half of the patients, *Pneumocystis carinii* pneumonia being most frequent. Rates of infection declined after the first 6 posttransplant months. Two thirds of all infections primarily involved the transplanted lung. One fourth of infections were disseminated.

The average patient in this study contracted three infections within 6 months after heart-lung transplantation. It seems best to restrict the procedure to centers having extensive experience in managing transplant patients. Monitoring by means such as bronchial lavage and new means of preventing and treating systemic viral infections hold promise.

▶ The care of patients following heart-lung transplantation remains uniquely complex. Transplanted lungs are very susceptible to infection whether bacterial, viral, or protozoal. An aggressive approach to diagnosis is extremely important. It is interesting in this series that lung biopsy was used in only seven patients, and in one of these it was actually misleading. No doubt, further experience will refine the indications for lung biopsy and improve the accuracy of diagnosis.—J.J. Collins, Jr., M.D.

The Effects of Donor Pretreatment on the Transmission of Murine Cytomegalovirus With Cardiac Transplants and Explants
Eileen J. Wilson, Donald N. Medearis, Leslie V. Barrett, Atul Bhan, and Robert H. Rubin (Massachusetts Gen. Hosp., Boston, and Harvard Med Univ.)
Transplantation 41:781–782, June 1986   5–45

The clinical course of cardiac transplant patients is often complicated by cytomegalovirus (CMV) infection acquired from the donor heart. Virus can be reactivated after transplantation, and potentially lethal disseminated CMV infection may ensue in the immunosuppressed recipient. It is not known, however, whether the virus is present within the cardiac muscle itself, or resides in passenger leukocytes that are not structural constituents of the heart. The distinction is an important one because, if passenger leukocytes are the source of virus, strategies aimed at eliminating such cells prior to transplantation might alleviate the CMV problem. If cardiac tissue itself is involved, prevention must be directed at the recipient. In this study, pretreatment of the donor with high-dose cyclophosphamide and total body irradiation of the donor were used in an attempt to distinguish the source of CMV infection in mice given cardiac tissue explants from CMV-infected donors.

Cyclophosphamide pretreatment resulted in a significant fall in peripheral white blood cells in donor mice. When cardiac tissue from these mice was transplanted into immunosuppressed CMV-seronegative recipients, lethal disseminated CMV infection resulted. Similar results occurred when tissue from irradiated donors or infected tissue from untreated donors was used. There were also no differences in recovery of active virus from any of the groups of mice when cardiac tissue was cultured.

These results indicate that pretreatment of the donor tissue does not eliminate the virus and does not enhance graft survival. Therefore, the major site of viral latency may be in intrinsic cardiac tissue. Efforts to control CMV infections in recipients must be directed entirely at treatment or prophylaxis of the recipient rather than pretreatment of the donor.

▶ This interesting animal study suggests that the problem of CMV transmission will continue to be a substantial one in cardiac and cardiopulmonary transplant recipients.—J.J. Collins, Jr., M.D.

Xenografts: Review of the Literature and Current Status

American Medical Assoc. Council on Scientific Affairs (Chicago)
JAMA 254:3353–3357, Dec. 20, 1985   5–46

Xenografting, or transplantation across species, has intrigued physicians for many years. Early attempts failed almost uniformly, although some organ function was observed for a brief period of time in a few cases. The work of Medawar and associates in the 1950s established the immunologic nature of graft rejection. In turn, this suggested ways in which such rejection might be minimized through immunosuppression, leading to a resurgence of interest in xenografting. Because human organ donors are relatively scarce and their availability is a chance occurrence, the use of xenografts promised easy and consistent availability of organs so that surgical procedures could be done in an organized, elective fashion. In the last two decades, various clinical and experimental programs have been undertaken with various donor-recipient combinations to delineate the mechanisms of rejection and the role of immunosuppression in graft survival.

Renal xenografts from chimpanzee to man were done by Reemtsma and associates in the early 1960s. After using immunosuppression and local irradiation of the graft, prompt renal function was seen in all cases. However, most of the grafts failed within 2 months. It was believed that the performance of these xenografts did not differ substantially from that of human allografts transplanted during that period. The rejection processes appeared to be qualitatively similar in both cases, although the severity varied. The advantage of the chimpanzee rested in its close similarity to man based on comparative studies of serum proteins, hemoglobin, and major histocompatibility systems. All patients receiving such grafts had serum cytotoxins and hemagglutinins that were correlated with the timing of rejection.

Baboon to human xenografts were attempted because of the expense and scarcity of chimpanzees. The baboon is a more distant relative of man, however, and the tissue match is less satisfactory. Some function was obtained immediately after transplantation with such grafts, but survival ranged only from 19 to 98 days. Even with immunosuppression and graft irradiation, repeated, vigorous rejection episodes occurred. The aggressive immunosuppression that then was required led to lethal infections in most cases. Pathologic changes and rejection episodes were more severe than in the case of the chimpanzee xenografts, and rejection was probably a result of both humoral and cellular immune reactions.

Chimpanzee to human xenografts of liver and heart have also been attempted. Liver transplants were done in two children, and even though some temporary function was attained, both died soon after operation. Rejection of such liver transplants was not as severe and histologic changes were not marked. Both baboon and chimpanzee hearts have been transplanted with generally poor results. Once again, some function was attained initially, but rejection soon followed. Thus, even though the rejection process is qualitatively similar for both xenografts and allografts, the severity of the process depends on the genetic disparity between donor and recipient.

The mechanism of rejection in chimpanzee and human allografts is mediated primarily by cellular processes; the humoral system comes into play as genetic disparity increases between donor and recipient. In these cases, heterospecific antibodies attack the vascular system of the graft, causing thrombosis and ischemic injury. Such processes are also seen with human allografts in which there is major blood group incompatibility or performed antibody. When the two involved species are widely divergent, graft rejection is rapid and severe and cannot be altered by treatment with immunosuppressive agents. Hyperacute rejection is characterized by a dense mononuclear cell infiltrate combined with fibrinoid vascular necrosis and hemorrhage. Humoral components of rejection include the complement and coagulation systems. Immunosuppressive regimens, including azathioprine, steroids, actinomycin C, antilymphocyte globulin, cyclosporin A, and local graft irradiation, enhance graft survival to some degree. Other methods include lymphoid irradiation of the recipient, use of complement system inhibitors, coagulation system inhibitors, and pretransplant donor blood transfusions. The objective is to render the host less reactive to the foreign antigens present on the donor organ. Some success has been seen in animal models, but clinical trials have not been attempted at this time.

The lack of full understanding of histocompatibility barriers and the mechanisms of rejection, coupled with a lack of adequate means to overcome those barriers, are major unresolved problems in the area of xenografting. Recent evidence has also shown that animal and human transplant organs may harbor viruses or other infectious agents that can cause serious infection in the immunosuppressed recipient.

▶ This interesting review may be particularly useful for persons beginning an involvement with cardiac and cardiopulmonary transplantation. It provides excellent background information and references for an appreciation of the current status of xenograft experience.—J.J. Collins, Jr., M.D.

Tumors

Intra-Atrial Extension of Renal and Adrenal Tumors: Diagnosis, Management, and Prognosis
Thomas B. Hugh, Robert M. Jones, and Mark X. Shanahan (St. Vincent's Hosp., Sydney)
World J. Surg. 10:488–495, June 1986   5–47

Venous invasion and the formation of a tumor thrombus in the inferior vena cava, sometimes with extension into the right atrium, arising from a renal or adrenal tumor, is a serious complication. The incidence rate for invasion of renal tumors may be as high as 4%. The incidence rate is extremely low for invasion of adrenal tumors. Three patients with intra-atrial tumor extension were seen; two had adrenal cortical carcinoma and one had a renal cell carcinoma.

Woman, 43, had a 12-month history of increasing shortness of breath, ankle edema, abdominal distention, and amenorrhea. Physical examination disclosed mild bilateral edema of the legs, distention of the superficial abdominal veins, and a prominent jugular venous pulsation in the neck. There were also signs of mild virilization, and a large abdominal mass was palpable on the right side. Computed tomography demonstrated the presence of a large mass above the right kidney, a thrombus in the adjacent vena cava, and a tumor thrombus in the right atrium. Serum androgen levels were markedly elevated. Venography confirmed the presence of caval occlusion and demonstrated the presence of a mushroom-shaped mass in the right atrium.

At operation, a tumor 15 cm in diameter was found in the right adrenal gland adherent to the right kidney. Tumor thrombus was palpable within the inferior vena cava. Cardiopulmonary bypass was initiated, and hepatic inflow through the portal vein and hepatic artery was occluded when the temperature of the liver reached 30C. The intracaval tumor extension was removed by atriotomy and cavotomy. Histopathologic examination confirmed the diagnosis of moderately differentiated adrenocortical carcinoma. The patient's recovery was complicated by bilateral pulmonary lower lobe collapse and a minor deep vein thrombosis in the right leg. However, she recovered completely and all venous obstructive symptoms disappeared.

▶ The use of cardiopulmonary bypass to expedite surgery for tumors or other conditions outside the thorax remains unusual, but it is more frequent than in the past. The proclivity of renal and adrenal tumors to intravascular extension into the right atrium makes this group of neoplasms especially suitable for combined thoracoabdominal resection involving the use of cardiopulmonary bypass. Resection of the primary neoplasm is safer and more complete, and there is better control of the possible complication of tumor embolization. Cardiac surgeons should stand ready to assist in such operations. The long-term results are not yet evident, but relief of life-threatening vascular complications is clearly possible. Vaislic et al. suggest that 5-year survival (in the absence of detectable metastases) may reach 75% in these patients (*J. Thorac. Cardiovasc. Surg.* 91:604–609, 1986).—J.J. Collins, Jr., M.D.

6 Hypertension

Introduction

In the area of hypertension, 1986 was characterized by controversy over the appropriateness of the stepped-care approach to treatment. More precisely, the role of the diuretic as a preferred step-one drug was questioned by many, largely because of safety issues. In the Multiple Risk Factor Intervention Trial (*JAMA* 248:1465–1477, 1982) the subgroup of hypertensive men with abnormal resting ECGs treated with a diuretic experienced what appeared to be an unusually high incidence of unexpected sudden death, suggesting arrhythmia from hypokalemia. Some large trials have failed to show any benefit of treatment with diuretic on coronary events, and this has been attributed, possibly, to an increase in the serum levels of cholesterol and triglycerides observed in some patients treated with diuretics. The 1984 report of the Joint National Committee (*Arch. Intern. Med.* 144:1045–1057, 1984) for the first time recommended a choice between two step-one drugs, either a diuretic or a β blocker. The latter drugs also cause adverse metabolic effects. Now, calcium channel blocking agents and the converting enzyme inhibitors are challenging the diuretics and β blockers as initial monotherapy in managing hypertension. In 1986 the second converting enzyme inhibitor, enalapril, was marketed and, in early 1987, the first calcium channel blocking agent was approved for treating hypertension (sustained-release verapamil). Consequently, considerable space has been devoted in this review to these two relatively new agents. It should be noted that not only do converting enzyme inhibitors have a role in managing hypertension, but they also may be helpful in the diagnosis of renovascular hypertension.

There were numerous publications describing the effects of atrial natriuretic peptide (or factor) on cardiovascular and renal hemodynamics. Whether this substance will ever have an important therapeutic role remains to be determined.

New insights into the relationship between sodium and hypertension are included in this review. Not every patient with hypertension responds adversely to a sodium load, or benefits from dietary sodium reduction. Hollenberg and co-workers attribute nonresponse to sodium in some hypertensive patients to failure of angiotensin II to regulate renal blood flow and aldosterone secretion appropriately ("nonmodulators").

For the first time evidence has been presented that left ventricular hypertrophy (LVH) observed on echocardiography has an ominous prognostic significance, even in the absence of ECG evidence of LVH.

The role of calcium in the treatment and pathogenesis of essential hypertension is still being debated, with no satisfactory resolution forthcoming. Calcium channel blocking agents have been available for the treatment of angina pectoris and certain supraventricular arrhythmias for several years, but until early 1987 none had been approved for the treatment of hypertension, for which they are very effective. In early 1987, sustained-release verapamil was approved for marketing for use in the management of hypertension. It is anticipated that the other preparations will be approved for the same indication later in 1987.

There are three classes of calcium channel blocking agents: the diphenylalkylamines (e.g., verapamil) have a greater effect on myocardial contractility and atrioventricular conduction than the others. The dihydropyridines (nifedipine, nitrendipine) are potent peripheral vasodilators but have only a minimal effect on the myocardium and conduction. The benzothiazepines (diltiazem) occupy an intermediate position between the other two, both with regard to cardiac effects and peripheral vasodilating effects. All are effective in the treatment of angina pectoris and in the treatment of hypertension.

Ray W. Gifford, Jr., M.D.

Calcium Channel Blocking Agents

Nitrendipine, A Calcium-Entry Blocker: Renal and Humoral Effects in Human Arterial Hypertension

Roberto Pedrinelli, Fetnet M. Fouad, Robert C. Tarazi, Emmanuel L. Bravo, and Stephen C. Textor (Cleveland Clinic Found.)

Arch. Intern. Med. 146:62–65, January 1986   6–1

Nitrendipine, a dihydropyridine calcium-entry blocker, is an effective antihypertensive agent. To evaluate its effects on renal hemodynamics, body fluid volume, and humoral factors in patients with arterial hypertension, 13 patients aged 30–65 years were given nitrendipine, 20 mg twice daily for 2 weeks. Twelve patients had essential hypertension and one had bilateral adrenal hyperplasia; all had normal renal function.

Nitrendipine significantly decreased the mean arterial pressure (MAP) from 137 mm Hg to 119 mm Hg, a mean decrease of 12.6% ($P < .01$); this was related to the decreased mean total peripheral resistance (from 49 units per sq m to 42 units per sq m; $P < .05$). Renal blood flow, glomerular filtration rate (GFR), and cardiac output were not significantly altered during nitrendipine therapy. Plasma catecholamines and plasma renin activity increased, but the plasma aldosterone level did not change significantly. No correlation was found between either MAP or cardiac output and changes in renal blood flow. Neither body weight nor plasma volume was significantly changed during nitrendipine therapy, but greater decrements in MAP tended to be associated with greater increases in plasma volume. Furthermore, the percent decrease in MAP was inversely correlated with basal renin levels and directly associated with age.

Long-term calcium-entry blockade by nitrendipine does not alter renal blood flow or reduce GFR in hypertensive patients despite decreased renal perfusion pressure. In addition, nitrendipine causes mild activation of the renin-angiotensin system without effecting aldosterone secretion. These findings explain the lack of plasma volume expansion or fluid retention in association with the reduction in blood pressure. Nitrendipine may be more effective in older patients and in the presence of low renin values.

Immediate and Short-Term Hemodynamic Effects of Diltiazem in Patients With Hypertension
Celso Amodeo, Isaac Kobrin, Hector O. Ventura, Franz H. Messerli, and Edward D. Frohlich (Alton Ochsner Med. Found., New Orleans)
Circulation 73:108–113, January 1986   6–2

Diltiazem is a calcium channel blocker that is widely used in the management of angina pectoris and is currently under investigation for the management of hypertension. Its hypotensive effect probably results from inhibition of calcium entry into vascular smooth muscle, consequently producing arteriolar dilatation. The drug's hemodynamic effects on systemic and regional blood flow were assessed in eight men and two women with mild to moderate hypertension. The group included seven blacks. One white male had primary aldosteronism.

Diltiazem was first administered in three intravenous doses of 0.06 mg/ kg, 0.06 mg/kg and 0.12 mg/kg, respectively; patients were then treated for 4 weeks with daily doses ranging from 240 mg to 360 mg. Diltiazem therapy immediately dropped the mean arterial pressure from 115 mm Hg to 96 mm Hg via a decrease in the total peripheral resistance index (from 37 units per sq m to 23 units per sq m) that was associated with an increase in heart rate from 66 beats per minute to 77 beats per minute and an increased cardiac index (from 3.3 L/minute/sq m to 4.3 L/minute/sq m). These changes were not associated with alterations in plasma levels of catecholamines or aldosterone, or changes in plasma renin activity. After 4 weeks the substantial drop in mean arterial pressure was observed to persist, and there still were no alterations in the humoral substances or plasma volume. The renal blood flow index increased from 368 ml/minute/ sq m to 462 ml/minute/sq m, and the renal vascular resistance decreased from 0.37 units per sq m to 0.26 units per sq m; splanchnic hemodynamics did not change. The left ventricular mass dropped markedly from 242 gm to 217 gm. The fall in arterial pressure produced by diltiazem was associated with improved renal hemodynamics and a reduced left ventricular mass without expansion of intravascular volume or alterations in circulating humoral substances.

Renal Effects of Diltiazem in Primary Hypertension
Sobha Sunderrajan, Garry Reams, and John H. Bauer (Univ. of Missouri)
Hypertension 8:238–242, March 1986   6–3

Diltiazem, a calcium channel blocker, is effective in lowering blood pressure in patients with primary hypertension. However, its effect on renal function, salt and water excretion, and body fluid composition in such patients has not been assessed. A study was conducted to evaluate the short-term effects of diltiazem monotherapy on the above-cited parameters in 18 men with primary hypertension first studied after 2–4 weeks of placebo treatment followed by an 8-week course of diltiazem given in dosages ranging from 240 mg/day to 480 mg/day. After completion of the placebo period, renal function was assessed by means of 24-hour urine collection, volume studies, and timed clearances. These tests were repeated after completion of the diltiazem study period.

Diltiazem monotherapy was effective in reducing both systolic and diastolic blood pressure in 16 of the 18 patients. Seven patients required 120 mg of diltiazem twice daily for adequate blood pressure control, four required 180 mg twice daily, and five required 240 mg twice daily. Renal function and hemodynamics were not altered significantly, as indicated by creatinine and inulin clearance, effective renal plasma flow, or renal blood flow. Nevertheless, a 22% reduction in renal vascular resistance was noted. Diltiazem given as monotherapy is effective in the treatment of mild to moderate hypertension. Because renal function was unchanged or improved, it is expected that diltiazem will assume a permanent role as first-step therapy in the treatment of hypertensive diseases.

▶ The papers by Pedrinelli et al., Amodeo et al., and Sundarrajan et al. (Abstracts 6–1, 6–2, and 6–3) are in general agreement that reduction of blood pressure in hypertensive patients using diltiazem or nitrendipine preserves renal blood flow and the glomerular filtration rate. Subtle differences are noted. Sundarrajan et al. and Amodeo et al., using diltiazem, noted a reduction in renal vascular resistance, whereas Pedrinelli et al., using nitrendipine, found no change in renal vascular resistance. Amodeo et al. reported a significant increase in renal blood flow after short-term therapy with diltiazem, whereas the other two groups found no significant change in renal blood flow. These differences are probably not clinically important; rather, the important finding is that, despite significant decreases in mean arterial pressure, renal hemodynamics are not disturbed by these calcium channel blocking agents. Similar findings have been reported for verapamil (Kubo et al.: *J. Clin. Hypertens.* 3:38s, 1986). It is important to note that the patients selected for these three studies all had normal renal function. Drug effects on normal renal hemodynamics cannot always be translated to what happens in the patient with chronic renal failure.

Pedrinelli et al. found that two weeks of therapy with nitrendipine significantly increased plasma renin activity and the plasma catecholamine concentration. On the other hand, plasma renin activity and plasma catecholamines were not affected by therapy with diltiazem in the report by Amodeo et al. This is consistent with previous studies that have shown that nitrendipine and nifedipine both tend to increase plasma renin activity and plasma catecholamine levels, but the other two classes of calcium channel blockers do not. Plasma volume was unaffected by therapy with calcium channel blockers in all three of these studies.—R.W. Gifford, Jr., M.D.

A Comparison of the Haemodynamic Effects of Nifedipine, Nisoldipine and Nitrendipine in Man

N. M. G. Debbas, S. H. D. Jackson, and P. Turner (St. Bartholomew's Hosp., London)

Eur. J. Clin. Pharmacol. 30:393–397, June 1986   6–4

In vitro and animal studies demonstrate comparable effects of nifedipine, nisoldipine, and nitrendipine in terms of potency and duration of action. In a placebo-controlled, double-blind, crossover study, the hemodynamic effects of nisoldipine, 10 mg, and nitrendipine, 20 mg, were determined and compared with those of nifedipine, 10 mg, in eight normal volunteers.

Compared with placebo, all active drugs produced a fall in blood pressure, preejection time (PEP), PEP/left ventricular ejection time (LVET), and electromechanical systole index (QS2 index), as well as a rise in the LVET index. Compared with nifedipine, nisoldipine had a significantly lesser effect on pulse, PEP, PEP/LVET, and the QS2 index; nitrendipine produced a significantly lesser effect on pulse, LVET index, and PEP/LVET. Compared with nitrendipine, nisoldipine was significantly less effective in decreasing the QS2 index, but was significantly more effective in reducing the diastolic blood pressure. All active drugs were associated with headache and flushing. Nifedipine, nisoldipine, and nitrendipine have a positive inotropic effect in normal persons, with nifedipine being the most active drug.

▶ This is a comparison of the effects of three dihydropyridine calcium channel blockers on blood pressure and systolic time intervals in *normotensive* individuals. It is generally agreed that calcium channel blocking agents have very little hypotensive effect in normotensive individuals. Although there were some differences, perhaps because of dosage or absorption of the drug, the findings are consistent with a positive inotropic effect in normal persons, with nifedipine being more active than nisoldipine or nitrendipine. Whether this is a direct positive inotropic effect or the result of reflex stimulation of the sympathetic nervous system induced by vasodilatation and a decrease in blood pressure cannot be differentiated here. It is my opinion that it is because of reflex sympathetic stimulation similar to that observed after the administration of hydralazine. It is known that the dihydropyridine group of calcium channel blockers, which includes all three of the drugs tested here, causes an increase in plasma catecholamine levels. Although unusual, a significant increase in heart rate is more likely to occur during chronic therapy with one of the dihydropyridine calcium channel blockers than with diltiazem or verapamil.—R.W. Gifford, Jr., M.D.

Similarities and Differences in the Antihypertensive Effect of Two Calcium Antagonist Drugs, Verapamil and Nifedipine

Enrico Agabiti-Rosei, Maria L. Muiesan, Giuseppe Romanelli, Maurizio Castellano, Marina Beschi, Luigi Corea, and Giulio Muiesan (Univ. of Brescia and Univ. of Perugia, Italy)

J. Am. Coll. Cardiol. 7:916–924, April 1986   6–5

The effects of the calcium antagonists verapamil and nifedipine, used to treat hypertension, were compared in 53 patients aged 22–58 years with primary hypertension and in 15 healthy normotensive individuals. All patients had a diastolic blood pressure of at least 95 mm Hg. An acute study compared verapamil in a single oral dose of 160 mg with 10 mg of nifedipine sublingually. Patients in a controlled hospital study received 80 mg of verapamil or 10 mg of nifedipine orally three times daily in a crossover design for 8 days each. The effect of doses of 80 mg and 160 mg of verapamil three times daily was compared with that of 10 mg of nifedipine orally three times daily in a chronic study for 2–4 months.

A single sublingual dose of nifedipine reduced the blood pressure in hypertensive patients more rapidly than did a single oral dose of 160 mg of verapamil. No fall in pressure occurred in normotensive individuals. Nifedipine increased the plasma norepinephrine level in both hypertensive and normotensive individuals. The two drugs produced similar blood pressure reductions in hospitalized hypertensive patients on a fixed sodium and potassium intake. The heart rate and plasma catecholamine level increased only after nifedipine. Neither treatment altered plasma volume, aldosterone, or plasma renin activity. Ambulatory treatment with both drugs produced changes similar to those found in the hospital study. No serious side effects occurred during long-term treatment, and there were no ECG abnormalities.

Verapamil and nifedipine both are effective and safe treatments for essential hypertension. Blood pressure is reduced by peripheral vasodilation, without significant renin stimulation or fluid retention occurring. Adverse effects from adrenergic stimulation by nifedipine may be limited by using a sustained-release preparation. Calcium antagonists may be especially useful in hypertensive patients with ischemic heart disease. They also can be used in patients with peripheral vascular insufficiency or chronic airway disease.

▶ The results of this study are not surprising. The antihypertensive effects of the calcium channel blocking agents are similar. Side effects are not. Close perusal of this report indicates that patients given nifedipine had more symptomatic side effects than those given verapamil, and the two patients who had to withdraw because of side effects (headache and tachycardia) were receiving nifedipine. Palpitations, facial flushing, headache, and sometimes ankle edema are fairly common side effects with nifedipine. Verapamil tends to decrease the pulse rate somewhat, although not as much as β blockers usually do, whereas nifedipine tends to increase the pulse rate somewhat. In this study we again see that nifedipine increases the plasma catecholamine activity, whereas verapamil does not. Plasma renin activity increased with nifedipine, although not statistically significantly so, whereas plasma renin activity was unchanged with verapamil. The differing effects of calcium channel blockers on plasma catecholamines may have some implication with respect to their potential for cardioprotective effects.

The prompt reduction of blood pressure after administration of sublingual doses of nifedipine is not surprising (see Abstract 6–6).—R.W. Gifford, Jr., M.D.

Management of Perioperative Hypertension Using Sublingual Nifedipine: Experience in Elderly Patients Undergoing Eye Surgery
Alan G. Adler, John J. Leahy, and Michael D. Cressman (Jefferson Univ. and Wills Eye Hosp., Philadelphia)
Arch. Intern. Med. 146:1927–1930, October 1986   6–6

The sublingual administration of nifedipine holds promise as a safe, convenient approach to perioperative hypertension because of its predictably rapid onset of action and a relatively long effect. Use of this drug was evaluated in 19 patients aged 60 years and older who became hypertensive during ophthalmologic surgery. The 13 women and 6 men had an average age of 76 years. All patients but one had a history of hypertension, and all but three were taking medication before admission. Extensive cardiovascular complications generally were present; two patients had chronic renal failure. Local anesthesia was used in all but two patients. Hypertension usually developed shortly before or at the beginning of the operative procedure. A 10-mg sublingual dose of nifedipine was given, with a second dose if necessary.

The mean systolic blood pressure fell from 225 mm Hg to 155 mm Hg after treatment; the mean diastolic pressure fell from 121.5 mm Hg to 78 mm Hg. No reflex tachycardia was observed. The pulse rate rose only insignificantly during the peak antihypertensive response. All patients had a prompt fall in blood pressure, and the response lasted longer than 2 hours in all but 1 patient. Two patients were retreated. No serious side effects followed treatment with nifedipine.

Sublingual administration of nifedipine is an effective, safe treatment for perioperative hypertension in elderly patients with cardiovascular problems. Although the findings may be applicable to other types of surgery, careful trials are needed to confirm the safety of nifedipine when it is used in association with general anesthesia.

▶ Although sublingual nifedipine is being widely used throughout the world in the management of hypertensive crises, this report is unique in that the average age of these patients was 76 years. There has always been some trepidation about reducing blood pressure abruptly in elderly patients. It must be presumed that these patients were supine when they received nifedipine sublingually, and the authors mentioned that local anesthesia was used in all but two. Bertel et al. (*Br. Med. J.* 286:19–21, 1983) reported that the magnitude of fall in blood pressure after administration of nifedipine orally was proportional to the pretreatment blood pressure. This group also demonstrated that cerebral blood flow actually increased as blood pressure decreased after the administration of nifedipine orally.

Nifedipine can be given sublingually by piercing the end of the capsule with a pin and squeezing the contents under the patient's tongue. Alternatively, the patient can chew the capsule and retain the liquid nifedipine in the oral cavity until it is absorbed. Some investigators believe that blood pressure will respond just as rapidly if the capsule is swallowed, but it is my firm conviction that sublingual administration produces a more rapid onset of antihypertensive activity.—R.W. Gifford, Jr., M.D.

Relative Potency of a Beta-Blocking and a Calcium Entry Blocking Agent as Antihypertensive Drugs in Black Patients
J. R. M'Buyamba-Kabangu, B. Lepira, R. Fagard, P. Lijnen, M. Ditu, K. A. Tshiani, and A. Amery (Univ. of Leuven, Belgium, and Univ. Hosp. of Kinshasa, Zaïre)
Eur. J. Clin. Pharmacol. 29:523–527, January 1986   6–7

β Blockers are highly effective as first-line treatment for hypertension. However, black persons respond less well to these drugs, as do patients with low renin levels. In contrast, the calcium channel entry blockers reportedly are more effective in blacks and low-renin individuals. Because blacks from Zaïre have low renin levels, the effectiveness of a β blocker was tested against a calcium channel blocker in this population. The β blocker used was acebutolol, a cardioselective agent with intrinsic sympathomimetic activity; the calcium channel blocker was nitrendipine. The dose of acebutolol was 200 mg/day, and that of nitrendipine was 20 mg/day. There was a 4-week placebo run-in period prior to drug administration. Treatment was for 6 weeks; 22 patients were given nitrendipine and 18 received acebutolol.

Nitrendipine treatment reduced recumbent systolic blood pressure by 13% and diastolic pressure by 14% after 2 weeks of treatment. No further decrease occurred during the 6-week study. In contrast, patients treated with acebutolol had a progressive decline in blood pressure, the systolic falling by 5% and the diastolic by 10% within 6 weeks. In some patients, the drug dosage was increased during the study; the nitrendipine-treated patients had a further fall in blood pressure, whereas those who had increases in the acebutolol dosage had no further reduction. The pulse rate increased only in the nitrendipine-treated group, as did the plasma renin level. Blood pressures were significantly lower in patients given nitrendipine, compared with those given acebutolol after 2 weeks of treatment. At 6 weeks, only the difference in standing systolic pressure remained significant.

A daily dose of 20 mg of nitrendipine was sufficient for most patients in this study. The increase in pulse rate, which has been reported after treatment with other compounds chemically similar to nitrendipine, may result from reflex sympathetic stimulation. The same mechanism could be responsible for the increased plasma renin level in this group. Body weight was reduced with nitrendipine treatment; the drug does not cause fluid retention and may even exert a slight diuretic effect. Acebutolol caused a progressive hypotensive effect that was of smaller magnitude than that produced by nitrendipine. More patients required an increase in the dose, but a corresponding fall in blood pressure did not occur. Pulse rates and plasma renin activity did not change, probably because of the intrinsic sympathomimetic activity of acebutolol. Because blacks have both a tendency for lack of adequate response to β blockers and a low plasma renin level, a calcium channel blocker such as nitrendipine appears to be an effective first-line antihypertensive agent in those with mild to moderate hypertension.

▶ There is evidence, which has not been confirmed by all studies, that race can be used as a guide to select first-step agents for the management of hypertension. Presumably, black hypertensive patients respond better to diuretics and calcium channel blockers than they do to converting enzyme inhibitors and β blockers. The report by M'Buyamba-Kabangu et al. does little to settle this dispute. Although the authors imply that the black patients in their study responded better to the calcium channel blocker nitrendipine than a comparable group did to the β blocker acebutolol, their data are not convincing. At 2 weeks there was a statistically significant difference in recumbent and standing diastolic and systolic blood pressures, favoring nitrendipine. However, at the end of 6 weeks, the statistical significance was lost except for the systolic blood pressure in the standing position. Although it is true that at the 6-week interval the average blood pressure of the patients receiving nitrendipine was lower than that in patients receiving acebutolol, the differences were not very remarkable and in fact there was practically no difference in the recumbent diastolic pressure. Incidentally, the patients receiving nitrendipine had a significant increase in plasma renin activity.—R.W. Gifford, Jr., M.D.

Felodipine Vs. Hydralazine: A Controlled Trial as Third Line Therapy in Hypertension
D. Maclean and members of the Co-Operative Study Group (Ninewells Med. School, Dundee, Scotland, and other institutions in the U.K.)
Br. J. Clin. Pharmacol. 21:621–626, June 1986   6–8

Because hydralazine may induce lupus, its value as a third-line drug in the treatment of hypertension is limited; rather, calcium antagonists are used increasingly. Felodipine, a calcium antagonist having pronounced antihypertensive effects, is more potent and has a longer elimination half-life than nifedipine. The efficacy of felodipine and hydralazine was compared in hypertensive patients who had not responded to a β-adrenoceptor blocker/diuretic regimen.

The series included 57 men and 44 women aged 28–74 years who had a supine diastolic blood pressure of at least 100 mm Hg after 2–4 weeks of treatment with atenolol (100 mg daily) plus chlorthalidone (25 mg daily). The patients were divided into two groups: One group received atenolol plus chlorthalidone plus felodipine placebo, and the second group was given atenolol plus chlorthalidone plus hydralazine placebo, twice daily for 2 weeks or 4 weeks. If the supine diastolic blood pressure still exceeded 110 mm Hg after 2 weeks of treatment, patients were randomized to receive the additional vasodilator (felodipine, 5 mg twice daily, or hydralazine, 25 mg twice daily). If after 2 weeks of treatment with the three drugs the supine diastolic blood pressure was still more than 90 mm Hg, the vasodilator dose was doubled for the next 2 weeks, and doubled again, if needed, for the next 2 weeks.

After 6 weeks of treatment, the supine and erect systolic blood pressure was lower with felodipine treatment than with hydralazine; more patients reached their target blood pressure with felodipine therapy than with hydralazine, and fewer required dose increments when given felodipine. Side effects included ankle swelling and flushing (more frequent in the felodipine group), and headache and nausea (more common in the hydralazine group).

In this short-term trial, felodipine was more effective as a third-line antihypertensive agent than hydralazine was. However, the long-term efficacy and acceptability of felodipine have not yet been established.

▶ Felodipine is a new dihydropyridine calcium channel blocker similar to nifedipine and nitrendipine. This short-term study showed that felodipine was more effective than hydralazine when added as a third-step drug to the regimen of patients whose hypertension was resistant to a combination of diuretic and β blocker. I have used calcium channel blocking drugs as third-step agents in the manner described and, although they were effective, I have not been impressed that they were consistently more effective than hydralazine. The lupus syndrome associated with hydralazine therapy is rare indeed if the total daily dose is kept below 300 mg. Furthermore, hydralazine is much less expensive than calcium channel blocking drugs. Nevertheless, for patients whose hypertension has not responded to a combination of a diuretic and a β blocker, a calcium channel channel blocker should be considered as an alternative to hydralazine, especially if hydralazine proves to be ineffective or if intolerable side effects result from its use.—R.W. Gifford, Jr., M.D.

Exercise Hemodynamics and Oxygen Delivery in Human Hypertension: Response to Verapamil
Robert J. Cody, Spencer H. Kubo, Andrew B. Covit, Franco B. Müller, Jorge Lopez-Ovejero, and John H. Laragh (New York Hosp.–Cornell Univ. Med. Ctr.)
Hypertension 8:3–10, January 1986   6–9

To clarify the impact of vasoconstriction on the heart and peripheral circulation, the hemodynamic characteristics of hypertensive patients must be evaluated. However, resting hemodynamics only provide a static profile of these patients and do not identify the cardiovascular changes that occur with daily activity. In addition, although noninvasive assessment of exercise performance offers additional information, it does not completely assess ventricular loading conditions, peripheral vascular responses, or changes in oxygen delivery and use during maximal exercise. Because of this, it is necessary to obtain more extensive invasive assessments of cardiac performance and peripheral vascular responses to exercise. Calcium channel blockers have provided a new approach to the therapy of hypertension and appear to decrease blood pressure by reducing peripheral vascular

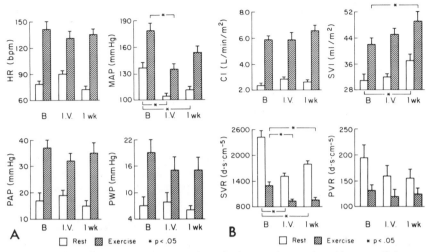

Fig 6–1.—Hemodynamic responses to exercise and subsequent intervention with verapamil therapy. The values shown represent baseline measurements (B), the immediate response to intravenous verapamil infusion (IV), and the response to 1 week of orally given verapamil therapy. HR = heart rate, MAP = mean arterial pressure, PAP = pulmonary artery pressure, PWP = pulmonary wedge pressure, CI = cardiac index, SVI = stroke volume index, SVR = systemic vascular resistance, and PVR = pulmonary vascular resisitance. (Courtesy of Cody, R.J., et al.: Hypertension 8:3–10, January 1986. By permission of the American Heart Association, Inc.)

resistance. However, a potential problem with this class of vasodilators is the possibility of a negative inotropic effect, which could limit cardiac performance. An attempt was made to characterize the hemodynamic response to exercise and the effects of calcium channel antagonism in ten hypertensive patients with moderate to severe hypertension.

Invasive exercise hemodynamics were performed in the baseline state after the intravenous infusion of verapamil and after 5–7 days of verapamil orally. In addition, oxygen delivery and use were also assessed, as was the response of the sympathetic nervous system, by measuring plasma norepinephrine levels at rest and during exercise. Both routes of drug administration were associated with significant reductions in mean arterial pressure and systemic vascular resistance at rest and peak exercise (Fig 6–1). The changes in heart rate were not statistically significant. After the oral administration of verapamil, the stroke volume increased markedly in both the resting and exercise states. However, the pulmonary-wedge pressure did not increase; in fact, the Frank-Starling relationship of cardiac performance actually was improved. Furthermore, oxygen delivery and use were not altered with either route of drug administration, and there was no significant difference in rest and exercise plasma norepinephrine levels after verapamil therapy.

Verapamil therapy led to a significant reduction in mean arterial pressure, mediated by a significant reduction of systemic vascular resistance, after both intravenous and short-term oral administration. This decrease occurred without expression of left ventricular dysfunction and not at the expense of increased oxygen use or enhanced sympathetic nervous systemic activity.

▶ I selected this paper because I am often asked which of the antihypertensive drugs have the least effect on exercise hemodynamics. We all know that the β blockers notoriously impair exercise performance by limiting the increase in heart rate and cardiac output that normally accompanies maximal exercise. Because verapamil has a negative inotropic effect similar to that of β blockers, it is surprising to find that, not only does it not interfere with the normal hemodynamic response to exercise, but it actually improves cardiac performance during exercise. Cardiac output increases appropriately during exercise, but because the total systemic vascular resistance decreases significantly, both during rest and exercise, the blood pressure does not rise as much with exercise as it did before verapamil was administered. Keep in mind that all of these patients had moderate to severe hypertension. I am disappointed that the authors did not mention the subjective reaction of these patients to exercise. I have always been impressed that patients taking β blockers experience a sensation of fatigue during exercise that is out of proportion to the physiologic derangement that can be measured objectively. It is interesting that single doses of nifedipine have been reported to impair maximal exercise tolerance in normal individuals (Chick, T.W., et al.: *Chest* 89:641–646, 1986). For more on calcium channel blocking agents, see Halperin, A.K., Kubeddu, L.X.: *Am. Heart J.* 111:363–382, 1986, and Ferlinz, J.: *Ann. Intern. Med.* 105:714–729, 1986.—R.W. Gifford, Jr., M.D.

Converting Enzyme Inhibitors

Double-Blind Comparison of Captopril and Enalapril in Mild to Moderate Hypertension

Peter H. Vlasses, Dale P. Conner, Heschi H. Rotmensch, Richard J. Fruncillo, Janice R. Danzeisen, Kenneth J. Shepley, and Roger K. Ferguson (Thomas Jefferson Univ., Philadelphia)
J. Am. Coll. Cardiol. 7:651–660, March 1986   6–10

A clinical trial was conducted involving 20 patients with mild to moderate essential hypertension to compare the antihypertensive effects of captopril and enalapril, both alone and in combination with hydrochlorothiazide (HCTZ). All had normal renal function. They received no treatment for the first 2 weeks and refrained from adding salt to their diets. They were randomly assigned to two parallel, double-blind treatment groups. Each group received a placebo for 1 day, followed by either 200 mg of captopril every 12 hours (9 patients) or 20 mg of enalapril maleate every 12 hours (11) during treatment days 1–14. On day 16, 25 mg of HCTZ every 12 hours was added to each group's regimen for treatment days 16–28. Captopril and enalapril were coadministered alone on day 15 and in combination with HCTZ on day 29 to learn whether further decreases in blood pressure would take place.

There were no clinically or statistically significant differences between the antihypertensive effects of captopril and enalapril. The addition of HCTZ further decreased blood pressure in each group, but coadministration of captopril and enalapril did not further reduce blood pressure. The antihypertensive effects and mechanisms of both drugs appear to be similar.

The Role of Renal Hemodynamics in the Antihypertensive Effect of Captopril
Katsuyuki Ando, Toshiro Fujita, Yasushi Ito, Hiroshi Noda, and Kamejiro Yamashita (Univ. of Tsukuba, Ibaraki, Japan)
Am. Heart J. 111:347–352, February 1986   6–11

The long-term effect of captopril on renal hemodynamics was evaluated and its relationship to decreased blood pressure after converting enzyme inhibition was assessed in 12 patients aged 21–57 years with mild to moderate essential hypertension. During the 2 weeks prior to the study, all antihypertensive medications were discontinued. All patients then received captopril, 37.5 mg/day, for 14 days. On day 15, patients were given 12.5 mg of captopril and hemodynamic parameters were measured 60–75 minutes later.

A significant decrease in mean blood pressure occurred together with a decrease in vascular resistance after captopril administration. However, cardiac output was not changed. Forearm vascular resistance was not altered, but renal vascular resistance decreased significantly. In addition, there was a highly significant correlation between changes in mean blood pressure and renal vascular resistance. After captopril treatment, the plasma renin activity was found to have increased as the plasma aldosterone value decreased, but the plasma norepinephrine level increased only slightly. The changes in renal vascular resistance correlated significantly with pretreatment levels of plasma renin activity. In essential hypertension, suppression of the renin-angiotensin system induces selective vasodilation in the renal vasculature that may play an important part in the long-term antihypertensive effect of captopril.

Low-Dose Captopril in Mild to Moderate Geriatric Hypertension
M. L. Tuck, L. A. Katz, W. M. Kirkendall, P. R. Koeppe, G. E. Ruoff, and D. G. Sapir (VA Med. Ctr., Sepulveda, Calif., VA Hosp., New York, Univ. of Houston, Univ. of Texas at Galveston, Westside Family Practice Clinic, Kalamazoo, Mich., and Wyman Park Hosp., Baltimore)
J. Am. Geriatr. Soc. 34:693–696, October 1986   6–12

Hypertension in the elderly is a significant risk factor for stroke, congestive heart failure, and coronary artery disease. The antihypertensive efficacy of low doses of captopril in elderly persons with mild to moderate hypertension was examined in a multicenter study of 99 patients older than age 60 years who had initial sitting diastolic pressures of 92–110 mm Hg. A 2-week placebo phase was followed by 6 weeks of active drug therapy, starting with 25 mg of captopril twice daily. The dose was doubled or captopril was combined with 15 mg of hydrochlorothiazide if the diastolic blood pressure remained above 90 mm Hg.

Fifty-one percent of patients were controlled with captopril alone. Seventy-six percent of patients had a diastolic pressure of less than 90 mm Hg or a fall of more than 10% with captopril, alone or combined with a diuretic, at the end of the trial. Black and white patients responded similarly to treatment. The incremental change in diastolic pressure was greater in patients who were given combined treatment. Treatment was well tolerated; the withdrawal rate was 5%. No significant laboratory abnormalities were noted.

Captopril is effective and well tolerated in the treatment of older patients who have mild to moderate diastolic hypertension. The concomitant use of a diuretic may be necessary. Patients accept the treatment well because of a general lack of symptomatic side effects and adverse metabolic effects.

The Contribution of PGI$_2$ to the Effects of Captopril in Conscious Dogs in Differing States of Sodium Balance

Michael L. Watson and Robert L. Jones (Univ. of Edinburgh)
Clin. Sci. 71:533–538, November 1986   6–13

The ability of captopril to reduce blood pressure in various low-renin states indicates that it may have hypotensive actions other than inhibition of angiotensin II synthesis. The possible role of prostaglandins in the hypotensive and renal vasodilating effects of captopril was studied by estimating the urinary excretion of 6-keto-PGF$_1$ after administration of captopril to salt-loaded and salt-depleted conscious dogs. Systemic hemodynamics and renal functions were monitored simultaneously. Foxhounds with a carotid arterial loop in the neck were used.

Captopril reduced blood pressure more in sodium-depleted animals. A transient rise in effective renal plasma flow and urinary excretion of metabolites occurred in the same animals, and there was a large but transient rise in plasma renin activity. A small reduction in blood pressure occurred in sodium-replete animals, with transient increases in renal plasma flow and urinary excretion of 6-keto-PGF$_1$, as well as progressive increases in plasma renin activity and urinary excretion of sodium.

Increased prostacyclin synthesis may contribute to a transient decrease in renal vascular resistance after administration of captopril. This effect is small, however. The chief effect probably is related to removal of the effect of angiotensin II on the renal vasculature. Decreased systemic blood pressure probably is not mediated by altered synthesis of prostacyclin.

▶ A second converting enzyme inhibitor, enalapril, was introduced in the United States in 1986. As shown in the study by Vlasses et al. (6–10), the two agents are equally effective whether as monotherapy or in combination with a diuretic. The doses used in this study are higher than ordinarily recommended.

The initial doses for patients with mild to moderate hypertension are in the range of 5 mg daily for enalapril and 12.5 mg twice daily for captopril. Enalapril is usually effective with once a day dosing because it has a longer duration of action than captopril has.

It is surprising that low-dose captopril was found to be so effective in managing mild to moderate hypertension in elderly patients (Tuck et al., Abstract 6–12). It has generally been accepted that converting enzyme inhibitors are more effective in young patients than in old patients and in white patients than in black patients. This was found to be true in a multicenter, double-blind trial comparing hydrochlorothiazide and enalapril (Vidt, D.G.: *J. Hypertension* 2:81–88, 1984). In the double-blind study by Vlasses et al., white patients responded better to converting enzyme inhibitors than did black patients.

Captopril (and enalapril) produce selective renal vasodilatation so that renal blood flow is preserved in spite of the decrease in blood pressure. Yet forearm vascular resistance does not drop significantly (Ando et al., Abstract 6–11). It is postulated by Ando et al. that this selective renal vasodilatation may play an important role in the long-term antihypertensive effect of captopril. More recent studies have shown that converting enzyme inhibitors dilate efferent arterioles of the glomeruli, thus increasing or maintaining renal blood flow but at the same time reducing intraglomerular pressure. This may explain why converting enzyme inhibitors decrease proteinuria in diabetic animals and man with diabetic glomerulosclerosis (Zatz, R., et al.: *J. Clin. Invest.* 77:1925–1930, 1986; Taguma, Y., et al.: *N. Engl. J. Med.* 313:1617–1620, 1985).

The major mechanism of antihypertensive action of converting enzyme inhibitors appears to be reduction of angiotensin II, but these drugs are effective even when the plasma renin level is low, and angiotensin II does not seem to be playing a role in maintaining the hypertension. The same enzyme that converts angiotensin I to angiotensin II also degrades bradykinin, so when it is inhibited it is only natural that the vasodilator bradykinin might accumulate and play a role in the vasodilating action of the converting enzyme inhibitor. Furthermore, treatment with converting enzyme inhibitors increases the synthesis of vasodilating renal prostaglandins as well as prostacyclin. Whatever the mechanism, it is not necessary to measure plasma renin activity to select patients for treatment with converting enzyme inhibitors. Converting enzyme inhibitors can be used as monotherapy to begin antihypertensive treatment, but they are much more expensive than diuretics, which have been the traditional step-one drug for many years.

Converting enzyme inhibitors also have a role in the diagnosis of renovascular hypertension (see Abstract 6–14).—R.W. Gifford, Jr., M.D.

The Captopril Test for Identifying Renovascular Disease in Hypertensive Patients

Franco B. Muller, Jean E. Sealey, David B. Case, Steven A. Atlas, Thomas G. Pickering, Mark S. Pecker, Jacek J. Preibisz, and John H. Laragh (New York Hosp.–Cornell Med. Ctr.)
Am. J. Med. 80:633–644, April 1986   6–14

The relationships between plasma and renal vein renin values in patients with essential hypertension and in those with unilateral and bilateral renovascular disease have been defined, and plasma renin assays have become more reliable. A simple screening test was developed by defining criteria for the plasma renin and/or blood pressure response to captopril to differentiate between essential and renovascular hypertension.

A retrospective review was made of data on 317 outpatients who were given a single oral dose of captopril as part of their evaluation for hyper-

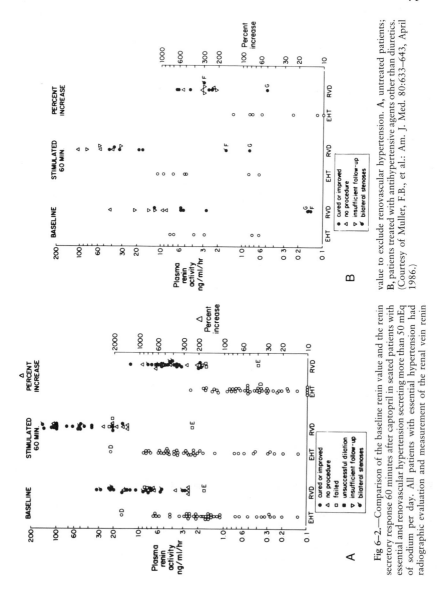

Fig 6–2.—Comparison of the baseline renin value and the renin secretory response 60 minutes after captopril in seated patients with essential and renovascular hypertension secreting more than 50 mEq of sodium per day. All patients with essential hypertension had radiographic evaluation and measurement of the renal vein renin value to exclude renovascular hypertension. A, untreated patients; B, patients treated with antihypertensive agents other than diuretics. (Courtesy of Muller, F.B., et al.: Am. J. Med. 80:633–643, April 1986.)

tension. Subsequently, 71 patients were excluded from the study on clinical grounds. Of the remaining 246 patients, 171 were studied while not taking any antihypertensive medication; the other 75 received a variety of antihypertensive drugs. The patients were further subdivided according to renal function. Plasma renin activity was measured 60 minutes after captopril administration by standard methodology.

Of 200 hypertensive patients without evidence of renal dysfunction, all 56 with renovascular disease were correctly identified by their renin secretory responses following captopril administration (Fig 6–2). Falsely positive results were found in only 2 of 112 patients with essential hypertension and in 6 with secondary hypertension. The captopril test is a useful screening tool for identification of patients with unilateral or bilateral renovascular disease. Moreover, the test is much simpler, less expensive, more specific, and less invasive than are older screening procedures, e.g., intravenous pyelography, arteriography, nuclear and isotope scanning, and the saralasin test.

Differential Renal Function During Angiotensin Converting Enzyme Inhibition in Renovascular Hypertension
Bruce Jackson, Barry P. McGrath, P. Geoffrey Matthews, Clem Wong, and Colin I. Johnston (Monash Univ. and Prince Henry's Hosp., Melbourne)
Hypertension 8:650–654, August 1986   6–15

Angiotensin converting enzyme inhibitors offer promise as an alternative to renovascular surgery in patients with atheromatous disease, especially when operative risks are high, but treatment has been associated with acutely deteriorating renal function in patients with renovascular hypertension. A prospective study was performed to assess split renal function by computed radionuclide renography in 32 patients with proved renovascular hypertension who took captopril for at least 3 days. In 11 subsequent patients renal function was studied before and 1–6 weeks after the start of captopril or enalapril therapy. Renal function was assessed by ^{99m}Tc-diethylenetriamine penta-acetic acid renography, and differential glomerular filtration rates were computed.

Six of the first 32 patients had acute deterioration of renal function when given captopril. These included 3 of 11 patients with bilateral renal artery stenosis and 3 of 8 with a single kidney and renal artery stenosis. These patients had higher baseline serum creatinine concentrations, but the blood pressure response to angiotensin converting enzyme inhibition was similar to that in other patients. Radionuclide clearance decreased in most kidneys with stenosed arteries during ACE inhibition. The serum creatinine concentration returned to baseline after withdrawal of angiotensin converting enzyme inhibitor therapy in all patients with acute renal failure. In two of the prospectively studied patients, angiotensin converting enzyme inhibition was discontinued, and both had a return of function to baseline in the kidneys with stenosed arteries.

Oral angiotensin converting enzyme inhibitor therapy reduces renal function in kidneys with markedly stenosed renal arteries. The functional impairment is reversible, but the long-term effects are unknown, and irreversible parenchymal damage or thrombosis cannot presently be excluded.

Effect of Captopril on ^{99m}Tc-Diethylenetriamine Pentaacetic Acid Renograms in Two-Kidney, One Clip Hypertension

Joseph V. Nally, Jr., Harry S. Clarke, Jr., George P. Grecos, Mark Saunders, Michael L. Gross, William J. Potvin, and Joe P. Windham (Med. College of Ohio)

Hypertension 8:685–693, August 1986   6–16

An attempt was made to improve the noninvasive detection of renal artery stenosis by studying the effects of angiotensin converting enzyme inhibition with captopril on computer-aided ^{99m}Tc-diethylenetriamine penta-acetic acid (DTPA) renal flow studies in a canine model of two-kidney, one-clip hypertension. Clearances of inulin and para-aminohippurate were determined in the stenotic and contralateral kidneys before and after captopril, given in an intravenous dose of 1.5 mg/kg and followed by a 60-minute infusion of 1.5 mg/minute. Scanning was repeated 3 days after operation.

The DTPA renal flow study with captopril was more sensitive in detecting unilateral renal artery stenosis than was the radionuclide study alone. Captopril-related changes were most evident in the 15-minute ^{99m}Tc-DTPA renal flow study, which showed markedly blunted uptake and excretion of technetium activity. The changes were reversed during a recovery study without captopril and were not observed when the blood pressure was lowered with nitroprusside to the level found with captopril. The captopril flow study correlated with a decrease in glomerular filtration rate in the kidney with a stenotic artery only. Effective renal plasma flow did not change significantly in either kidney after captopril administration. The filtration fraction decreased in both kidneys after captopril treatment.

The captopril-aided ^{99m}Tc-DTPA renal flow study unmasked angiotensin II-dependent renal functional and hemodynamic changes in a kidney with a stenotic renal artery in this canine model of two-kidney, one-clip hypertension. The approach may hold promise in detecting renovascular hypertension.

▶ Muller et al. (Abstract 6–14) have reported that captopril stimulates renin production more in patients with renovascular hypertension than in those with essential hypertension, and they have used this as a criterion for screening for renovascular hypertension before subjecting patients to renal angiography. The response of the blood pressure to a test dose of captopril was much less specific and sensitive in detecting patients with renovascular hypertension than was the response of peripheral plasma renin activity. Blood pressure is measured and blood is drawn for plasma renin activity before and 60 minutes after the administration of 25 mg or 50 mg of captopril, crushed and dissolved in 10 ml of water immediately prior to administration. In patients with normal renal function, and excluding two patients with renovascular disease and plasma renin activity of less than 1 ng/ml/hour, all patients with renovascular disease were identified (sensitivity, 100%) by using the following criteria: (1) stimulated plasma renin activity of at least 12 ng/ml/hour; (2) an absolute increase in plasma renin activity of at least 10 ng/ml/hour; and (3) a percent increase in plasma renin activity of at least 150, or of at least 400 if baseline plasma renin activity is less than 3 ng/ml/hour. Of 158 patients without classic renovascular disease, 8 had positive results, giving a specificity of 95%.

When patients with severe renal artery stenosis are given a converting enzyme inhibitor, either captopril or enalapril, renal function deteriorates in the kidney supplied by the stenotic artery, presumably because under such circumstances renal blood flow and the glomerular filtration rate are maintained by angiotensin II. Clinically, this has been recognized in patients with severe bilateral renal artery stenosis or severe stenosis in the artery to a solitary kidney, when administration of a converting enzyme inhibitor will lead to acute renal failure. However, this is more difficult to recognize clinically when renal artery stenosis is unilateral and the opposite kidney is normal. It is now being proposed that a technetium renal flow scan following administration of captopril may be more sensitive in picking up unilateral renal artery disease than the flow scan alone. Nally et al. (Abstract 6–16) have demonstrated this in a dog model. Jackson et al. (Abstract 6–15), reporting a series of patients with unilateral or bilateral renal artery disease, have shown that functional impairment is reversible when the converting enzyme inhibitor is withdrawn. Prior administration of a converting enzyme inhibitor may well enhance the diagnostic reliability of the technetium renal flow scan in the diagnosis of renovascular hypertension. Until there has been more experience with the captopril renin stimulation test as a screening procedure for renovascular hypertension, I would be unwilling to accept a negative test as absolute evidence for ruling out renovascular disease. It should be pointed out that 62 of the patients in the series reported by Muller et al. did not have renal arteriograms to rule out renal artery stenosis.—R.W. Gifford, Jr., M.D.

Metabolic Side Effects of Diuretics and Beta Blockers

Propranolol or Hydrochlorothiazide Alone for the Initial Treatment of Hypertension: IV. Effect on Plasma Glucose and Glucose Tolerance
E. A. Ramírez and F. N. Talmers, for the Veterans Administration Cooperative Study Group on Antihypertensive Agents (VA Med. Ctr., San Juan, P.R., and participating centers throughout the United States)
Hypertension 7:1008–1016, November–December 1985   6–17

Thiazide diuretics in therapeutic doses used for the treatment of hypertension are associated with elevated blood glucose levels and impaired glucose tolerance in many patients. β-Blockers have been proposed as an alternative to thiazides in the treatment of hypertension. The short-term and long-term effectiveness of propranolol was compared with that of hydrochlorothiazide in the monotherapy of hypertension.

The study included 683 hypertensive men aged 21–65 years who were randomly assigned to treatment with propranolol (340 men) or hydrochlorothiazide (343 men) in titrated twice-daily divided doses for 1 year. Patients were selected for the study after a prerandomization, single-blind placebo period of 4 weeks to obtain baseline data and assess eligibility. Excluded from the study were patients with unstable diabetes, diabetes of preadult onset, or diabetes requiring insulin treatment. A 2-hour glucose tolerance test was administered to a subset of 191 patients.

Overall, both drugs increased the average fasting plasma glucose level and impaired glucose tolerance regardless of age, initial fasting plasma glucose level, race, or weight changes. After 10 weeks of treatment, 2-hour glucose tolerance tests were increased significantly to a greater degree in the group treated with hydrochlorothiazide than in those given propranolol. However, the most important difference between the two drugs was the fact that elevated fasting plasma glucose levels persisted in patients treated with propranolol after tapering and discontinuation of the drug, but these levels returned to baseline in patients treated with hydrochlorothiazide after similar periods. Both drugs have mildly diabetogenic effects when given in therapeutic doses, and both should be given in the lowest effective dosage. If necessary, either drug can be combined with other medications in an effort to obtain optimum antihypertensive effectiveness.

Relationship of Diuretic Therapy and Serum Magnesium Levels Among Participants in the Multiple Risk Factor Intervention Trial

Lewis Kuller, Noel Farrier, Arlene Caggiula, Nemat Borhani, and Signe Dunkle (Univ. of Pittsburgh and Univ. of California at Davis)
Am. J. Epidemiol. 122:1045–1059, December 1985   6–18

Thiazide diuretics cause increased magnesium excretion in the urine. Because low serum and tissue magnesium levels have been noted in diuretic users, the relationship between serum magnesium levels and diuretic therapy was studied during the fourth or fifth year of the Multiple Risk Factor Intervention Trial in two different centers.

Included were men aged 35–57 years at the time of entry into the trial between 1972 and 1974. During 1980 and 1981, serum samples were obtained from most of the study participants during two consecutive, regularly scheduled, 4-month interval visits to the centers. The participants were divided into two groups depending on whether or not they were currently taking antihypertensive medication, primarily chlorthalidone. Magnesium levels as well as other parameters, including serum potassium and cholesterol levels, were measured according to standard methodology.

About 15% of diuretic users had persistently lower serum magnesium levels than nondiuretic users had. No correlation was found between serum potassium and magnesium levels. The results suggest that, within similar populations, low serum magnesium levels are rarely encountered.

The Cardiovascular Risks of Thiazide Diuretics

Edward D. Freis (Georgetown Univ.)
Clin. Pharmacol. Ther. 39:239–244, March 1986
6–19

The antihypertensive response to diuretics is closely related to reduction of extracellular fluid and plasma volumes. Much attention is given to avoiding hypokalemia, but the extracellular hypokalemia caused by diuretics is not associated with a parallel fall in the intracellular potassium concentration. This is not a serious concern unless heart disease is present. Recent ECG monitoring studies have shown no association between hypokalemia and ventricular arrhythmias. Thiazides are widely thought to increase fatal arrhythmias in some patients with minor ECG abnormalities, but the evidence for this is questionable. Many physicians are concerned that fatal arrhythmias are more likely to develop in the setting of AMI if a patient has received a thiazide diuretic, but there is also little confirmatory evidence for this. Infusion of glucose, insulin, and potassium fails to reduce the occurrence of ventricular tachycardia and fibrillation in patients with AMI.

There is concern that elevations in the serum cholesterol level may, over a long period, exacerbate coronary artery disease in diuretic-treated patients. A modest rise in the serum cholesterol level does occur after use of a thiazide diuretic, but the baseline level usually returns during long-term dosing. Like the alleged adverse cardiovascular effects of thiazide diuretics, an elevation in the serum cholesterol level does not seem to be cause for serious concern.

Diuretics continue to be the most useful antihypertensive drugs, both alone and in combination with other agents. Replacing them with less effective drugs or reducing their dosage to a marginally effective level would compromise control of hypertension.

▶ Since the publication of the results of the Multiple Risk Factor Intervention Trial (MRFIT) (*JAMA* 248:1465–1477, 1982), diuretics have come under rather fierce criticism, much of which is undeserved in my opinion.

Kuller et al. (Abstract 6–18), who participated in the MRFIT trial, report serum magnesium levels among participants who were receiving diuretics and those who were not. The results are not dramatic, although as one would expect, those who were receiving diuretics on the average had slightly lower serum magnesium levels, the significance of which is not apparent. As the authors mention in the discussion, serum magnesium may not reflect total body magnesium, and there are those who believe that only tissue levels of magnesium as determined from muscle biopsy specimens are reliable guides to magnesium balance. It is interesting that in this study there was no relation between the levels of serum magnesium and the levels of serum potassium, although it is generally believed that patients with low serum magnesium levels are to be found only among those who have low serum potassium levels. In other words, it is not worthwhile measuring plasma for magnesium if the serum potassium level is normal. What interested me most about this article from the MRFIT group was a statement that there were relatively few low serum potassium levels among the diuretic users. In the discussion they state that, "These results suggest that lower serum magnesium levels are not a major problem among long-term diuretic users who have had their potassium levels carefully monitored and controlled as in the Multiple Risk Factor Intervention Trial." Yet, the critics of diuretics attribute the excess deaths among men in the Special Intervention Group with abnormal resting ECGs who received diuretics to cardiac arrhythmias from diuretic-induced hypokalemia!

The Veterans Administration Cooperative Study Group (Abstract 6–17) reported their results of the effect of propranolol or hydrochlorothiazide on the plasma glucose level and glucose tolerance. This is a sequel to a study published several years ago (*JAMA* 248:1996–2003, 2004–2011, 1982), comparing the effects on blood pressure of propranolol and hydrochlorothiazide studied in a double-blind fashion. It is of concern that both propranolol and hydrochlorothiazide led to elevations of the fasting plasma glucose level and a decrease in glucose tolerance, as manifested by an increase in the plasma glucose level (over control levels) 2 hours after an oral glucose load compared with pretreatment values. In the group receiving hydrochlorothiazide, the average increase in the fasting plasma glucose level was about 4.5 mg/dl, and about 6.4 mg/dl for propranolol. The increase in the 2-hour blood glucose level in patients taking hydrochlorothiazide averaged 18 mg/dl at 10 weeks and 25.9 mg/dl at 58 weeks. For propranolol, comparable figures were 0.4 mg/dl at 10 weeks and 18.1 mg/dl at 58 weeks. The onset of impaired glucose tolerance appeared later in those receiving β blockers than in those receiving hydrochlorothiazide. The fasting plasma glucose level returned to normal within 1 month after discontinuing hydrochlorothiazide therapy, but remained elevated 1 month after the dose of propranolol was tapered and 2 weeks after it was discontinued. In defense of the diuretics, it must be pointed out that very large doses of both propranolol and hydrochlorothiazide were used in this study (up to 640 mg of propranolol daily and up to 200 mg of hydrochlorothiazide daily). The hyperglycemic effects were dose related, being greater in patients taking more than 320 mg of propranolol or more than 50 mg of hydrochlorothiazide daily. Doses of hydrochlorothiazide of more than 50 mg a day are no longer recommended. Berglund and Andersson (*Lancet* 1:744–747, 1981) found no adverse effect of bendroflumethiazide, 2.5–5 mg daily, on the fasting blood glucose level or glucose tolerance in 49 men who had received the drug for 6 years.

The article by Freis (Abstract 6–19) is a defense of thiazide diuretics. Fairly citing both sides of the question from the literature, he concludes that the dangers of diuretic-induced hypokalemia and increased serum cholesterol levels have been overstated. I would add that oral diuretics or β blockers have been used in all of the major trials that have shown a reduction in cardiovascular morbidity and mortality, and no other classes of drugs have been subjected to such rigorous testing.—R.W. Gifford, Jr., M.D.

Cardiovascular Effects of Atrial Natriuretic Factor in Anesthetized and Conscious Dogs

Hollis D. Kleinert, Massimo Volpe, Geoffrey Odell, Donald Marion, Steven A. Atlas, Maria J. Camargo, John H. Laragh, and Thomas Maack (Cornell Univ.)
Hypertension 8:312–316, April 1986   6–20

Atrial natriuretic factor (ANF) is a peptide or group of peptides with both natriuretic and vascular actions; it is likely that the natriuretic effect of ANF results from its renal hemodynamic actions. Atrial natriuretic factor inhibits both receptor-mediated and nonreceptor-mediated vaso-constriction of isolated rabbit aorta, in addition to carbachol-induced con-traction of chick intestinal smooth muscle. Whether the consistent blood pressure-lowering effect of ANF during steady state results from a decrease in peripheral vascular resistance, cardiac output, or both, was examined in normotensive female mongrel dogs.

Four awake dogs previously instrumented with electromagnetic flow probes for measurement of cardiac output and catheters for systemic hemo-dynamic and cardiac dynamic measurements were investigated. After a 30-minute control period, a 24-residue synthetic ANF bolus, 3 µg/kg, followed by 0.3 µg/minute/kg, was infused for 30 minutes, followed by a recovery period of 1 hour. The mean arterial pressure fell markedly during infusion and was accompanied by a slight but significant bradycardia. In addition, there were substantial reductions in cardiac output and stroke volume, and a maximum increase in rate of change of left ventricular systolic pressure. There were no significant changes in total peripheral resistance or central venous pressure, although the latter tended to decrease during infusion. A similar pattern of observations was noted in six pen-tobarbital-anesthetized dogs, except that infusion of ANF did not induce bradycardia. The mean arterial pressure is lowered in these models by a mechanism other than reduction in total peripheral resistance, specifically by a reduction in cardiac output.

Long-Term Hypotensive and Renal Effects of Atrial Natriuretic Peptide
Joey P. Granger, Terry J. Opgenorth, Javier Salazar, J. Carlos Romero, and John C. Burnett, Jr. (Mayo Clinic and Found.)
Hypertension 8 (Suppl. II):II-112–II-116, June 1986   6–21

Short-term administration of atrial natriuretic peptide (ANP) to dogs affects renal hemodynamics, sodium excretion, and arterial pressure, and suppresses the renin-angiotensin system and aldosterone. The long-term effects of ANP were examined in chronically instrumented, conscious fe-male dogs, six of which were treated with a bolus injection of synethetic rat ANP. Blood samples were taken 30 minutes after ANP infusion and measured for plasma inulin, sodium, potassium, ANP, and aldosterone levels. Plasma renin activity was assessed at the midpoint of each clearance period. Another six dogs were given intravenous infusions of ANP for 5 days continuously. Blood was drawn daily and studied for the same pa-rameters as in the short-term study. Daily measurements were taken of arterial pressure and the 24-hour urinary excretion of sodium, potassium, and water, urine osmolality, 24-hour water intake, and the glomerular filtration rate (GFR) also were determined.

Short-term ANP plasma level increases resulted in marked increases in the GFR and sodium excretion but in only small reductions in mean arterial pressure. In contrast, long-term ANP plasma level increases resulted in greater reductions in mean arterial pressure but had no significant long-term effects on the GFR or sodium excretion. The lack of a sustained effect on the GFR during long-term ANP plasma level increases may result from the large reduction in mean arterial pressure. The data suggest that two different mechanisms may be responsible for the short-term and long-term effect of ANP infusion on arterial pressure.

▶ Of the many publications concerning ANF and ANP that appeared in 1986, these two were selected because they show some of the problems of studying hemodynamic effects of this recently discovered atrial peptide, which has both natriuretic and hypotensive activity. The Cornell group (Abstract 6–20) report that a 30-minute infusion of ANF into both conscious and anesthetized dogs reduced blood pressure by reducing cardiac output. On the other hand, the Mayo group (Abstract 6–21) found that a 45-minute infusion of ANP into conscious dogs reduced arterial blood pressure only slightly but increased the GFR significantly. Both groups reported significant natriuresis with the acute infusions. The Cornell group did not measure the GFR and did not report a chronic study. The Mayo group reported that, after 5 days of continuous intravenous infusion of ANP, there was a significant decrease in mean arterial pressure but no change in the GFR. It is interesting that this peptide reduces blood pressure, presumably by decreasing cardiac output because of venodilatation and a reduction in venous return to the heart. Yet, there is no reflex tachycardia and plasma renin activity is not increased. Whether cardiac output or total peripheral resistance, or both, are decreased during long-term administration of ANP is as yet unknown. What role ANP plays in human homeostasis and what future it has as a therapeutic agent in man remain to be determined.— R.W. Gifford, Jr., M.D.

Sodium and Hypertension

Excessive Sodium Retention as a Characteristic of Salt-Sensitive Hypertension
Harriet P. Dustan, Gloria Valdes, Emmanuel L. Bravo, and Robert C. Tarazi (Cleveland Clinic Found.)
Am. J. Med. Sci. 292:67–74, August 1986   6–22

Salt excess is an important factor in certain patients with essential hypertension. The effects of salt deprivation and loading on arterial pressure, the renin-angiotensin-aldosterone system, and plasma volume were examined in 20 patients (15 men), aged 21–64 years, with essential hypertension. Six were black. A 10-mEq sodium diet was given for 4 days, following mercuhydrin therapy to insure a negative sodium balance. A 3-

day salt-loading period using 0.9% saline infusion followed. The salt load was 3.9 mEq/kg daily.

Ten patients rapidly became normotensive during sodium deprivation; in the other ten, blood pressure was unchanged. The responders retained more sodium during salt loading than did the other patients, and this could not be ascribed to a measurable decrease in filtered sodium load or to differences in plasma renin activity or aldosterone excretion. Sodium excretion did not correlate with arterial pressure except in nonresponders on the last day of salt loading. Responders had a higher plasma volume after salt loading, but this did not explain their increased sodium retention.

The increase in arterial blood pressure that results from salt loading in patients with essential hypertension is not explained by responses of the renin-angiotensin-aldosterone system. Salt-sensitive hypertension is characterized by greater sodium retention when a salt load follows salt deprivation. Efforts are needed to determine whether salt-sensitive hypertensives retain more sodium than do other hypertensives when a salt load is given without previous salt depletion.

Abnormal Renal Sodium Handling in Essential Hypertension: Relation to Failure of Renal and Adrenal Modulation of Responses to Angiotensin II
Norman K. Hollenberg, Thomas Moore, Dolores Shoback, Jamie Redgrave, Steven Rabinowe, and Gordon H. Williams (Harvard Univ. and Brigham and Women's Hosp., Boston)
Am. J. Med. 81:412–418, September 1986   6–23

Patients with essential hypertension vary in their sensitivity to sodium intake, but at present there is no consensus on what causes this variation. Renal vascular and adrenal responses to a volume challenge are both abnormal in such patients, and these abnormalities are linked to their response to angiotensin II. The impact of the abnormal control of sodium handling in the kidney and adrenal gland was studied in patients with essential hypertension during sodium restriction and sodium loading after balance was achieved with a low-sodium diet.

The study included 60 controls and 61 patients with normal-renin essential hypertension. Two protocols were used: In study A, sodium balance was achieved with a daily sodium intake of 10 mEq, whereas in study B, the shift in sodium intake from 10 mEq to 200 mEq daily resulted in rapid, progressive increase in sodium excretion in the two groups of patients. Angiotensin II was infused to classify persons with essential hypertension into modulator (i.e., normal renal responsiveness to angiotensin II) and nonmodulator (i.e., abnormal renal responsiveness) subgroups. The nonmodulator group in study B demonstrated a delayed rate at which external sodium balance was achieved, had a greater cumulative positive sodium balance, experienced more weight gain, and had a greater frequency of blood pressure increase.

The abnormality in the rate at which external sodium balance is achieved in patients with nonmodulating essential hypertension results in a difference in total body sodium that varies with sodium intake. This may well contribute to, or cause, sodium-sensitive hypertension.

Renal and Endocrine Response to Saline Infusion in Essential Hypertension
Linea L. Rydstedt, Gordon H. Williams, and Norman K. Hollenberg (Harvard Univ. and Brigham and Women's Hosp., Boston)
Hypertension 8:217–222, March 1986   6–24

Earlier findings indicated that a reduction in the rate of sodium excretion is associated with significant delay in suppression of the renin-angiotensin-aldosterone system in about half of the hypertensive patients studied. These results raised the possibility that excessive intrarenal angiotensin II concentrations are responsible for that phenomenon. The response to a sodium load was reassessed after treatment with enalapril, a converting enzyme inhibitor, in 21 patients with essential hypertension. The series included 16 with normal renin hypertension (who formed the basis of this study) and 5 with low renin hypertension who served as positive controls. The study also included nine normotensive controls. The patients ranged in age between 23 and 67 years.

All antihypertensive medications were withdrawn for at least 2 weeks prior to the study, and all patients were on isocaloric diets containing 10 mEq of sodium and 100 mEq of potassium. The daily fluid intake was maintained at 2,500 ml. All patients were given a 1-hour infusion containing 60 mEq of sodium. The patients with low-renin hypertension experienced the expected transient, exaggerated natriuresis without a rise in blood pressure, whereas those with normal renin levels had either a normal or a blunted natriuretic response. The 16 hypertensive patients with normal renin levels were then given enalapril in increasing daily doses for 72 hours.

Enalapril significantly increased the renal plasma flow in hypertensive patients with normal renin levels and the natriuretic response to the sodium load returned to normal. Blunted natriuresis is a common feature of essential hypertension in patients with controlled prior sodium intake and normal renin levels, whereas exaggerated natriuresis is associated with low renin levels.

▶ Patients with primary hypertension can be classified into those whose blood pressure responds favorably to sodium deprivation (sodium responders) and those who do not (nonresponders). Similarly, sodium loading does not necessarily raise the blood pressure in hypertensive patients unless they are sodium sensitive. It has generally been assumed that patients with so-called low renin hypertension are sodium responders, whereas those with normal or high renin hypertension are less responsive to sodium deprivation. However, Dustan and colleagues (Abstract 6–22) found no statistically significant difference between plasma renin activity in ten patients whose hypertension responded to sodium deprivation compared with ten patients whose blood pressure did not respond to sodium deprivation. Nor was there any significant difference between aldosterone excretion rates in the two groups.

In a group of normal renin essential hypertensive patients, Hollenberg et al. (Abstract 6–23) have demonstrated in an elegant study that those in whom angiotensin II infusion reduced para-aminohippurate clearance by more than 125 ml/minute/1.73 sq m on a high sodium diet were not sensitive to sodium loading with respect to a change in blood pressure. These were called "modulators." In nonmodulating patients there was a substantial reduction in the response of para-aminohippurate clearance to angiotensin II infusion. Compared with modulators, nonmodulators took longer to reach equilibrium when placed on a 10-mEq sodium intake and had a delayed natriuretic response to sodium loading. Nonmodulators also had an abnormal response of aldosterone to angiotensin II infusion compared with modulators who had a significantly greater plasma aldosterone concentration after angiotensin infusion than did nonmodulators. Sodium loading led to more weight gain and a greater frequency of blood pressure rise in nonmodulators than in modulators. It was their conclusion that this could be explained on the basis of the abnormal renal and adrenal responses to angiotensin II. It is interesting that modulators and nonmodulators had equal hypotensive responses to a 10-mEq sodium diet.

In a related study, Rydstedt et al. (Abstract 6–24) found that enalapril, a converting enzyme inhibitor, corrected the blunted natriuretic response to saline infusion in patients with normal renin hypertension. This suggests an abnormality in control of the intrarenal angiotensin II concentration underlying the blunted natriuretic response. It should be noted that arterial blood pressure did not change during or after the saline load in these patients. This observation helps explain why chronic treatment with converting enzyme inhibitors does not lead to fluid retention. Suppression of aldosterone secretion is another factor.—R.W. Gifford, Jr., M.D.

Cation Transport Abnormalities *in Vivo* in Untreated Essential Hypertension

Nicholas A. Boon, Jeffrey K. Aronson, Keith F. Hallis, and David G. Grahame-Smith (Radcliffe Infirmary, Oxford, England)
Clin. Sci. 70:611–616, June 1986   6–25

Abnormal transmembrane cation transport in cells of patients with essential hypertension has been reported previously in association with the hypothesis that hypertension may develop in response to increased concentrations of a circulating sodium, potassium-dependent adenosine triphosphatase (Na^+,K^+-ATPase) inhibitor. Because these studies were mostly done in vitro, cation transport in vivo was examined in patients with untreated essential hypertension by measuring changes in plasma and intraerythrocytic rubidium concentrations after oral administration of rubidium chloride (RbCl). Rubidium chloride was chosen for the study because it is transported into cells mainly through the action of Na^+,K^+-ATPase, thus it could be expected that a reduction in activity of this enzyme

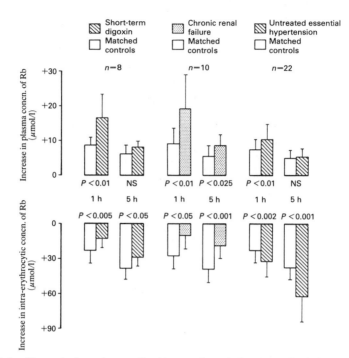

Fig 6–3.—Changes in plasma *(top panel)* and intra-erythrocytic *(bottom panel)* rubidium concentrations in patients taking short-term digoxin therapy, patients with chronic renal failure, patients with untreated essential hypertension, and their respective matched controls. The data are given as the means ± SD. Statistical testing was by Student's two-tailed, unpaired *t*-test. NS, not significant. (Courtesy of Boon, N. A., et al.: Clin. Sci. 70:611–616, 1986.)

would lead to reduced clearance of rubidium from plasma and to increased rubidium plasma concentrations.

The study was done in 22 patients with untreated essential hypertension and in 22 matched normotensive controls. The study also included ten chronic renal failure patients and eight taking digoxin, both groups with respective matched controls. A separate evaluation was made of the disposition of ^{42}KCl in five men with untreated essential hypertension and five matched controls.

The measured changes in plasma and intraerythrocytic rubidium concentrations suggest a generalized reduction in activity of Na^+,K^+-ATPase in patients taking digoxin and in patients with chronic renal failure, but increased Na^+,K^+-ATPase activity in patients with essential hypertension (Fig 6–3). These findings are at variance with results of previously reported studies. The study of ^{42}K disposition after ^{42}KCl administered intravenously shows that net cation transport is enhanced in erythrocytes of patients with untreated essential hypertension.

Effect of Serum From Patients With Essential Hypertension on Sodium Transport in Normal Leukocytes

H. H. Gray, P. J. Hilton, and P. J. Richardson (St. Thomas' Hosp. and King's College Hosp., London)
Clin. Sci. 70:583–586, June 1986   6–26

Leukocytes of patients with essential hypertension have both abnormal sodium transport and an elevated intracellular sodium concentration. These abnormalities are reversed with diuretic treatment and can be induced in hormonal leukocytes by incubation in serum from hypertensive patients (cross-incubation effect). It was thus hypothesized that there is a circulating inhibitor of sodium transport that may be of mechanistic importance in essential hypertension. An attempt was made to confirm the cross-incubation effect and to investigate its relationship to blood pressure in 27 patients with essential hypertension (mean blood pressure, 179/108 mm Hg) and 27 normotensive controls (mean blood pressure, 126/80 mm Hg).

Comparison of leukocyte sodium transport in normal cells incubated in the serum of a hypertensive patient, and that of the hypertensive patient's own cells, demonstrated a significant relationship. Both the total and ouabain-sensitive sodium efflux rate constants of the leukocytes incubated in hypertensive serum were observed to be positively correlated with the total and ouabain-sensitive rate constant of the hypertensive's own cells. The cross-incubation effect also correlated with the hypertensive's own ouabain-sensitive rate constant, suggesting that this effect was caused by a factor in the hypertensives' own serums and was not an experimental artifact. The serum of those patients with the highest diastolic blood pressures had the greatest inhibitory effect on sodium transport by normal leukocytes. The systolic blood pressure showed a weak negative correlation with the cross-incubation effect.

Serum from patients with essential hypertension inhibits sodium transport and elevates intracellular sodium in normal human leukocytes, and the magnitude of this effect is positively correlated with diastolic blood pressure in hypertensive patients. The extent of sodium transport inhibition is correlated with the abnormal sodium transport in the hypertensive's own leukocytes. These results confirm the presence of a serum inhibitor of sodium transport in essential hypertension and suggest that the relationship between the inhibitory effect and severity of hypertension may be of mechanistic importance.

▶ Boon et al., (Abstract 6–25) using rubidium chloride, failed to demonstrate any decrease in Na^+,K^+-ATPase activity in patients with primary hypertension. The authors point out that their study was done in vivo, whereas other studies that have shown decreased Na^+,K^+-ATPase activity in hypertensives have been in vitro. On the other hand, Gray et al. (Abstract 6–26) have demonstrated that the serum from hypertensive patients inhibited sodium transport in leukocytes taken from normotensive individuals. How to resolve the differences between these two studies is not clear. One study used the rubidium concentration in erythrocytes in vivo, and the other used the efflux of radioactive sodium from leukocytes in vitro. Presumably, rubidium transport is dependent upon Na^+,K^+-ATPase. Perhaps the difference is that some hypertensive patients have a reduction in Na^+,K^+-ATPase activity and others do not.—R.W. Gifford, Jr., M.D.

Calcium and Hypertension

Serum Calcium Fractions in Essential Hypertensive and Matched Normotensive Subjects

Aaron R. Folsom, Charles L. Smith, Ronald J. Prineas, and Richard H. Grimm (Univ. of Minnesota)
Hypertension 8:11–15, January 1986   6–27

It has been proposed that elevations in intracellular calcium are involved in the pathogenesis of essential hypertension. In addition, recent studies suggest that extracellular calcium concentrations may also differ between hypertensive and normotensive persons. There are three extracellular calcium fractions—ionized, protein-bound, and complexed calcium. These serum calcium fractions were compared in 28 mildly hypertensive patients and 28 normotensive controls matched for race, sex, and age.

The mean levels of serum total calcium were not different between the two groups. However, hypertensive patients had lower mean serum levels of ultrafilterable calcium (-0.32 mg/dl), ionized calcium (-0.07 mg/dl), and complexed calcium (-0.23 mg/dl), and higher levels of protein-bound calcium ($+0.36$ mg/dl). The estimated dietary calcium intake was similar in the hypertensive and normotensive groups. These findings add to the evidence that essential hypertension is associated with perturbations in calcium metabolism. An epidemiologic study of hypertension should be undertaken to measure in one population serum levels of calcium, renin, and parathyroid hormone, as well as calcium intake and excretion.

Effects of Calcium Infusion on Blood Pressure in Hypertensive and Normotensive Humans

David H. Ellison, Robert Shneidman, Cynthia Morris, and David A. McCarron (Oregon Health Sci. Univ., Portland)
Hypertension 8:497–505, June 1986   6–28

The metabolism of calcium may be abnormal in hypertensive persons and could influence the control of blood pressure. However, there are many variables to be considered, including dietary calcium and sodium intake, which may interact. Some studies have suggested that effects that appear to be dependent on sodium chloride may be mediated directly by changes in the systemic calcium balance. Experiments were designed to compare the hemodynamic and metabolic responses to short-term calcium infusion in normal individuals and in persons with essential hypertension. The dietary intake of both calcium and sodium was controlled and altered in steps to evaluate interactions between calcium response and sodium intake. Seven normal controls and seven hypertensives participated. Antihypertensive medications were withdrawn prior to the study. There were 3 test days during which calcium was infused; each took place after the participants had followed a diet having varying amounts of sodium for 4 days.

During the study, the dietary sodium intake did not alter the baseline blood pressure in either group. Calcium infusion raised systolic pressure in both groups; dietary sodium affected this response differently in each group. In normal individuals, systolic pressure increased during calcium infusion at the higher levels of sodium intake; in hypertensive patients, the cardiovascular effects of calcium occurred regardless of sodium intake. Serum ionized calcium did not correlate with the systolic pressure response in either group, however. Diastolic pressure increased during higher dietary sodium intake when calcium was infused in the hypertensive patients. The mean arterial pressure rose significantly and independently of dietary sodium intake in the hypertensive patients during calcium infusion, but not in normal controls. The mean arterial pressure rose during calcium infusion and remained elevated even as serum calcium levels began to fall in the recovery period. Inulin and para-aminohippuric acid (PAH) clearances were similar in both groups and were not affected by dietary sodium intake. Fractional sodium excretion was similar in both groups, but fractional potassium excretion was significantly higher in normal persons. Calcium infusion did not affect inulin or PAH clearance in either group. The fractional excretion of sodium was increased by calcium infusion, but there was no effect on fractional potassium excretion. The hypertensive patients tended to have higher fractional calcium excretion, but the effect was not significant. Calcium infusion increased serum calcium and fractional calcium excretion in both groups, but reduced urinary cyclic adenosine monophosphate excretion.

Hypertensive patients excreted more cyclic adenosine monophosphate than did normal persons, even when dietary sodium and calcium intake was controlled. Alteration of dietary sodium intake altered the cardiovascular response to infused calcium, an effect that was more acute in the hypertensive group. These abnormalities of sodium and calcium handling may contribute to the pathogenesis of essential hypertension. The enhanced parathyroid activity in patients with essential hypertension may be related to increased urinary calcium excretion in this group. In addition, hypertensive patients reportedly consume less calcium than do normal persons. Increased dietary sodium can induce a state of negative calcium balance by increasing urinary calcium excretion. The short-term infusion of calcium increases blood pressure by increasing systemic vascular resistance, an effect that may be mediated by calcium. Hypertensive patients may be more sensitive to these effects of calcium than are nonhypertensive persons under certain dietary conditions. However, the acute effects of calcium on blood pressure are quite different from more prolonged exposure; dietary loading with calcium may prevent increases in blood pressure by blocking slow calcium channels and decreasing the calcium permeability of vascular smooth muscle cell membranes. Such downregulation of calcium's effect by calcium itself may be consistent with the results seen in this study. The findings are compatible with a state of relative calcium deficiency that may contribute to the enhanced calcium sensitivity seen in hypertensive patients.

▶ The role of calcium in the pathogenesis and treatment of hypertension has been the subject of numerous reports in the last 3 or 4 years. High serum levels of calcium, associated with primary hyperparathyroidism, are associated with a higher than usual prevalence of hypertension. On the other hand, McCarron and colleagues (*Science* 224:1392–1398, 1984) reported that blood pressure is inversely related to calcium intake, and that hypertensive patients on the average have lower serum calcium levels than normotensive patients. Yet, calcium channel blocking agents definitely reduce blood pressure. How can we put all this together? Klatsky et al. (Abstract 6–29) reported a positive relationship between systolic pressure and total serum calcium. Folsom et al. (Abstract 6–27) report no difference in mean levels of serum total calcium between hypertensive and normotensive persons. However, when the serum calcium was fractionated, the hypertensive patients had lower mean serum levels of ultrafiltrable calcium, ionized calcium, and complexed calcium and higher levels of protein-bound calcium than normotensive persons. Using acute infusions of calcium, Ellsion et al. (Abstract 6–28) have shown an increase in systolic blood pressure in both hypertensive and normotensive volunteers. In the hypertensive group, systolic blood pressure rose during calcium infusion irrespective of sodium intake. Diastolic pressure rose with calcium infusion only when the patients were receiving high sodium diets. In normotensive individuals systolic blood pressure rose when a high sodium diet was taken, but diastolic blood pressure did not rise irrespective of the dietary sodium. Although this reflects an interaction between calcium and sodium, it does very little to clarify the role of calcium in the genesis or treatment of hypertension.— R.W. Gifford, Jr., M.D.

Alcohol and Hypertension

The Relationships Between Alcoholic Beverage Use and Other Traits to Blood Pressure: A New Kaiser Permanente Study

Arthur L. Klatsky, Gary D. Friedman, and Mary Anne Armstrong (Kaiser Permanente Med. Care Program, Oakland)
Circulation 73:628–636, April 1986   6–29

Although an empiric link between the regular use of alcoholic beverages and the development of hypertension has been shown in numerous previous studies, a proven mechanism for this link has not been identified. A study was conducted with many controlled parameters, including adiposity, coffee or tea use, and plasma concentrations of calcium, potassium, glucose, cholesterol, and uric acid. Data were collected from approximately 80,000 persons of several races who had undergone a multiphasic health examination during a 4-year period. As part of the examination the group completed a detailed questionnaire.

Analysis of the data confirmed a positive relationship between alcohol use and elevated blood pressure (Fig 6–4). In men, whites, and persons

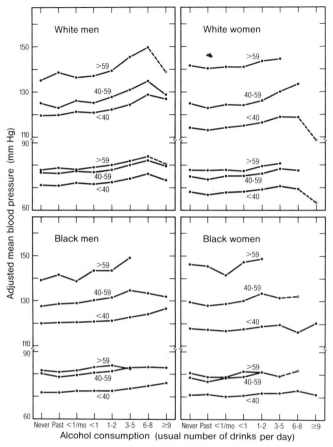

Fig 6–4.—Adjusted mean systolic and diastolic blood pressures (mm Hg) according to alcohol consumption by three age groups *(top left,* white men; *lower left,* black men; *top right,* white women; *lower right,* black women). Dashed lines and open circles indicate 10 < n < 25. Data omitted from figure for categories with n < 11 (white women aged 40–59 years, nine or more drinks/day and age > 59 years, six to eight and nine or more drinks/day; black men aged > 59 years, six to eight and nine or more drinks/day; black women aged 40–59 years, nine or more drinks/day and age > 59 years, three to five, six to eight, and nine or more drinks/day). (Courtesy of Klatsky, A.L., et al.: Circulation 73:628–636, April 1986. By permission of the American Heart Association, Inc.)

aged 55 years and older a slightly stronger relationship was observed. Among men who had several alcoholic drinks daily, a slight increase in blood pressure was noted; this increase continued steadily as drinking levels became higher. However, in women an increase in blood pressure occurred only when three or more drinks were taken daily. Only minor differences in blood pressure were associated with the various types of alcoholic beverages. Past drinking of alcoholic beverages had no relationship to blood pressure in current abstainers, supporting earlier data that alcohol-associated hypertension is totally reversible.

Smoking and drinking coffee or tea were not associated with higher blood pressure findings. There was a positive relationship between systolic pressure and the total serum calcium level, and an inverse relationship between systolic pressure and the serum potassium level. Diastolic pressure showed little relationship to these blood constituents. Alcohol-associated hypertension has substantial public health implications.

The Pressor and Metabolic Effects of Alcohol in Normotensive Subjects

John F. Potter, Robert D. S. Watson, Wendy Skan, and D. Gareth Beevers (Dudley Road Hosp., Birmingham, England)
Hypertension 8:625–631, July 1986
6–30

A clinical study was conducted in normotensive persons to examine the acute effects of alcohol and placebo on blood pressure and to assess the relationship to possible pressor mechanisms. The series included 16 male medical students, including 8 with a family history of hypertension; ages ranged from 20 to 30 years. The students, who drank up to 200 gm of alcohol per week, were studied twice, with an interval of at least 1 week between tests. All were in good health and not taking any medication at the time of the study. They were given 600 ml of either alcohol-free or alcohol-containing beer according to a double-blind, random, crossover design. Blood samples, taken prior to and for 5 hours after beer administration, were tested for plasma catecholamines, renin activity, cortisol, and calcium levels. Changes in blood pressure and pulse rate were also recorded.

Both systolic and diastolic blood pressure rose after alcohol consumption in parallel with the rise in the blood alcohol level but not with placebo ingestion. There was no significant difference in systolic and diastolic blood pressure between those who had a family history of hypertension and those who did not. Pulse rates were significantly higher after alcohol consumption in all 16 students, and they continued to go up throughout the study. No difference was noted in plasma norepinephrine or epinephrine levels between alcohol and placebo phases in those with a family history for hypertension, but significantly higher plasma norepinephrine levels were seen in those without a positive family history during both placebo and alcohol phases. Plasma renin activity were unchanged, but plasma cortisol levels fell during both phases. Alcohol ingestion appears to cause a rise in systolic and diastolic blood pressure that is unrelated to a family history of hypertension.

▶ Potter et al. (Abstract 6–30) demonstrated that acute administration of alcohol to normotensive medical students leads to a significant increase in systolic and diastolic blood pressure compared with the effect of placebo. The rise in blood pressure following alcohol ingestion was no greater in those students who had a family history of hypertension than in those who did not. Klatsky et al. (Abstract 6–29) confirmed previous findings that there is a positive relationship between the use of alcohol and elevated blood pressure. For men there was a linear relationship between the amount of alcohol consumed and the blood pressure up to the level of six to eight drinks daily. This relationship was true for women over 40 years of age.

In evaluating the hypertensive patient it is important to obtain a history of alcohol consumption. Excessive use of alcohol can make a borderline hypertensive definitely hypertensive and can be responsible for resistance to antihypertensive therapy. Reduction of alcohol consumption to less than two or three drinks a day is an important step in the nonpharmacologic treatment of hypertension. It may be as effective as weight control and perhaps more effective than sodium restriction for some patients. For patients who are already taking antihypertensive therapy, decreasing the alcohol intake may reduce the dose requirements for medication and in some cases may make it possible to eliminate pharmacologic therapy entirely.

It is interesting that in the paper by Klatsky et al. there was a positive correlation between systolic pressure and the total serum calcium level.—R.W. Gifford, Jr., M.D.

Hypertension and Obesity

The Role of Weight in the Positive Association Between Age and Blood Pressure
Wen-Harn Pan, Serafim Nanas, Alan Dyer, Kiang Liu, Arline McDonald, James A. Schoenberger, Richard B. Shekelle, Rose Stamler, and Jeremiah Stamler (Northwestern Univ., Rush Presbyterian-St. Luke's Med. Ctr., Chicago, and Univ. of Texas at Houston)
Am. J. Epidemiol. 124:612–623, October 1986   6–31

A relationship between age and blood pressure is evident in many cross-sectional and longitudinal population-based studies. However, in some preliterate societies and some subgroups in industrialized countries, this association is absent. Cross-sectional data (collected in 1967–1973) on 19,704 white men and 13,895 white women in the Chicago Heart Association Detection Project in Industry were reviewed to determine whether the association between age and blood pressure can be explained by body weight. Mean blood pressure and hypertension were studied in groups stratified by age and relative weight.

In men a positive association between age and systolic blood pressure was apparent only after ages 35–44 years in most weight groups. Similar results were obtained for women, but the age effect was seen after ages 25–34 years. A curvilinear relationship between age and systolic pressure was seen in both sexes in all relative weight groups. The relationship between age and diastolic pressure was linear for women and curvilinear for men, apparently because of the large sample size. Weight alone cannot explain the relationship between age and diastolic pressure. Age trends of hypertension were not consistent across relative weight groups.

In the absence of overweight, age and blood pressure generally are associated in persons living in the United States. There is considerable evidence that differences in life-styles (e.g., intake of sodium and physical fitness) account for apparent aging effects on blood pressure in industrialized societies.

Obesity and Hypertension: Demonstration of a "Floor Effect"

Neill Cohen and Walter Flamenbaum (Beth Israel Med. Ctr., New York)
Am. J. Med. 80:177–181, February 1986 6–32

Weight loss appears to have a role in the treatment of essential hypertension; supplemented fasting produces a hypotensive response, but it may be caused by factors other than weight loss. This study was undertaken to examine blood pressure changes in morbidly obese hypertensive patients who achieved weight reduction by supplemental fasting. The relationship between weight loss and blood pressure was studied, as well as whether absolute or relative weight change was a more accurate predictor of the hypotensive effect. Of the 129 patients, 30 were not taking medication for hypertension.

Both weight and blood pressure changed significantly in these patients during the study. After a mean of 10.6 weeks of supplemental fasting, patients went from a mean of 56.8% over ideal weight to 28.3% over ideal weight for untreated patients. Patients taking antihypertensive medication were able to reduce their number of medications from a mean of 1.9 to a mean of 0.4. Weight reduction was similar in both groups, but the patients who had not been taking medication had a 10 mm Hg greater decline in diastolic blood pressure. By the end of the fast, reductions in blood pressure in the two groups were similar, however. When realimentation was done, weight and blood pressure measurements remained constant for the untreated patients. Those taking medication had a slightly additional weight loss on realimentation, but no further change in blood pressure or number of medications. In this group, blood pressure went from 139.6/88.6 mm Hg at baseline to 127.2/81.5 mm Hg at conclusion of the fast. Analysis showed positive correlations between weight loss and reduction in blood pressure for both groups. When patients were stratified by upper and lower halves of amount of weight lost, there were no significant differences in the blood pressure reductions between the two strata for untreated patients. For treated patients, however, those who lost more weight had greater reductions in blood pressure and a slightly greater reduction in the number of medications taken.

Thus, weight loss can lead to clinically meaningful reductions in blood pressure and number of antihypertensive medications in obese persons with essential hypertension. Prior medical therapy reduced the blood pressure lowering response, but this could have been because of the fact that the group given medication was a mean of 8 years older, may have been hypertensive longer, and may have had a greater volume component than in the nonmedicated group. More weight was lost by the untreated patients also. The blood pressure declines appeared to be caused by the weight loss itself, as realimentation did not alter pressure responses. The relationship between weight loss and blood pressure is not linear; a floor effect may be present when there is a degree of weight loss beyond which further reductions in blood pressure will not occur. Therefore, because it may be difficult for morbidly obese persons to reach their ideal body weight, emphasis should be put on moderate weight reductions that may achieve the same goals with respect to blood pressure reduction.

Associations of Body Mass Index and Waist:Hip Ratio With Hypertension

Franklin M. M. White, Linda H. Pereira, and J. Barry Garner (Dalhousie Univ., Halifax)

Can. Med. Assoc. J. 135:313–320, Aug. 15, 1986   6–33

The association between relative weight and hypertension has been documented in several studies, although the correlation is low. It is important to determine the risk of hypertension associated with overweight by subgroups of age and sex. The anatomical distribution of excess weight is also a factor in determining which persons are more susceptible to hypertension. Data from the Canada Fitness Survey for persons aged 20–69 years were used to examine the relationships among age, relative weight, location of body fat, weight distribution, and hypertension in a sample of 10,724 individuals.

Diastolic hypertension was more prevalent in men than in women younger than age 50 years. Rates increased consistently with age, except for a slight decrease in men aged 60–69 years. Correlations of body mass index, waist:hip ratio, and skinfold measurements with diastolic hypertension varied with age and sex. In men, hypertension was more closely correlated with the body mass index; for women in some age groups, the subscapular skinfold measurement had the greatest correlation with hypertension. Overall, in women, the subscapular skinfold measurement was somewhat less useful as a measure of excess fat or excess weight. The sum of the five skinfold measurements gave no additional information over the subscapular measurement alone. In men there was a steady rise in the incidence of hypertension as body mass index increased; the highest prevalence was 46.1%, occurring in men 50–59 years of age with a body mass index of 28 or more. This relationship was not seen in women unless the body mass index was 35 or more. The highest prevalence rate among women, 41.7%, was for those aged 60–69 years with a body mass index of 35 or more. As the waist:hip ratio increased, so did the incidence of hypertension. The highest rates were in men aged 40–59 and women aged 40–69. The three most important factors in the development of hypertension were age, waist:hip ratio, and body mass index.

These data probably underestimate the prevalence of hypertension because those who refused participation in the study might have done so based on excess weight or ill health. Both weight and amount of body fat increase with age. Other studies corroborate the value of the subscapular skinfold measurement and show that measurements of body density are not superior to weight measurements. However, body mass index and waist:hip ratio are simpler than skinfold measurements, and provide much of the same informational and predictive value. The waist:hip ratio is a strong independent predictor, but is secondary to that of body mass index. In light of concerns about the side effects of long-term antihypertensive drug therapy, weight reduction should be considered as a treatment for hypertension. Some studies have shown that an individual does not need to reach "ideal weight" to experience the benefits of weight-reduction and blood pressure reduction. The present results suggest that in evaluating the appropriateness of weight loss as a treatment, age, sex, body mass index, and predominant location of body fat need to be taken into account.

Evidence for an Association of High Blood Pressure and Hyperinsulinemia in Obese Man

V. Manicardi, L. Camellini, G. Bellodi, C. Coscelli, and E. Ferrannini (Hosp. of Guastalla, Regional Hosp. of Parma, and Univ. of Pisa, Italy)

J. Clin. Endocrinol. Metab. 62:1302–1304, June 1986   6–34

A previous study has suggested that insulin resistance may be a common pathophysiologic factor of obesity, glucose intolerance, and hypertension. A study was conducted to determine whether obese patients with essential hypertension and normal glucose tolerance are more insulin resistant than are normotensive persons matched for age and degree of obesity.

The study included 10 women and 25 men who weighed between 25% and 75% more than desirable weight according to standard life insurance tables. All had normal glucose tolerance and were not taking any medications. Eighteen had a diastolic blood pressure of at least 95 mm Hg, and 17 were normotensive. After an overnight fast, all of the patients were given a standard oral glucose tolerance test, and plasma glucose and insulin levels were measured before, 1 hour, and 2 hours after glucose ingestion. The groups were matched for sex, age, and degree of obesity.

The mean plasma glucose levels were significantly higher in the hypertensive group than in the normotensive group. Although insulin levels were similar for both groups in the fasting state, they rose twice as high in the hypertensive as compared with the normotensive persons in response to glucose ingestion. However, glucose levels also increased to higher levels in the hypertensive group, indicating more severe insulin resistance. There was a strong positive correlation between systolic blood pressure and the 2-hour plasma insulin level in the hypertensive group, but not in the normotensive group. In obese persons, hypertension is also accompanied by hyperinsulinemia and insulin resistance, but these parameters are independent of impaired glucose tolerance.

▶ The evidence is overwhelming that obese persons have higher blood pressure and a higher prevalence of hypertension than do nonobese individuals. There is equally good evidence that weight reduction of 20 lb or more in obese patients with hypertension will lead to a decrease in blood pressure, although not necessarily to normal. In fact, weight reduction for obese patients is a more reliable and consistent method of reducing blood pressure than is sodium restriction.

In so-called low blood pressure populations, blood pressure does not rise with age, but neither does body weight, whereas in the industrialized acculturated societies weight and blood pressure both increase with age. The question then arises: Does blood pressure not rise with age because weight does not rise with age, or are there other factors? The paper by Pan et al. (Abstract 6–31) addresses this issue. At least in the United States, blood pressure tends to rise with age even when body weight is normal.

In the paper by Cohen and Flamenbaum (Abstract 6–32), weight reduction reduced blood pressure significantly for morbidly obese hypertensive patients whether or not they were taking medication. However, the relationship between weight loss and blood pressure was not linear. Among patients who were not receiving antihypertensive medications, those who lost an average of 68.1 lb had blood pressures similar to those who lost only 28.3 lb. In patients taking antihypertensive medication, the group that lost more than 40 lb had a 7.3-mm Hg greater decrease in systolic pressure and a 5.6-mm Hg greater decrease in diastolic blood pressure than those who lost less than 40 lb. This suggests a "floor effect," implying that it isn't necessary to achieve ideal body weight to achieve a significant reduction in blood pressure as a result of obesity control.

The paper by White et al. (Abstract 6–33) indicates that body mass index is the best independent predictor of hypertension, followed closely by the waist:hip ratio. Either is a better predictor than are skinfold measurements.

Manicardi et al. (Abstract 6–34) report that obese hypertensive persons have higher plasma insulin levels following a glucose load than do obese normotensive persons. Although both the normotensive and hypertensive groups had normal glucose tolerance tests, the plasma glucose level was statistically significantly higher after an oral glucose load in the hypertensive than in the normotensive group, indicating insulin resistance. There was a statistically significant correlation between the 2-hour plasma insulin level and systolic blood pressure in the hypertensive patients but not in the normotensive group. It thus appears that there is some association between insulin resistance and hypertension in obese patients even when glucose tolerance is normal. It would be interesting to observe whether insulin resistance disappears with significant weight reduction.

Whereas calorie restriction is an attractive alternative to drug therapy for obese hypertensive patients, the limiting factor is adherence. Many patients will lose weight initially if they are highly motivated, but few will maintain the weight reduction for more than a year or two.—R.W. Gifford, Jr., M.D.

Hypertension in the Elderly

Efficacy of Antihypertensive Drug Treatment According to Age, Sex, Blood Pressure, and Previous Cardiovascular Disease in Patients Over the Age of 60

A. Amery, W. Birkenhäger, R. Brixko, C. Bulpitt, D. Clement, M. Deruyttere, A. De Schaepdryver, C. Dollery, R. Fagard, F. Forette, J. Forte, R. Hamdy, J. F. Henry, J. V. Joossens, G. Leonetti, P. Lund-Johansen, K. O'Malley, J. C. Petrie, T. Strasser, J. Tuomilehto, and B. Williams (European Working Party on High Blood Pressure in the Elderly)
Lancet 2:589–592, Sept. 13, 1986   6–35

Previous trials have suggested that antihypertensive measures may be less helpful in women. The findings of the European Working Party on High Blood Pressure in the Elderly that were reported in 1985 were analyzed in relation to age, sex, blood pressure, and previous cardiovascular disease. In this study, a total of 840 patients aged 60 years and older who had initial sitting blood pressures of 160–239/90–119 mm Hg received hydrochlorothiazide plus triamterene or a matching placebo. Methyldopa was added to the active regimen if the blood pressure remained elevated.

Cardiovascular mortality increased with advancing age and with increasing systolic blood pressure at presentation, but not with increasing diastolic pressure. Treatment was effective after adjusting for age, sex, cardiovascular complications, and systolic and diastolic pressures at randomization. Reductions in mortality were more marked in men than in women, but were similar in patients with and those without cardiovascular complications at randomization. Effects of treatment may have declined with advancing age. Little benefit was apparent in persons who were older than age 80 years, most of whom were women.

Antihypertensive drug therapy was effective in this trial regardless of the presenting blood pressure or the presence or absence of cardiovascular complications. Benefit was most evident in those at highest risk, including men and patients who had cardiovascular complications at randomization.

Systolic Hypertension in the Elderly Program (SHEP): Antihypertensive Efficacy of Chlorthalidone
Stephen B. Hulley, Curt D. Furberg, Barry Gurland, Robert McDonald, H. Mitchell Perry, Harold W. Schnaper, James A. Schoenberger, W. McFate Smith, and Thomas M. Vogt (SHEP Res. Group, San Francisco Gen. Hosp. and various other medical institutions in the United States)
Am. J. Cardiol. 56:913–920, Dec. 1, 1985   6–36

Although the 1984 report from the Joint National Committee on the Detection, Evaluation and Treatment of High Blood Pressure issued a comprehensive set of policy guidelines on the management of diastolic hypertension, it has not been established whether isolated systolic hypertension should also be treated with drugs. If so, the question is whether such treatment is safe, and whether it will prevent some or all of the twofold to threefold excess risk of cardiovascular mortality associated with isolated systolic hypertension. This question was the subject of the Systolic Hypertension in the Elderly Program.

The study included 551 men and women older than 60 years with isolated systolic hypertension who were randomly assigned in double-blind fashion to receive daily either one capsule of 25 mg of chlorthalidone (443 persons) or matching placebo (108). A patient who did not respond adequately to this step-one drug after 4 weeks was first given two capsules of chlorthalidone daily for another 8 weeks, and was given step-two drugs or placebo if the desired systolic blood pressure was still not attained. The step-two drugs consisted of twice-daily administration by random assignment of 0.05 mg of reserpine, 50 mg of metoprolol, 25 mg of hydralazine, or matching placebo.

The mean systolic blood pressure in the chlorthalidone group decreased from 172 mm Hg to 146 mm Hg during the first month of treatment, with a small further decline during the year of follow-up. At the 1-year follow-up visit, 83% of the chlorthalidone group and 80% of the placebo group were still taking their medications as prescribed. At that time, 88% of those still taking chlorthalidone had reached desired blood pressure levels without the need for progression to a step-two drug, and most had responded to the 25 mg/day dose. Statistical analysis showed no major differences in blood pressure response in various age, race, and sex subgroups. Side effects consisted mostly of asymptomatic lowering of serum potassium levels and increased serum uric acid and creatinine levels. Chlorthalidone is safe and effective in lowering the blood pressure in elderly patients with systolic hypertension.

Dissociation of 24-Hour Catecholamine Levels From Blood Pressure in Older Men

Naftali Stern, Elizabeth Beahm, Dennis McGinty, Peter Eggena, Michael Littner, Michael Nyby, Robert Catania, and James R. Sowers (Univ. of California at Los Angeles)
Hypertension 7:1023–1029, November–December 1985   6–37

Aging is associated with a gradual increase in plasma norepinephrine levels as well as with a tendency for rising blood pressure. Although increased sympathetic outflow has been implicated in the induction of early "neurogenic" essential hypertension, the age-dependent increase in norepinephrine is observed in normotensive persons. However, it is not known whether the observed increment in circulating norepinephrine is related to the age-associated rise in blood pressure or to the increased incidence of hypertension in aging human beings. The state of plasma norepinephrine, epinephrine, and dopamine levels was examined in older hypertensive and normotensive men.

The study population consisted of 25 men older than age 55 years, 12 of whom had essential hypertension; the other 13 were age-matched normotensive controls. Blood samples were obtained at bihourly intervals from 9:00 AM to 10:00 PM, and every 30 minutes from 10:00 PM to 9:00 AM. Sleep and breathing were monitored continuously. Both groups displayed a circadian rhythm of plasma epinephrine levels but not plasma norepinephrine or dopamine levels. During the 24-hour cycle, the plasma epinephrine level, but not the norepinephrine or dopamine levels, was positively related to mean arterial blood pressure. The mean 24-hour plasma norepinephrine level was 377 pg/ml in hypertensive persons vs. 455 pg/ml in the controls; the mean epinephrine level was 34 pg/ml in the hypertensive group vs. 45 pg/ml in controls; the dopamine level was 40 pg/ml in the hypertensive group vs. 62 pg/ml in the normotensive controls. Although the catecholamine levels were lower in the hypertensive group, the two groups did not differ in parameters known to affect catecholamine secretion, e.g., body weight, sodium intake, sleep efficiency, or sleep-related breathing disorders. The mean 24-hour plasma norepinephrine level was inversely related to the 24-hour mean arterial blood pressure.

High norepinephrine levels in the elderly may reflect decreased baroreceptor sensitivity as well as a compensatory response to decreased β-adrenergic receptor sensitivity. However, it is not known why elderly hypertensive persons, unlike younger hypertensive persons, have lower plasma catecholamine levels than do elderly normotensive persons.

▶ Hypertension in the elderly is receiving increasing attention because the above-65 age group is the fastest growing segment of our population and 60% of patients aged 65–74 years have hypertension (Working Group on Hypertension in the Elderly: *JAMA* 256:70–74, 1986).

The report by Amery et al. (Abstract 6–35) concerning the European Working Party on High Blood Pressure in the Elderly (EWPHE) trial is a sequel to their first publication (*Lancet* 1:1349–1354, 1985), which showed a reduction in cardiovascular mortality in elderly patients receiving a diuretic compared with those given placebo in a single-blind trial. This is one of the few controlled clinical trials that showed a significant decrease in mortality from myocardial infarction. It is interesting that cardiovascular mortality and the cardiovascular study-terminating events were significantly related to systolic but not diastolic blood pressure. Moreover, the beneficial effect of treatment was not observed in the small group of patients over age 80 years when the trial started.

It should be noted that all elderly patients in the EWPHE trial had diastolic blood pressures of 90 mm Hg or more at entry; other trials have also shown that elderly patients with diastolic blood pressures of 90 mm Hg or more benefit from antihypertensive therapy (Management Committee of the National Heart Foundation of Australia: *Med. J. Aust.* 2:398–402, 1981; Hypertension Detection and Follow-up Program Cooperative Group: *JAMA* 242:2572–2577, 1979). There is still no evidence from controlled trials that treatment of isolated systolic hypertension (systolic blood pressure of at least 160 mm Hg, diastolic blood pressure of less than 90 mm Hg) in the elderly will reduce cardiovascular morbidity and mortality. The Systolic Hypertension in the Elderly Program is a double-blind, placebo-controlled trial sponsored by the National Heart, Lung, and Blood Institute and the Institute of Aging. This trial is just getting underway and data on morbidity and mortality cannot be expected for several years. In a feasibility trial that lasted for 1 year, reported by Hulley et al. (Abstract 6–36), chlorthalidone was significantly more effective than placebo in reducing systolic blood pressure in elderly patients with isolated systolic hypertension. Symptomatic side effects were no more frequent in those receiving chlorthalidone than in those receiving placebo. In this short trial, morbidity and mortality data were too meager to draw any conclusions regarding the beneficial effect of treatment.

The study by Stern et al. (Abstract 6–37) is interesting because it showed that in men older than 55 years of age, plasma norepinephrine is not related to mean arterial blood pressure. In fact, normotensive men in this age group had significantly higher plasma norepinephrine levels than did hypertensive men. This would suggest that the sympathetic nervous system does not play a key role in the pathogenesis of hypertension in older men, and therefore that adrenergic inhibiting agents might not be effective in managing hypertension in this age group. Although it is true that β blockers do not seem to be as effective in treating hypertension in elderly patients as they are in younger patients, our clinical experience would indicate that when given with a diuretic, methyldopa or clonidine is usually effective in elderly patients.—R.W. Gifford, Jr., M.D.

A Regimen for Resistant Hypertension

Minoxidil, Nadolol, and a Diuretic: Once-A-Day Therapy for Resistant Hypertension
Samuel Spitalewitz, Jerome G. Porush, and Ira W. Reiser (Brookdale Hosp. Med. Ctr., Brooklyn)
Arch. Intern. Med. 146:882–886, May 1986   6–38

Poor patient compliance is a common cause of inadequate blood pressure control in hypertensive patients. A once-a-day antihypertensive regimen was tested for its effectiveness and side effects in 55 patients aged 27–77 years who had resistant hypertension. Included were 47 patients with evidence of end-organ damage and 12 with mild renal insufficiency. Forty-six patients were given nadolol with chlorthalidone or furosemide once daily. In 34 patients blood pressure control was not achieved after 4 weeks, and minoxidil was added to the regimen. The other patients were given a combination of nadolol, a diuretic, and minoxidil because of the severity of their initial blood pressure elevation. Compliance was assessed by counting left-over pills at each visit.

At the time of follow-up, blood pressure control had been achieved in 46 of 55 patients (84%). In the other nine (16%), blood pressure remained elevated and could not be controlled with the triple-drug regimen. At a later follow-up, blood pressure remained controlled in all 46 patients, but 6 had to discontinue treatment with this regimen because of severe side effects. Only relatively infrequent and mild side effects were noted in the other 40 patients. The regimen was therapeutically successful in 40 of 55 patients, for an overall success rate of 73%.

▶ It is not surprising that a combination of a diuretic, nadolol, and minoxidil would be effective in patients with previously resistant hypertension, because this is a very potent combination. What is surprising is that blood pressure control was accomplished in 84% of these patients on a once-a-day regimen. Except for six patients who had to discontinue treatment because of side effects, the regimen remained effective during a follow-up of 43 ±5 weeks. This is a rational regimen for patients with resistant hypertension.—R.W. Gifford, Jr., M.D.

Ketanserin

Ketanserin and Prazosin: A Comparison of Antihypertensive and Biochemical Effects
G. S. Stokes, B. A. Mennie, and J. F. Marwood (Sydney Hosp., and Royal North Shore Hosp., Sydney)
Clin. Pharmacol. Ther. 40:56–63, July 1986   6–39

The mechanism of antihypertensive action of the serotonin receptor antagonist ketanserin is unknown. To compare ketanserin with the α_1-adrenoceptor blocker prazosin, equidepressant doses of these two drugs were used to treat 16 patients who had mild to moderate essential hypertension. The ten men and six women were aged 28–58 years and had initial standing diastolic blood pressures of 92–111 mm Hg. A randomized crossover design was used, with two 4-week periods of active treatment. Prazosin was given in an initial dosage of 2 mg daily and a peak dosage of 4 mg daily. The dosage of ketanserin was begun at 40 mg daily and was raised to 80 mg daily when the diastolic pressure remained above 90 mm Hg.

Supine blood pressure was satisfactorily controlled in 9 of 12 patients who completed the prazosin phase of the study and in 11 of 15 who completed the ketanserin phase. Pressure responses to the drugs were similar. Neither drug significantly altered the pulse rate, body weight, plasma renin activity, urinary excretion of aldosterone, or serum concentration of triglycerides. The serum level of cholesterol was lowered only by prazosin. Side effects were similar with the two drugs, but three patients withdrew during the prazosin phase.

Ketanserin is a useful drug in treating mild to moderate essential hypertension. Neither drug altered plasma renin activity in the present series, and urinary excretion of aldosterone also was unchanged.

▶ The similar effect of these two drugs on blood pressure without affecting heart rate, plasma renin activity, urinary excretion of aldosterone, or body weight does not necessarily prove that they should have the same mechanism of antihypertensive action. Ketanserin is an investigational drug that has anti-serotonin properties, whereas prazosin is a well-known selective α_1 blocking agent. Nevertheless, as the authors point out, α_1 adrenoreceptors and 5-HT$_2$ receptors have been reported to overlap in vascular smooth muscle cells. Hemodynamic studies with prazosin indicate that it reduces blood pressure by reducing systemic vascular resistance without changing cardiac output, whereas at least one study with ketanserin indicated that it reduced blood pressure by decreasing cardiac output without a change in systemic vascular resistance (Omvik, P., et al.: *J. Hypertension* 1:405–412, 1983).—R.W. Gifford, Jr., M.D.

Nonsteroidal Anti-inflammatory Drugs

Prostaglandin E$_2$ but not I$_2$ Restores Furosemide Response in Indomethacin-Treated Rats

Kent A. Kirchner, Chris J. Martin, and John D. Bower (Univ. of Mississippi)
Am. J. Physiol. 250:F980–F985, June 1986   6–40

Indomethacin can blunt the natriuretic, chloruretic, and diuretic response to furosemide. The mechanism involved is thought to be inhibition of the furosemide-induced activation of the renal prostaglandin system because other prostaglandin inhibitors have much the same effect as in-

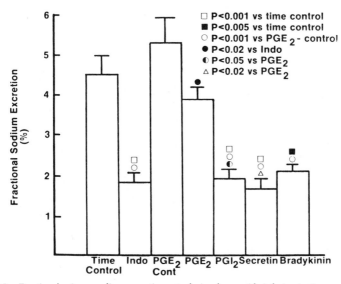

Fig 6–5.—Fractional urinary sodium excretion rate during furosemide infusion in time-control, prostaglandin (PG) E_2-control, and indomethacin (Indo)-treated rats during intra-aortic infusions of PGE_2, PGI_2, secretin, bradykinin, or vehicle for their administration (Indo control). (Courtesy of Kirchner, K.A., et al.: Am. J. Physiol. 250:F980–F985, June 1986.)

domethacin. The drug has other pharmacologic actions that might cause such an effect, however, which has led some investigators to question this proposed mechanism. The effects of intraaortic infusions of prostaglandin E_2 (PGE_2), prostaglandin I_2 (PGI_2), or the vasodilators secreton and bradykinin were examined in rats with respect to their effects on the furosemide response in indomethacin-treated animals. If indomethacin's anticyclooxygenase effect is responsible for the blunting of furosemide's effect, prostaglandin infusion should restore the response in indomethacin-treated animals.

As shown in Figure 6–5, both absolute and fractional sodium excretion rates produced by furosemide were less in indomethacin-treated rats than in controls. Infusion of PGE_2 restored absolute and fractional sodium excretion rates after furosemide to levels similar to those in controls and greater than those seen in rats receiving indomethacin alone. Infusion of PGE_2 alone did not potentiate the furosemide response, however. The PGI_2 had no effect on the indomethacin-blunted furosemide response in rats, nor did bradykinin or secretin have any effect, although the latter did lower renal vascular resistance. The prostaglandins did not alter inulin clearance, the serum sodium level, or mean arterial pressure.

The mechanism behind PGE's restoration of indomethacin-blunted furosemide responses is not the result of a synergistic natriuretic effect, as they are limited to indomethacin-treated rats. Others have hypothesized that indomethacin inhibits prostaglandin-mediated changes in renal hemodynamics. In this scenario, PGE_2 could maintain furosemide's potency by counteracting the indomethacin effect. Alternatively, the slightly greater renal blood flow in indomethacin and PGE$_2$-treated rats might account for the failure of indomethacin to attenuate furosemide's effects. This possibility is unlikely because rats treated with PGI$_2$ and secretin also had increased renal blood flows, but the furosemide effect was not restored. The data suggest that PGE$_2$ restores furosemide's effects through mechanisms other than alterations in renal hemodynamics. The PGE$_2$ can inhibit sodium chloride reabsorption in the loop of Henle and the collecting tubule, and could restore the furosemide effect in this manner. It does not appear that restoration of furosemide activity is caused by increased delivery of the drug to its active site. Although the doses of prostaglandins used in this study were pharmacologic and not physiologic, it does appear as if the effect of PGE$_2$ infusion is to counteract the prostaglandin synthesis inhibition produced by indomethacin. The restoration of the furosemide natriuretic response seems to be independent of renal vasodilatation, as well.

▶ It is a frequently described clinical observation that administration of nonsteroidal anti-inflammatory drugs (NSAIDs) will counteract the antihypertensive effect of most antihypertensive drugs and will decrease the effectiveness of diuretics. This study lends credence to the theory that the cause of this interaction, at least with diuretics, is because of inhibition of secretion of the vasodilating prostaglandin PGE$_2$. In my experience, some NSAIDs are more likely to interact with diuretics and antihypertensive agents than are others. Indomethacin, ibuprofen, and piroxicam are more likely than the others to have this effect. Sulindac is least likely to cause problems with antihypertensive drugs and diuretics.—R.W. Gifford, Jr., M.D.

Prognostic Importance of the Echocardiogram

Value of Echocardiographic Measurement of Left Ventricular Mass in Predicting Cardiovascular Morbid Events in Hypertensive Men

Paul N. Casale, Richard B. Devereux, Mark Milner, Gerardo Zullo, Gregory A. Harshfield, Thomas G. Pickering, and John H. Laragh (New York Hosp.–Cornell Med. Ctr.)

Ann. Intern. Med. 105:173–178, August 1986   6–41

Echocardiography of left ventricular (LV) mass is a much more sensitive tool in assessment of ventricular hypertrophy than in ECG or chest radiography; consequently, it is suggested that echocardiography could be a useful predictor of increased risk for morbidity and mortality in hypertensive patients. This theory was tested in 140 males aged 17–68 years with borderline or established essential hypertension; all had undergone echocardiography as part of their first evaluation. Initial findings included normal LV mass measurements in 111 patients and hypertrophy in 29 patients. All were contacted after a mean of 4.8 years and evaluated again by echocardiography, as well as for current blood pressure and other clinical characteristics.

Follow-up visits showed that of the 111 males with a normal LV mass, 7 (6%) had experienced morbid events including death, myocardial infarction, stroke, and coronary bypass surgery. Of the 29 males with LV hypertrophy, 7 (24%) experienced similar morbid events. In males with mild, uncomplicated hypertension, echocardiography is useful in the detection of patients at high risk for cardiovascular morbid events.

▶ Data from Framingham have shown that ECG evidence of LV hypertrophy (LVH), especially when there are accompanying ST-T changes, has an ominous prognostic significance in hypertensive patients. No such data have previously been reported with respect to echocardiographic evidence of LVH, which can be found before there is ECG evidence of it. This paper by Casale et al. clearly demonstrates that, even in the absence of ECG-LVH, echocardiographic evidence of LVH carries an ominous prognosis with regard to cardiovascular morbid events. Of the seven men with echocardiographic evidence of increased LV mass who had morbid events, only two had ECG-LVH by the Cornell voltage criteria. This evidence supports the contention that the echocardiogram should be part of the routine evaluation of the hypertensive patient. This would be cost effective only if it could be shown either that medical management should be altered in patients with echocardiographic evidence of LVH so that it would reduce mortality, or that some patients without echocardiographic evidence of LVH could be safely managed nonpharmacologically, or both.—R.W. Gifford, Jr., M.D.

The Role of the Sympathetic Nervous System

Cardiac Mass in Glucocorticoid-Hypertensive Rats With and Without Circulating Adrenaline

James F. Burris, Bernard Waeber, and Hans R. Brunner (Centre Hospitalier Universitaire, Lausanne, Switzerland)
Cardiovasc. Res. 19:734–736, December 1985   6–42

Although sustained arterial hypertension often results in the genesis of myocardial hypertrophy, there is evidence that β-adrenoceptor stimulation by catecholamines can play a trophic role in the process. An experimental study was conducted in Wistar rats with glucocorticoid-induced hypertension to compare cardiac mass in the absence of circulating epinephrine with cardiac mass in equally hypertensive rats able to release epinephrine normally. The 29 adrenalectomized Wistar rats and 31 sham-operated controls had initial weights of approximately 250 gm. The adrenalectomized rats were made hypertensive with methylprednisolone. Experiments were done within 12–16 days after initial surgery.

There was no significant difference between the two groups in intra-arterial mean blood pressure, heart rate, or body weight. Although the heart weight in adrenalectomized rats was significantly lower than in the sham-operated rats, the heart weight to body weight ratio was comparable. The presence or absence of circulating epinephrine apparently does not significantly affect regulation of cardiac mass in rats with glucocorticoid-induced hypertension.

▶ The differing effects of antihypertensive agents on preventing or reversing left ventricular hypertrophy (LVH) have received considerable attention recently. It was thought originally that only sympatholytic agents (methyldopa, β blockers) reversed LVH, whereas nonsympatholytic agents (diuretics, hydralazine, minoxidil) did not. The implication is that sympathetic activity does indeed have a role in the development of cardiac hypertrophy, although this thesis was not supported by the findings in the above report. Now it has been shown that calcium channel blockers and converting enzyme inhibitors, neither of which inhibit the sympathetic nervous system, also prevent or reverse LVH. In my opinion, however, this study does not rule out the possibility of a relationship between the sympathetic nervous system and cardiac hypertrophy.—R.W. Gifford, Jr., M.D.

Blood Pressure and Catecholamines Following Exercise During Selective Beta-Blockade in Hypertension
R. Vandongen, B. Margetts, L. J. Beilin, N. deKlerk, and P. Rogers (Univ. of Western Australia, Perth, and Royal Perth Hosp., Australia)
Eur. J. Clin. Pharmacol. 30:283–287, May 1986   6–43

The effects of β-blocking drugs on plasma epinephrine and norepinephrine are important considering the varied properties of the many β blockers on the market. Some are cardioselective and others are nonselective. If peripheral β-receptors are blocked, exercise-induced sympathetic stimulation may cause a pressor effect by stimulation of unopposed α-receptors. Despite this theoretical prediction, several studies have failed to show an advantage of cardioselective agents over nonselective drugs in this respect. Therefore, the effects of equipotent doses of metoprolol and propranolol were compared during cardiovascular responses to exercise in 13 patients with essential hypertension. Plasma norepinephrine and epinephrine concentrations were also measured. Propranolol, 80 mg or 160 mg, or metoprolol, 100 mg or 200 mg, was given twice daily for 2 weeks each; a third group of patients received placebo on the same dose schedule. Patients were then crossed over to the other treatments. Exercise was by bicycle ergometer.

Immediately after exercise, the systolic blood pressure and heart rate increased to the same extent in both drug groups. Diastolic pressure in the metoprolol group did not change, and it rose in the propranolol-treated group. Thus, the change in systolic and diastolic blood pressure immediately and 20 minutes after exercise was consistently smaller during metoprolol treatment. The differences were particularly notable at 20 minutes after exercise. The plasma norepinephrine and epinephrine levels both increased after exercise and returned to baseline levels at 20 minutes. The levels of these compounds were higher during propranolol and metoprolol treatment, compared with placebo. There were no differences between the two drugs in these parameters.

Thus, both the plasma norepinephrine level and epinephrine release are enhanced by β-blockers after exercise. Further, the effect does not appear to be related to cardioselectivity, as similar increases occurred with both propranolol and metoprolol. The mechanism for this increase may be related to a fall in cardiac output, altering blood flow to the liver and lungs, and decreasing norepinephrine and epinephrine elimination. The value of a selective β-blocker is seen by the blunted response to these catecholamine levels during metoprolol treatment as opposed to propranolol treatment. Other studies have shown conflicting results, but this may be because of methodological differences. The balance between dilator and constrictor activities is likely to be important when sympathoadrenal activity is stimulated, e.g., during exercise. With cardioselective agents, β_2 adrenoceptors in the periphery are stimulated and oppose the vasoconstrictor effects of norepinephrine. This may be an important consideration when treating the active hypertensive patient.

▶ Vandongen et al. have demonstrated that blood pressure rises less during bicycle exercise in patients with essential hypertension being treated with the cardioselective β blocker metoprolol than it does during treatment with the noncardioselective β blocker propranolol. However, the rise in blood pressure with exercise was less for propranolol than it was for placebo. Plasma epinephrine and norepinephrine levels increased during exercise more for patients receiving either of the β blockers than for those receiving placebo. Presumably, cardioselective β blockers interfere less with vasodilating β_2 receptors in peripheral arterioles than do nonselective β blockers, and therefore vasoconstriction from α receptors is less likely to be unopposed when the sympathetic nervous system is stimulated by exercise.—R.W. Gifford, Jr., M.D.

Function of the Autonomic Nervous System in Young, Untreated Hypertensive Patients
W. Schütz, H. Hörtnagl, and D. Magometschnigg (Univ. of Vienna)
Int. J. Cardiol. 10:133–140, February 1986   6–44

The role of the sympathetic nervous system in essential hypertension is not known. The literature provides evidence that plasma catecholamine levels are increased in essential hypertension in only a defined subgroup of young patients with established hypertension. In addition, there reportedly is an increased basal sympathetic tone associated with increased sympathetic reactivity. Reactivity of the sympathetic nervous system to various stimuli can be used as an additional parameter for classification of essential hypertension. This hypothesis was tested in ten asymptomatic, ambulatory men aged 24–35 years with labile hypertension. Reactivity of the sympathetic nervous system was studied in these patients and the findings compared with those in a normotensive age-matched control group.

On graded exercise on a constant-speed bicycle ergometer, the hypertensive patients reacted with an exaggerated blood pressure response and a significantly greater elevation in plasma epinephrine and epinephrine levels. In contrast, basal catecholamine levels were similar in both groups despite an intact baroreceptor reflex in the hypertensive group, as indicated by a normal hemodynamic response to angiotensin II. This apparent discrepancy may be explained by an enhanced uptake of epinephrine during stress into the neuron, where it acts as a cotransmitter and facilitates the release of norepinephrine via presynaptic β_2 adrenoceptors. In addition, similar blood pressure and heart rate responses to isoproterenol and atropine were found for both groups. Thus, hypertensive patients have normal β adrenoceptor sensitivity and vagal nerve activity.

Young adult patients with labile hypertension can be differentiated from normotensive, age-matched controls by testing the reactivity of the sympathetic nervous system to graded exercise. These results support the "epinephrine hypothesis" of essential hypertension.

▶ In this group of young men with labile hypertension, resting catecholamine levels were similar to those observed in a normotensive age-matched control group. However, after exercise on a bicycle ergometer, the hypertensive patients had an exaggerated blood pressure response and a significantly greater elevation in plasma catecholamine activity than did the controls. It would appear that young hypertensive or prehypertensive individuals have a hyperresponsive sympathetic nervous system to exercise, cold pressor test, or mental arithmetic. More longitudinal studies are needed to determine whether, indeed, this trait is a reliable predictor of the ultimate development of hypertension.—R.W. Gifford, Jr., M.D.

Blood Pressure Response to Exercise as a Predictor of Hypertension
Jochanan Benbassat and Paul Froom (Hadassah Univ., Jerusalem)
Arch. Intern. Med. 146:2053–2055, October 1986   6–45

Variable responses of blood pressure to exercise may reflect the heterogeneity of the populations studied and a lack of standardization of the protocols for exercise testing as well as differing definitions of "response." It is possible, however, that the blood pressure response to exercise may be a better predictor of hypertension than is the resting blood pressure. Review was made of 11 English-language articles concerning the blood pressure response to exercise.

These reports suggested a 10% to 61% incidence of hypertensive responses to exercise in currently normotensive persons and a 10% to 49% incidence of normotensive responses in currently hypertensive individuals. In most studies the sensitivity of a hypertensive response for future hypertension was 16% to 46%, and the specificity was 87% to 95%.

These findings do not justify routine exercise testing for screening purposes in view of the relatively low prevalence of hypertension that was anticipated in young adults during the following years. The use of exercise testing to predict hypertension remains in need of experimental development and validation. Exercise protocols must be rigidly standardized. The cutoff point should be defined according to age, sex, and physical fitness. The effects of repeated testing of the same patients must be considered.

Controlled longitudinal studies are needed to determine the prognostic significance of abnormal blood pressure responses to exercise.

▶ Benbassat and Froom have reviewed the literature with regard to blood pressure response to exercise as a predictor of future hypertension and concluded that, because of the low anticipated prevalence of hypertension in young adults, routine exercise testing for screening purposes cannot be justified.— R.W. Gifford, Jr., M.D.

Diuretic Treatment Alters Clonidine Suppression of Plasma Norepinephrine
Thomas P. Hui, Lawrence R. Krakoff, Katherine Felton, and Karen Yeager (City Univ. of New York)
Hypertension 8:272–276, April 1986   6–46

The combination of clonidine and a diuretic in the treatment of hypertension results in a greater reduction in arterial pressure than when either drug is administered alone. It is thought that clonidine inhibits sympathetic tone to a higher degree by acting on central α_2-adrenergic receptors in patients who are treated with diuretics. This hypothesis was tested in five men and three women with mild essential hypertension who were given a combination of 50 mg of hydrochlorothiazide and 5 mg of amiloride once daily. Potassium supplements or other medications were not permitted. The patients were monitored for serum electrolyte levels and urine sodium and potassium excretion. A single oral dose of 0.3 mg of clonidine was given before and after 1 week of diuretic therapy. Mean arterial pressure, heart rate, plasma norepinephrine and epinephrine levels, and plasma renin activity were measured before and after clonidine suppression studies.

Significant weight loss, increased plasma renin activity, and reduced serum sodium, potassium, and chloride levels were noted with diuretic treatment. Urinary sodium excretion was unchanged, but potassium excretion was increased significantly. An absolute reduction in the mean arterial pressure caused by clonidine was not significantly altered by diuretic treatment, but the absolute clonidine-induced reduction in plasma renin activity was three times greater after diuretic treatment than before. Clonidine reduced norepinephrine levels significantly before, but not after, diuretic treatment. This difference from prediuretic changes was significant. Epinephrine levels were not altered significantly by diuretic or clonidine therapy. Diuretic treatment alters the clonidine-activated mechanism for reduction of arterial pressure by means of a shift from overall suppression of sympathetic tone to pathways more restricted to renal tone.

▶ The failure of a single oral dose of clonidine to suppress the plasma norepinephrine concentration after 1 week of diuretic therapy implies that the mechanism of action of the hypotensive response observed after diuretic therapy may be related more to a reduction in plasma renin activity than to overall suppression of the sympathetic nervous system. The authors correctly suggest that diuretic therapy might produce a false positive response when the clonidine suppression test is used to diagnose pheochromocytoma. Failure of the plasma norepinephrine level to fall after a single dose of clonidine would suggest the presence of a pheochromocytoma (Bravo et al.: *N. Engl. J. Med.* 305:623–626, 1981). Dr. Bravo and I have not observed this in our experience, and so far as I know there have been no reports of false positive responses to clonidine suppression from diuretic therapy. Nevertheless, clinicians should be aware of this possibility. It is surprising, at least to me, that prior diuretic administration did not alter the overall magnitude of the effect of clonidine on arterial pressure.—R.W. Gifford, Jr., M.D.

Community Control of Hypertension

Hypertension Control in Two Canadian Communities: Evidence for Better Treatment and Overlabelling

N. J. Birkett, C. E. Evans, R. B. Haynes, D. W. Taylor, D. L. Sackett, J. R. Gilbert, M. E. Johnston, S. A. Hewson, and L. A. Macdonald (McMaster Univ., Hamilton, Ontario)
J. Hypertension 4:369–374, June 1986   6–47

Blood pressure screening based on a single measurement might yield overestimated incidence rates of undetected hypertension because such data do not reflect the fact that the blood pressure tends to fall below initially elevated levels, nor do they reflect the clinical diagnostic approach of assessments over several visits, as applied by local family physicians. The prevalence and control of hypertension were surveyed in two Canadian cities that do not have university medical centers to learn whether local physicians are as effective at diagnosing and treating hypertension as mass screening programs initiated by university medical centers.

The survey was conducted for a 5-month period in two cities in southern Ontario located about 30 km from the nearest university medical center. In all, 6,258 adult residents between ages 30–69 years were included. Permanent residents of institutions were excluded. Home visits included an interview and blood pressure screening. Persons with untreated hypertension were followed up once or twice. Hypertension was defined as diastolic blood pressure of at least 90 mm Hg.

The survey identified 708 persons with hypertension, for a prevalence of 114/1,000, including 6% with undetected hypertension, 6% with detected but untreated hypertension, 17% with treated but uncontrolled hypertension, and 70% with treated and controlled hypertension. Blood pressure control was better among women and older persons. However, 143 of 1,000 persons who reported having been given a diagnosis of hypertension were in fact normotensive without medication. The rates of control found in this study show that family physicians can effectively detect and treat hypertension, but that they have a tendency to overlabel.

▶ The findings suggest that physicians may be telling patients that they have hypertension on the basis of one office visit. Fourteen percent of the population sample surveyed had been told that they had high blood pressure, but were actually normotensive without medication. It is impossible to determine how many of the 70% whose hypertension was treated and controlled might not have required treatment if blood pressure had been measured a sufficient number of times before making the determination to use pharmacologic therapy. The fact that only 12.6% of hypertensives were undetected, or detected and untreated, indicates that family physicians are doing a better job than they did 15 years ago when it was determined that 50% of the hypertensives were undetected and 25% were detected but untreated.—R.W. Gifford, Jr., M.D.

Psychological Factors

Anger-Coping Types, Blood Pressure, and All-Cause Mortality: A Follow-up in Tecumseh, Michigan (1971–1983)

Mara Julius, Ernest Harburg, Eric M. Cottington, and Ernest H. Johnson (Univ. of Michigan and Allegheny-Singer Res. Inst., Pittsburgh)
Am. J. Epidemiol. 124:220–233, August 1986   6–48

The suspicion exists that there is a relationship between anger-hostility behavior and cardiovascular disorders; this may be the underpinning of the well-known "type A" behavior profile and a predilection for coronary heart disease. In this study the interactions between anger coping styles, blood pressure, and all-cause mortality were examined in 696 persons, aged 30–69 years. Individuals were classified as "anger-in" or "anger-out" types, reflecting whether an anger-provoking situation resulted in pent-up hostility, or whether they expressed their anger openly upon provocation. Such responses were elicited by two structured situations: One involved an unjustified attack by an authority figure, a policeman, and the other involved such an attack by a spouse. Most of the participants were white, middle-class, employed, and had a high school education. Factors such as education, smoking, blood pressure, age, chronic bronchitis, and coronary heart disease were factored into the mortality results because these factors are significantly and independently related to all-cause mortality.

Suppressed anger was not directly related to higher blood pressure, nor were there any significant trends noted. Item analysis revealed that none of the specific anger-coping items had a relationship with mortality in the authority figure attack, but two of three items in the spousal attack did predict mortality risk. Persons who would hold in their anger toward a spouse were 2.4 times more likely to die during the follow-up period than were those who would express their anger. Although experiencing guilt in response to expressing anger to one's spouse did not predict mortality, the results were in the predicted direction. Those who would protest an unjustified attack by their spouse were 1.7 times more likely to die than were those who did protest. Various indices of suppressed anger were also associated with mortality. Those who scored highest on total suppressed anger for both situations were 1.6 times more likely to have died during the follow-up period, compared with those with moderate or low scores. There was no apparent difference, other than chance, that the relationships between anger-coping types and mortality were significantly different across age, sex, or educational status. There were, however, significant interactions between anger-coping types and systolic pressure. The suppressed anger indices showed signficantly higher mortality only for those persons with systolic pressure of at least 140 mm Hg; these persons were about five times as likely to have died, compared with those who expressed their anger in relation to an attack from a spouse. These patients also had a higher risk of dying than did hypertensives who expressed their anger.

There have been many studies showing an association between suppressed anger and increased risk of disease and death. Along with this study, these findings urge the importance of considering psychosocial and physiologic risk factors when identifying individuals at increased mortality risk. There is also reason to believe that the effects of suppressed anger may differ between the two sexes. The reason for the stronger influence of the spousal situation may result from the chronic nature of the marital interaction. When such anger processes interact with elevated blood pressure, a morbid condition and mortality may result. Women may have a more "reflective" response to anger, which defuses the attack and the resulting physiologic consequences. This relationship between anger expression and disease has been found for breast cancer patients also. In sum, these findings suggest that the health consequences of anger-response behaviors are broad and are consistent with the observation that suppressed anger significantly predicts all-cause mortality. Unfortunately, there are no standardized tests for anger behavior, causing methodological problems in interpretation of studies. Suppressed anger may act as a stressor in the body, disrupting the biochemical balance and precipitating disease.

▶ Psychiatrists and psychologists have been telling us for years that suppressing anger is a trait of hypertensives. This epidemiologic study from Tecumseh, Michigan, found no relationship between anger suppression and the prevalence of hypertension, but hypertensives who suppressed anger had a significantly higher mortality rate than normotensives or hypertensives who did not suppress anger. The $64 question is this: How practical and how successful are efforts to change anger-coping behavior?—R.W. Gifford, Jr., M.D.

Compliance with Relaxation Therapy

Home Relaxation Practice in Hypertension Treatment: Objective Assessment and Compliance Induction

Timothy J. Hoelscher, Kenneth L. Lichstein, and Ted L. Rosenthal (Duke Univ., Memphis State Univ., and Univ. of Tennessee)
J. Consulting Clin. Pathol. 54:217–221, April 1986   6–49

Relaxation training can be helpful in treating essential hypertension, but little is known about the relationship between the frequency of relaxation practice and the blood pressure response. Patients often overreport their compliance with home relaxation practice, and there is often little correlation between practice and blood pressure changes. Findings were reviewed in 50 hypertensive persons who were randomly assigned to individual relaxation training, group training, group training plus a contingency contract, and a waiting list group; evaluation was made of the compliance, efficacy, and value of various demographic variables in predicting compliance and reported compliance. A monitoring device was used, unknown to the study participants, to provide an objective measure of compliance. All continued to take their regular medication during the study. The mean age was 51.1 years, and the mean baseline blood pressure was 149.4/96.0 mm Hg. The average duration of hypertension was more than 9 years. Further, 70% of the participants were taking antihypertensive medication at the beginning of the study. Blood pressure was determined weekly during the 3-week baseline, 4-week treatment period, and 6-week posttreatment period. Participants were instructed to practice relaxation techniques at least once daily, and they were given a tape recorder with the relaxation program permanently sealed inside. Total therapist contact for the individual training group was 5.5 hours, compared with 4 hours for the group training sessions. Those on a waiting list served as controls.

All three treatment groups had reduced blood pressure, compared with controls, but the groups did not differ from each other. None of the participants suspected the existence of the monitoring device. Only 32% averaged one practice per day; the mean was 100 minutes per week for a 16-minute taped relaxation program. Practice rates were higher in the group training participants, followed by the individual training participants. Those with group training plus behavioral contract did less well. Overestimation of practice was common in all groups and averaged 91% overall. Greater overestimation occurred in the final weeks of the study. Younger persons tended to overestimate more severely than did older ones. Those who practiced at least once a day had greater reductions in systolic, but not diastolic, blood pressure than did noncompliers. Self-reported relaxation practice correlated with systolic, but not with diastolic, pressure reductions. In this patient population, group instruction was more cost effective because it involved less therapist time and gave as good results as did individual instruction. Group training was more cost effective than group training plus a behavioral contract by a factor of two.

The results showing a greater effect with group training than with either individualized training or behavioral contracts were surprising and may indicate that noncompliance with this type of program will be difficult to remediate. More powerful methods of increasing compliance need to be developed. Noncompliance was common in all groups. Those who received individualized training had an advantage in maintenance of initial practice levels over time, however. The amount of practice was correlated with age, perceived self-efficacy, and pretreatment expectations of benefit. Clearly, objective measures of home relaxation practice are required to identify noncompliant persons and exaggerated self-reports.

► Compliance or adherence to a therapeutic regimen presents a major problem in any chronic disease. In my opinion, compliance is greater to nonpharmacologic modes of treating hypertension (sodium restriction, weight reduction, alcohol abstinence, and behavioral modification) than it is to pharmacologic treatment. In this study it was possible to monitor compliance with relaxation practice at home; only 32% of the participants averaged one practice session daily as they had been instructed and self-reporting exceeded documented practice by 91%. Those who practiced regularly had a greater decrease in systolic blood pressure than those who did not, but there was no significant difference in diastolic blood pressure change. For the entire group, the average reduction in systolic blood pressure was about 11 mm Hg and the average reduction in diastolic blood pressure was about 6 mm Hg. This is not a cost-effective way of treating hypertension because of the time required by the professional therapist to instruct and monitor the relaxation techniques. Nevertheless, for some patients who refuse to take drugs or want to avoid drugs at all costs, it is an alternative to be considered, providing that the blood pressure is monitored frequently to be certain that normotension is achieved and maintained.—R.W. Gifford, Jr., M.D.

Dissection of the Aorta

Effects of Chronic Hypertension on Vasa Vasorum in the Thoracic Aorta
Melvin L. Marcus, Donald D. Heistad, Mark L. Armstrong, and Francois M. Abboud (Univ. of Iowa)
Cardiovasc. Res. 19:777–781, December 1985   6–50

The outer half of the canine and human thoracic aorta contains vascular channels known as vasa vasorum. The vasa vasorum provide considerable blood flow to the outer layer of the thoracic aorta; they dilate during infusions of adenosine, constrict during hemorrhagic hypotension, and respond to neural stimuli. Preliminary experiments found that acute elevations of systemic pressure did not increase blood flow through the vasa vasorum, even though the metabolic needs of the aortic wall had probably risen. It was hypothesized that, during chronic hypertension, if vasodilator responses are impaired in the vasa vasorum as in other vessels, ischemia might occur and predispose the aortic wall to medial necrosis and dissecting aneurysm. An attempt was made to determine whether chronic hypertension decreases the vasodilator capacity of the vasa vasorum.

Flow and conductance in the vasa vasorum were measured in 12 awake dogs with renal hypertension (arterial pressure, 127 ± 4 mm Hg) and 9 normotensive controls (arterial pressure, 100 ± 3 mm Hg). At rest, the blood flow delivered via the vasa vasorum to the thoracic aorta was similar in hypertensive and normotensive dogs. Thus, it appears that, in hypertensive dogs, conductance of the vasa vasorum decreased to maintain the flow constant. During maximal dilatation induced by intravenously administered adenosine, flow delivered via the vasa vasorum increased by 100% in both hypertensive and normotensive dogs. Calculations of maximum conductance demonstrate that vasodilator capacity was decreased by 67% in the vasa vasorum of hypertensive dogs.

The vasodilator capacity of the vasa vasorum in the thoracic aorta is limited in chronic hypertension. It is possible that this abnormality contributes to the pathogenesis of medial necrosis and aortic dissection in hypertensive patients.

▶ Hypertension is an important risk for aortic dissection. In the absence of cystic medial necrosis associated with Marfan's syndrome and other conditions, most aortic dissections occur in hypertensive individuals. This study provides some insight into the possible mechanism for this. If hypertension limits the ability of the thoracic vasa vasorum to dilate, it could contribute to the development of ischemia and subsequent dissection of the aortic wall.—R.W. Gifford, Jr., M.D.

Subject Index

Author Index